# Advances in the Treatment of Kidney and Upper Urinary Tract Cancers

# Advances in the Treatment of Kidney and Upper Urinary Tract Cancers

Editors

**Łukasz Zapała**
**Pawel Rajwa**

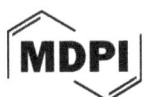

Basel • Beijing • Wuhan • Barcelona • Belgrade • Novi Sad • Cluj • Manchester

*Editors*
Łukasz Zapała
Medical University of Warsaw
Warsaw
Poland

Pawel Rajwa
Medical University of Silesia
Zabrze
Poland

*Editorial Office*
MDPI
St. Alban-Anlage 66
4052 Basel, Switzerland

This is a reprint of articles from the Special Issue published online in the open access journal *Biomedicines* (ISSN 2227-9059) (available at: https://www.mdpi.com/journal/biomedicines/special_issues/Upper_Urinary).

For citation purposes, cite each article independently as indicated on the article page online and as indicated below:

Lastname, A.A.; Lastname, B.B. Article Title. *Journal Name* **Year**, *Volume Number*, Page Range.

**ISBN 978-3-7258-0553-2 (Hbk)**
**ISBN 978-3-7258-0554-9 (PDF)**
doi.org/10.3390/books978-3-7258-0554-9

© 2024 by the authors. Articles in this book are Open Access and distributed under the Creative Commons Attribution (CC BY) license. The book as a whole is distributed by MDPI under the terms and conditions of the Creative Commons Attribution-NonCommercial-NoDerivs (CC BY-NC-ND) license.

# Contents

**Łukasz Zapała and Paweł Rajwa**
Advances in the Treatment of Kidney and Upper Urinary Tract Cancers
Reprinted from: *Biomedicines* 2024, *12*, 536, doi:10.3390/biomedicines12030536 . . . . . . . . . . . 1

**Piotr Domański, Mateusz Piętak, Barbara Kruczyk, Jadwiga Jarosińska, Anna Mydlak, Tomasz Demkow, et al.**
Adverse Events of Cabozantinib as a Potential Prognostic Factor in Metastatic Renal Cell Carcinoma Patients: Real-World Experience in a Single-Center Retrospective Study
Reprinted from: *Biomedicines* 2024, *12*, 413, doi:10.3390/biomedicines12020413 . . . . . . . . . . . 5

**Ljubinka Jankovic Velickovic, Ana Ristic Petrovic, Zana Dolicanin, Slavica Stojnev, Filip Velickovic and Dragoslav Basic**
Expression of Basal Compartment and Superficial Markers in Upper Tract Urothelial Carcinoma Associated with Balkan Endemic Nephropathy, a Worldwide Disease
Reprinted from: *Biomedicines* 2024, *12*, 95, doi:10.3390/biomedicines12010095 . . . . . . . . . . . 18

**Xinxin Li, Qihui Kuang, Min Peng, Kang Yang and Pengcheng Luo**
Basement Membrane-Associated lncRNA Risk Model Predicts Prognosis and Guides Clinical Treatment in Clear Cell Renal Cell Carcinoma
Reprinted from: *Biomedicines* 2023, *11*, 2635, doi:10.3390/biomedicines11102635 . . . . . . . . . . 27

**Liliana Eleonora Semenescu, Ligia Gabriela Tataranu, Anica Dricu, Gheorghe Vasile Ciubotaru, Mugurel Petrinel Radoi, Silvia Mara Baez Rodriguez and Amira Kamel**
A Neurosurgical Perspective on Brain Metastases from Renal Cell Carcinoma: Multi-Institutional, Retrospective Analysis
Reprinted from: *Biomedicines* 2023, *11*, 2485, doi:10.3390/biomedicines11092485 . . . . . . . . . . 47

**Jun Ito, Shigeki Sugawara, Takeo Tatsuta, Masahiro Hosono and Makoto Sato**
Catfish Egg Lectin Enhances the Cytotoxicity of Sunitinib on Gb3-Expressing Renal Cancer Cells
Reprinted from: *Biomedicines* 2023, *11*, 2317, doi:10.3390/biomedicines11082317 . . . . . . . . . . 65

**Mateusz Marcinek, Michał Tkocz, Kamil Marczewski, Robert Partyka, Leszek Kukulski, Krystyna Młynarek-Śnieżek, et al.**
Evaluation of Parameters Affecting the Occurrence of Systemic Inflammatory Response Syndrome in Patients Operated on Due to Kidney Tumors
Reprinted from: *Biomedicines* 2023, *11*, 2195, doi:10.3390/biomedicines11082195 . . . . . . . . . . 77

**Joanna Bialek, Stefan Yankulov, Felix Kawan, Paolo Fornara and Gerit Theil**
Role of Nivolumab in the Modulation of PD-1 and PD-L1 Expression in Papillary and Clear Cell Renal Carcinoma (RCC)
Reprinted from: *Biomedicines* 2022, *10*, 3244, doi:10.3390/biomedicines10123244 . . . . . . . . . . 93

**Ádám Széles, Petra Terézia Kovács, Anita Csizmarik, Melinda Váradi, Péter Riesz, Tamás Fazekas, et al.**
High Pretreatment Serum PD-L1 Levels Are Associated with Muscle Invasion and Shorter Survival in Upper Tract Urothelial Carcinoma
Reprinted from: *Biomedicines* 2022, *10*, 2560, doi:10.3390/biomedicines10102560 . . . . . . . . . . 107

**Łukasz Zapała, Aleksander Ślusarczyk, Rafał Wolański, Paweł Kurzyna, Karolina Garbas, Piotr Zapała and Piotr Radziszewski**
The Four-Feature Prognostic Models for Cancer-Specific and Overall Survival after Surgery for Localized Clear Cell Renal Cancer: Is There a Place for Inflammatory Markers?
Reprinted from: *Biomedicines* 2022, *10*, 1202, doi:10.3390/biomedicines10051202 . . . . . . . . . . 119

**Karolina Hanusz, Piotr Domański, Kacper Strojec, Piotr Zapała, Łukasz Zapała and Piotr Radziszewski**
Prostate Cancer in Transplant Receivers—A Narrative Review on Oncological Outcomes
Reprinted from: *Biomedicines* **2023**, *11*, 2941, doi:10.3390/biomedicines11112941 . . . . . . . . . . **133**

**Milena Matuszczak, Adam Kiljańczyk and Maciej Salagierski**
The Role of Focal Therapy and Active Surveillance for Small Renal Mass Therapy
Reprinted from: *Biomedicines* **2022**, *10*, 2583, doi:10.3390/biomedicines10102583 . . . . . . . . . . **150**

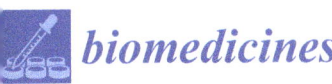 

*Editorial*

# Advances in the Treatment of Kidney and Upper Urinary Tract Cancers

Łukasz Zapała [1,*] and Paweł Rajwa [2,3,*]

1 Clinic of General, Oncological and Functional Urology, Medical University of Warsaw, 02-005 Warsaw, Poland
2 Department of Urology, Medical University of Silesia, 41-800 Zabrze, Poland
3 Department of Urology, Comprehensive Cancer Center, Medical University of Vienna, 1090 Vienna, Austria
* Correspondence: zapala.lukasz@gmail.com (Ł.Z.); pawelgrajwa@gmail.com (P.R.)

Citation: Zapała, Ł.; Rajwa, P. Advances in the Treatment of Kidney and Upper Urinary Tract Cancers. *Biomedicines* 2024, 12, 536. https://doi.org/10.3390/biomedicines12030536

Received: 6 February 2024
Accepted: 26 February 2024
Published: 27 February 2024

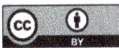

Copyright: © 2024 by the authors. Licensee MDPI, Basel, Switzerland. This article is an open access article distributed under the terms and conditions of the Creative Commons Attribution (CC BY) license (https://creativecommons.org/licenses/by/4.0/).

Kidney and upper tract urinary cancers (UTUC) are diseases of increasing population coverage, the treatment of which is undergoing a continuous process of evolution [1,2]. A characteristic feature of the picture comprising the results of renal cell cancer (RCC) treatment is the significant heterogeneity of patients (including different stages of local advancement and different locations of metastases) [3,4]. Importantly, it is estimated that up to 30% of newly diagnosed RCC cases are patients with disseminated disease at the time of diagnosis [4]. Therefore, predicting the response to modern treatment remains the unmet need of modern urologic oncology [5,6]. Recent advancements in systematic treatment, i.e., immunotherapy, shed additional light on adjuvant treatments to be implemented in new clinical scenarios, including localized disease [7,8].

This Special Issue aims to cover novel approaches in renal and urothelial cancers. We collected papers focused on novel approaches to urothelial cancers involving upper urinary tract and renal cancers that undertook original research focused on pre-clinical studies and biomarkers [9–12], prognostic models [13–15], the specific population of metastatic patients [16], and, finally, two narrative reviews [17,18].

Ito et al., in their paper, presented a novel concept for the search for anticancer drugs [9]. The authors had already reported that the treatment of globotriaosylceramide (Gb3)-expressing cells with catfish (Silurus asotus) egg lectin (SAL) increased the intracellular uptake of propidium iodide (PI) and sunitinib (SU). In their current paper, they tended to determine if SAL pretreatment affects the intracellular uptake and cytotoxic effects of molecular-targeted drugs in RCC cells using commercially available TOS1, TOS3, TOS3LN, and ACHN human RCC cell lines. They revealed that TOS1 cell viability decreased to 70% after treatment with 25 µM SU [18] alone and to 48% after pre-treatment with SAL (50 µg/mL), while there was a significantly enhanced SU uptake noted in SAL-treated TOS1 cells compared to control cells. Interestingly, SAL treatment did not increase PI uptake in normal renal cells. The authors concluded that adequate cytotoxic activity may be achieved even when SU is administered at a sufficiently low dose so as not to cause side effects in combination with SAL.

A recent paper by Szeles et al. [10] focused on the relevance of the circulating soluble levels (sPD-L1) of programmed death ligand-1 (PD-L1) in upper tract urothelial carcinoma (UTUC). The authors prospectively collected serum samples from 61 UTUC patients treated with radical nephroureterectomy (RNU), chemotherapy (CTX), or immune checkpoint inhibitor (ICI) therapy. It was reported that increased pre-operative sPD-L1 was associated with a higher tumor grade ($p = 0.019$) and stage ($p < 0.001$) and the presence of metastasis ($p = 0.002$) in the RNU group. Furthermore, high sPD-L1 levels were significantly correlated with poorer survival in both the RNU- and CTX-treated patients. Finally, the authors showed that ICI treatment caused a significant increase in sPD-L1 ($p < 0.001$). As a consequence, an increased pre-operative sPD-L1 level may act as a predictor of higher pathological tumor stage and worse survival in UTUC, while the specific sPD-L1 flare-up observed in UTUC seems to be therapy-specific, and its clinical relevance needs to be fully assessed.

On the other hand, Bialek et al. [11] investigated the response of renal carcinoma subtypes to the immune checkpoint inhibitor nivolumab in vitro using various RCC cell lines. Increasing doses of nivolumab increased the PD-1 levels in the analyzed cells and caused aggressive behavior in pRCC, but this induced contrary results in ccRCC. All cell lines exhibited a complex response to nivolumab treatment, so the authors summed concluded that there is definitely room for further studies to improve ICI-based therapy for RCC subtypes.

In the study by Velickovic et al. [12], the authors focused on the association of basal compartment and superficial markers, including CK5/6, CD44, CK20, and the pathological characteristics of UTUC associated with Balkan endemic nephropathy (BEN). The study enrolled 127 patients with UTUC who had undergone RNU and extended lymphadenectomy (54 tumors from the BEN region and 73 control UTUC). No significant differences between the expressions of the investigated markers in both groups were observed. The parameters with predictive influence on the expression of CD44 in BEN UTUC included growth pattern ($p = 0.010$), necrosis ($p = 0.019$), and differentiation ($p = 0.001$), and for the control UTUC, lymphovascular invasion ($p = 0.021$). Divergent squamous differentiation in BEN tumors ($p = 0.026$) and stage in control tumors ($p = 0.049$) had a predictive influence on the expression of CK5/6. The authors concluded that BEN and control tumors have a similar antigen presentation of the basal compartment and superficial layer, while the phenotypic characteristics of UTUC have a predictive influence on the expression of the basal compartment and superficial markers.

In the paper by Zapala L. et al. [13], the authors performed an analysis of the relevance of comorbidities and selected inflammatory markers on the survival of patients with primary non-metastatic localized cRCC. In a single-center retrospective cohort of patients post-renal surgery, they included the following parameters in the risk calculations, namely, tumor stage, grade, size, selected hematological markers (SIRI—systemic inflammatory response index; SII—systemic immune-inflammation index), and a comorbidities assessment tool (CCI—Charlson comorbidity index), and then further compared the new concept model with the existing prognostic tools. Four different features were included in the predictive models for CSS (grade, size, stage, and SII) and OS (grade, size, CCI, and SIRI), which were characterized by adequate or even superior accuracy when compared with existing prognostic tools. Here, the authors demonstrated the higher accuracy of their model in OS prediction compared to the commonly used Leibovich and GRANT models, and their model also outperformed the GRANT model in CSS prediction. The described scoring systems can be utilized for the stratification of patients into their respective risk groups for follow-up establishment or enrollment into clinical trials after prospective validation in a larger population.

In another study by Marcinek et al. [14], which included biomarkers in the prognostic models, the authors set out to determine any existing associations between systemic inflammatory reaction syndrome (SIRS) markers and post-operative complications occurrence in patients undergoing kidney tumor surgery and to determine if SIRS occurrence is dependent on age, sex, BMI (body mass index), comorbidities, patients' general condition before surgery, type of surgery, intraoperative blood loss, or intraoperative ischemia time. They found that BMI values, pre-operative general health status measured with the ASA scale, and the amount of intraoperative blood loss in patients undergoing surgery due to a kidney tumor can contribute to SIRS occurrence. On the other hand, the patient's sex, age, tumor size, type of surgery, operated side, and time of intraoperative ischemia do not affect SIRS occurrence.

Li et al. [15] focused on the identification of biomarkers of ccRCC and developed a risk model to assess patient prognosis based on the data from the Cancer Genome Atlas (TCGA). They developed a nomogram to predict the prognosis of ccRCC. GO, KEGG, and immunity analyses were used to explore differences in biological function. The authors prepared a risk model containing six BM-associated lncRNAs (LINC02154, IGFL2-AS1, NFE4, AC112715.1, AC092535.5, and AC105105.3), which have been proven to have higher diagnostic efficiency compared to clinical characteristics and can be used to forecast patient prognoses. Then, using RCC cell lines and tissue microarrays to verify the expression of lncRNAs in the risk model, they found that knocking down LINC02154 and AC112715.1 could inhibit the invasion ability of renal cancer cells. The authors concluded that the basement membrane-associated lncRNA risk model may accurately assess the prognosis of individuals with ccRCC.

Semenescu et al. [16] presented a unique cohort with neurosurgical treatment of brain metastases from RCC (BM RCC) ($n$ = 24 patients; 91.6% with cRCC and 37.5% after previous nephrectomy). Interestingly, only 29.1% of patients developed extracranial lesions, while 83.3% had a single BM RCC. Neurosurgical resection of the BM was carried out in 23 out of 24 patients. Prognostic factors included previous nephrectomy, having undergone systemic therapy, and a single BM RCC. The authors pinpointed that neurosurgery remains a cornerstone in the treatment of symptomatic BM RCC, being the solution for the quick reversal of neurological manifestations, which, in most cases, can be life-saving.

The recent review by Matuszczak et al. [17] summarized the current treatment options in the management of small renal masses. Briefly, despite the advances in focal methods that have been made in recent years, the NCCN guidelines recommend PN as the preferred method in patients with stage T1a tumors. AS is still recommended in sicker patients, especially the elderly, where surgery is high risk. The authors hypothesized that more long-term and larger cohort-based studies will help to confirm the clinical utility of these methods, together with minimally invasive ablative procedures, and to demonstrate their advantages over classical surgery.

Finally, links between kidney transplant patients and other tumors, e.g., prostate cancer, were presented in the narrative review by Hanusz et al., the first example of the planned thorough analyses on the immunosuppression of cancer patients in these Special Issues [18]. The association between PCa and transplantation is not entirely clear. The authors critically presented a perspective on a possible link between a more frequent occurrence of PCa and a worse prognosis in advanced or metastatic PCa.

In summary, we are witness to constant advances in the modalities used in the management of renal and urothelial cancers [2]. As emphasized in this editorial, the challenges posed by these diseases necessitate a multidimensional approach, including the investigation and integration of novel therapeutic options [4,19]. In the face of these facts, ongoing studies will hopefully lead to improved survival rates, better quality of life, and renewed hope for those affected by renal and urothelial cancers [20].

**Author Contributions:** P.R. and Ł.Z. supervised and conceived the topic and wrote the original manuscript. All authors have read and agreed to the published version of the manuscript.

**Funding:** This research received no external funding.

**Conflicts of Interest:** The authors declare no conflicts of interest.

## References

1. Trapani, D.; Curigliano, G.; Alexandru, E.; Sternberg, C.N. The global landscape of drug development for kidney cancer. *Cancer Treat. Rev.* **2020**, *89*, 102061. [CrossRef] [PubMed]
2. Chang, S.L.; Blute, M.L. The Progession Landscape of Diagnostic and Treatment Options for Kidney Cancer. *Urol. Clin. N. Am.* **2023**, *50*, xv–xvi. [CrossRef] [PubMed]
3. Iheanacho, K.; Vaishampayan, U. Perioperative approaches to kidney cancer. *Clin. Adv. Hematol. Oncol.* **2020**, *18*, 56–65. [PubMed]
4. Graham, J.; Heng, D.Y.C.; Brugarolas, J.; Vaishampayan, U. Personalized Management of Advanced Kidney Cancer. *Am. Soc. Clin. Oncol. Educ. Book* **2018**, *38*, 330–341. [CrossRef] [PubMed]
5. Stewart, G.D.; Klatte, T.; Cosmai, L.; Bex, A.; Lamb, B.W.; Moch, H.; Sala, E.; Siva, S.; Porta, C.; Gallieni, M. The multispeciality approach to the management of localised kidney cancer. *Lancet* **2022**, *400*, 523–534. [CrossRef] [PubMed]
6. Lv, Y.; Lin, S.Y.; Hu, F.F.; Ye, Z.; Zhang, Q.; Wang, Y.; Guo, A.Y. Landscape of cancer diagnostic biomarkers from specifically expressed genes. *Brief Bioinform* **2020**, *21*, 2175–2184. [CrossRef] [PubMed]

7. Autorino, R.; Porpiglia, F.; Dasgupta, P.; Rassweiler, J.; Catto, J.W.; Hampton, L.J.; Lima, E.; Mirone, V.; Derweesh, I.H.; Debruyne, F.M.J. Precision surgery and genitourinary cancers. *Eur. J. Surg. Oncol.* **2017**, *43*, 893–908. [CrossRef] [PubMed]
8. Bedke, J.; Stuhler, V.; Stenzl, A.; Brehmer, B. Immunotherapy for kidney cancer: Status quo and the future. *Curr. Opin. Urol.* **2018**, *28*, 8–14. [CrossRef] [PubMed]
9. Ito, J.; Sugawara, S.; Tatsuta, T.; Hosono, M.; Sato, M. Catfish Egg Lectin Enhances the Cytotoxicity of Sunitinib on Gb3-Expressing Renal Cancer Cells. *Biomedicines* **2023**, *11*, 2317. [CrossRef] [PubMed]
10. Szeles, A.; Kovacs, P.T.; Csizmarik, A.; Varadi, M.; Riesz, P.; Fazekas, T.; Vancsa, S.; Hegyi, P.; Olah, C.; Tschirdewahn, S.; et al. High Pretreatment Serum PD-L1 Levels Are Associated with Muscle Invasion and Shorter Survival in Upper Tract Urothelial Carcinoma. *Biomedicines* **2022**, *10*, 2560. [CrossRef] [PubMed]
11. Bialek, J.; Yankulov, S.; Kawan, F.; Fornara, P.; Theil, G. Role of Nivolumab in the Modulation of PD-1 and PD-L1 Expression in Papillary and Clear Cell Renal Carcinoma (RCC). *Biomedicines* **2022**, *10*, 3244. [CrossRef] [PubMed]
12. Velickovic, L.J.; Petrovic, A.R.; Dolicanin, Z.; Stojnev, S.; Velickovic, F.; Basic, D. Expression of Basal Compartment and Superficial Markers in Upper Tract Urothelial Carcinoma Associated with Balkan Endemic Nephropathy, a Worldwide Disease. *Biomedicines* **2024**, *12*, 95. [CrossRef] [PubMed]
13. Zapala, L.; Slusarczyk, A.; Wolanski, R.; Kurzyna, P.; Garbas, K.; Zapala, P.; Radziszewski, P. The Four-Feature Prognostic Models for Cancer-Specific and Overall Survival after Surgery for Localized Clear Cell Renal Cancer: Is There a Place for Inflammatory Markers? *Biomedicines* **2022**, *10*, 1202. [CrossRef] [PubMed]
14. Marcinek, M.; Tkocz, M.; Marczewski, K.; Partyka, R.; Kukulski, L.; Mlynarek-Sniezek, K.; Sedziak-Marcinek, B.; Rajwa, P.; Berezowski, A.; Kokocinska, D. Evaluation of Parameters Affecting the Occurrence of Systemic Inflammatory Response Syndrome in Patients Operated on Due to Kidney Tumors. *Biomedicines* **2023**, *11*, 2195. [CrossRef] [PubMed]
15. Li, X.; Kuang, Q.; Peng, M.; Yang, K.; Luo, P. Basement Membrane-Associated lncRNA Risk Model Predicts Prognosis and Guides Clinical Treatment in Clear Cell Renal Cell Carcinoma. *Biomedicines* **2023**, *11*, 2635. [CrossRef] [PubMed]
16. Semenescu, L.E.; Tataranu, L.G.; Dricu, A.; Ciubotaru, G.V.; Radoi, M.P.; Rodriguez, S.M.B.; Kamel, A. A Neurosurgical Perspective on Brain Metastases from Renal Cell Carcinoma: Multi-Institutional, Retrospective Analysis. *Biomedicines* **2023**, *11*, 2485. [CrossRef] [PubMed]
17. Matuszczak, M.; Kiljanczyk, A.; Salagierski, M. The Role of Focal Therapy and Active Surveillance for Small Renal Mass Therapy. *Biomedicines* **2022**, *10*, 2583. [CrossRef] [PubMed]
18. Hanusz, K.; Domanski, P.; Strojec, K.; Zapala, P.; Zapala, L.; Radziszewski, P. Prostate Cancer in Transplant Receivers—A Narrative Review on Oncological Outcomes. *Biomedicines* **2023**, *11*, 2941. [CrossRef] [PubMed]
19. Braun, D.A.; Bakouny, Z.; Hirsch, L.; Flippot, R.; Van Allen, E.M.; Wu, C.J.; Choueiri, T.K. Beyond conventional immune-checkpoint inhibition—Novel immunotherapies for renal cell carcinoma. *Nat. Rev. Clin. Oncol.* **2021**, *18*, 199–214. [CrossRef] [PubMed]
20. Hammers, H. Immunotherapy in kidney cancer: The past, present, and future. *Curr. Opin. Urol.* **2016**, *26*, 543–547. [CrossRef] [PubMed]

**Disclaimer/Publisher's Note:** The statements, opinions and data contained in all publications are solely those of the individual author(s) and contributor(s) and not of MDPI and/or the editor(s). MDPI and/or the editor(s) disclaim responsibility for any injury to people or property resulting from any ideas, methods, instructions or products referred to in the content.

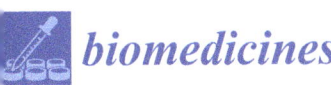 

*Article*

# Adverse Events of Cabozantinib as a Potential Prognostic Factor in Metastatic Renal Cell Carcinoma Patients: Real-World Experience in a Single-Center Retrospective Study

Piotr Domański [1,2,†], Mateusz Piętak [2,†], Barbara Kruczyk [2], Jadwiga Jarosińska [2], Anna Mydlak [3], Tomasz Demkow [2], Marta Darewicz [2], Bożena Sikora-Kupis [2], Paulina Dumnicka [4], Wojciech Kamzol [5] and Jakub Kucharz [2,*]

1. Department of Experimental Immunotherapy, Maria Sklodowska-Curie National Research Institute of Oncology, Roentgena 5, 02-781 Warsaw, Poland; piotr.domanski@nio.gov.pl
2. Department of Genitourinary Oncology, Maria Sklodowska-Curie National Research Institute of Oncology, Roentgena 5, 02-781 Warsaw, Poland
3. Department of Head and Neck Oncology, Maria Sklodowska-Curie National Research Institute of Oncology, Roentgena 5, 02-781 Warsaw, Poland
4. Department of Medical Diagnostics, Jagiellonian University Medical College, 31-008 Cracow, Poland
5. Department of Radiotherapy, Maria Sklodowska-Curie National Research Institute of Oncology, Roentgena 5, 02-781 Warsaw, Poland
* Correspondence: jakub.kucharz@nio.gov.pl; Tel.: +48-22-546-27-22
† These authors contributed equally to this work.

**Abstract:** Cabozantinib, an oral inhibitor targeting MET, AXL, and VEGF receptors, has become a key component of a sequential treatment strategy for clear cell renal cell carcinoma (ccRCC). The purpose of this work is to show that effective management of adverse events (AEs) during cabozantinib treatment and achieving a balance between AEs and treatment efficacy is crucial to achieving therapeutic goals. In this retrospective study, involving seventy-one metastatic RCC (mRCC) patients receiving second or subsequent lines of cabozantinib at the Department of Genitourinary Oncology, Maria Sklodowska-Curie National Research Institute of Oncology, we explored the impact of AEs on overall survival (OS) and progression-free survival (PFS). AEs were observed in 92% of patients. Hypothyroidism during treatment was significantly associated with prolonged OS and PFS (HR: 0.31; $p < 0.001$ and HR: 0.34; $p < 0.001$, respectively). The occurrence of hand–foot syndrome (HFS) was also linked to improved OS (HR: 0.46; $p = 0.021$). Patients experiencing multiple AEs demonstrated superior OS and PFS compared to those with one or no AEs (HR: 0.36; $p < 0.001$ and HR: 0.30; $p < 0.001$, respectively). Hypothyroidism and HFS serve as valuable predictive factors during cabozantinib treatment in ccRCC patients, indicating a more favorable prognosis.

**Keywords:** tyrosine kinase inhibitors (TKI); cabozantinib; metastatic renal cell carcinoma (mRCC); adverse events; predictive factor

## 1. Introduction

Renal cell carcinoma (RCC) is the most commonly diagnosed kidney cancers and accounts for 90% of all kidney malignancies [1]. Clear cell carcinoma (ccRCC) is a histological subtype responsible for about 70% of the diagnoses, and it usually develops on a background of different sporadic mutations, including VHL mutation [1]. The VHL mutation results in a loss of control of hypoxia-inducible factor (HIF) expression [1]. Under those circumstances, HIF proteins (HIF-1α, HIF-2α, and HIF-3α) accumulate and, through various molecular pathways, lead to the promotion of angiogenesis and cell proliferation, which play an essential role in carcinogenesis [2,3]. Therefore, it is considered an essential metabolic checkpoint in the development of renal tumors [2].

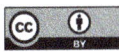

Understanding these pathways enabled the implementation of tyrosine kinase inhibitors (TKIs) in the systemic treatment of RCC [1]. Cabozantinib is an oral VEGF receptor (VEGFR) inhibitor that also inhibits other receptors and kinases such as RET, KIT, MET, AXL, and ROS1. TKIs targeting VEGFR cause an antiangiogenic effect [4] which limits the growth potential of tumors [1]. Moreover, as VEGF has some immunosuppressive properties, inhibition of VEGFR is responsible for the immunomodulatory properties of cabozantinib, such as decreasing the number of myeloid-derived suppressor cells (MDSC) and regulatory T-cells [5–7]. Furthermore, cabozantinib also affects the tumor's physiology and leads to mutated cell apoptosis, disrupted vascularization, and increased hypoxia within the tumor. Cabozantinib affects not only the tumor microenvironment but also directly acts on the tumor cells, making them more susceptible to immune-mediated killing [8]. These features are the reason for the occurrence of a synergistic effect with immune oncology (IO), which has been already described in various studies [9].

Following the publication of the CABOSUN study, cabozantinib emerged as a viable option for patients falling within the intermediate- and poor-risk categories, as defined by the International Metastatic RCC Database Consortium (IMDC) [10] and, subsequently, the METEOR study [4]. The most recent investigations have demonstrated cabozantinib's antitumor activity, even in cases where prior therapies involved immune checkpoint inhibitors (IO), combination IO regimens (IOIO), or IO in conjunction with vascular endothelial growth factor inhibitors (VEGFi)-IOVE [11–14]. The latest clinical guidelines issued by both the European Society for Medical Oncology (ESMO) [15] and the American Society of Clinical Oncology (ASCO) [16] recommend the utilization of combination therapy IO and VEGFi, such as the pairing of nivolumab and cabozantinib. Moreover, cabozantinib is the preferred initial treatment for patients with advanced papillary RCC when additional molecular testing is not deemed necessary [15].

In the treatment of ccRCC with tyrosine kinase inhibitors, AEs have been identified as valuable predictive factors. Previous research has substantiated that AEs such as hand–foot syndrome (HFS), hypothyroidism, or diarrhea are associated with improved overall survival (OS) and progression-free survival (PFS) [17]. Therefore, effectively managing AEs to maintain them at acceptable levels is crucial to ensure the therapeutic effectiveness of this approach. Achieving the right balance between therapeutic efficacy and management of adverse events requires reasonable dose modifications. This becomes particularly significant in the geriatric population. One must bear in mind that cabozantinib is often used as a second-line drug, which often means that there are more geriatric patients in this group than in the group receiving first-line drugs. In those patients, the reduced physiological reserves demand more frequent and delicate adjustments in dosing. The decline in functional reserves and muscle mass is a persistent and inevitable consequence of the ageing process. Furthermore, it affects drug metabolism in the liver and kidney excretion [18,19]. These factors collectively contribute to diminished treatment tolerance, compromised treatment response, and increased susceptibility to treatment-related toxicities.

The early detection of cancer and the implementation of effective radical treatments can delay the need for systemic therapies; therefore, when analyzing the details of cabozantinib treatment, it is imperative to consider all of these aforementioned factors.

## 2. Materials and Methods

### 2.1. Patients Collection

This retrospective analysis included seventy-one patients with biopsy-proven metastatic renal clear cell carcinoma (mRCC) undergoing cabozantinib treatment as a second-line, or further, treatment at the Department of Genitourinary Oncology of the Maria Skłodowska-Curie National Research Institute of Oncology in Warsaw. The database contained the data of patients with mRCC treated at the department between 30 January 2017 and 23 June 2021. This study was performed in line with the principles of the Declaration of Helsinki. Permission to conduct this study was granted by the Maria Sklodowska-Curie National Research Institute of Oncology Bioethics Committee (permission number 38/2018).

## 2.2. Data Collection

The database contained detailed information on age, gender, clinicopathological factors, laboratory results, comorbidities, adverse events, sites of metastases, ECOG performance score, International Metastatic RCC Database Consortium (IMDC), Memorial Sloan-Kettering Cancer Center (MSKCC) risk scores [10], and outcome data associated with individual patients. Characteristics of the studied group at the time of the start of the study are shown in Table 1. Clinical data were extracted from medical records and mortality data were obtained from the Polish national database. This study included patients ranging in age between 42 and 80 years who were treated with cabozantinib as second-line, or further, treatment. The previous lines of treatment are depicted in Table 2. The collected data comprised the date of treatment initiation, type of administered drug, drug dose, date of treatment discontinuation, and the reason behind it. Patients were classified into three MSKCC and IMDC groups: favorable-, intermediate-, and poor-risk. The required data were collected retrospectively, and the dataset consisted of patients' demographics, laboratory test results (including complete blood count (CBC), corrected calcium, LDH), treatment delays, treatment duration, and treatment outcomes. The complete blood counts were evaluated before starting the course of treatment. Hematology parameters were measured using Sysmex XN-1000. Laboratory tests were carried out by the Diagnostic Department of the National Research Institute of Oncology. PLR was calculated with the formula [platelet count/lymphocyte count] and NRL with [neutrophil count/lymphocyte count]. Counts of inflammatory cells were taken from laboratory results which were performed immediately prior to the treatment initiation. Detailed information about the laboratory test results at the baseline start can be found in Table 3.

**Table 1.** Characteristics of studied group at the start of the study (= start of cabozantinib treatment).

| Characteristic | Values Observed in mRCC Patients ($n$ = 71) |
|---|---|
| male sex, $n$ (%) | 46 (65) |
| mean age (SD), years | 63 (9) |
| median time from RCC diagnosis (Q1; Q3), years | 4.3 (2.0; 8.2) |
| mean BMI (SD), kg/m$^2$ | 28.1 (5.9) |
| morphology clear cell, $n$ (%) | 69 (97) |
| non-clear cell, $n$ (%) | 6 (8) |
| sarcomatoid differentiation, $n$ (%) | 11 (14) |
| nephrectomy, $n$ (%) | 69 (97) |
| Fuhrman grade | |
| 1, $n$ (%) | 6 (8) |
| 2, $n$ (%) | 33 (46) |
| 3, $n$ (%) | 21 (30) |
| 4, $n$ (%) | 11 (15) |
| MSKCC score | |
| 0, $n$ (%) | 19 (27) |
| 1, $n$ (%) | 36 (51) |
| 2, $n$ (%) | 15 (21) |
| 3, $n$ (%) | 1 (1) |
| IMDC prognostic score | |
| 0, $n$ (%) | 16 (23) |
| 1, $n$ (%) | 30 (42) |
| 2, $n$ (%) | 15 (21) |
| 3, $n$ (%) | 7 (10) |
| 4, $n$ (%) | 3 (4) |

Table 1. Cont.

| Characteristic | Values Observed in mRCC Patients (n = 71) |
|---|---|
| metastases | |
| lungs, n (%) | 53 (75) |
| bone, n (%) | 24 (34) |
| liver, n (%) | 12 (17) |
| pancreas, n (%) | 6 (8) |
| other sites, n (%) | 31 (44) |
| median number of sites (Q1; Q3) | 2 (2; 3) |
| ECOG performance score | |
| 0, n (%) | 19 (27) |
| 1, n (%) | 42 (59) |
| 2, n (%) | 9 (13) |
| 3, n (%) | 1 (1) |
| Karnofsky performance scale | |
| 100, n (%) | 10 (14) |
| 90, n (%) | 21 (30) |
| 80, n (%) | 37 (52) |
| <80, n (%) | 3 (4) |
| cabozantinib as 2nd-line treatment, n (%) | 30 (42) |
| cabozantinib as 3rd-line treatment, n (%) | 36 (50) |
| cabozantinib as 4th- or 5th-line treatment, n (%) | 5 (7) |

Table 2. Previous treatment (before the initiation of cabozantinib).

| | n (%) |
|---|---|
| 1st-line treatment | |
| TKI (sunitinib, pazopanib, sorafenib), n (%) | 65 (92) |
| other (immunotherapy), n (%) | 6 (8) |
| 2nd-line treatment | |
| TKI (axitinib, sunitinib, pazopanib, sorafenib), n (%) | 20 (28) |
| everolimus, temsirolimus, n (%) | 18 (25) |
| nivolumab, n (%) | 3 (4) |
| 3rd-line treatment | |
| TKI (sorafenib, pazopanib), n (%) | 4 (6) |
| nivolumab, n (%) | 1 (1) |
| 4th-line treatment (nivolumab), n (%) | 1 (1) |

Table 3. Results of laboratory test at the start at baseline.

| Laboratory Test | Values Observed in mRCC Patients (n = 71) |
|---|---|
| median hemoglobin (Q1; Q3), g/dL | 13.1 (11.0; 14.4) |
| median neutrophils (Q1; Q3), G/L | 3.80 (3.20; 5.30) |
| median lymphocytes (Q1; Q3), G/L | 1.73 (1.26; 2.30) |
| median platelets (Q1; Q3), G/L | 252 (198; 343) |
| median NLR (Q1; Q3) | 2.46 (1.53; 3.63) |
| median PLR (Q1; Q3) | 137 (98; 214) |

2.3. Adverse Events

The initial dosing of cabozantinib was 60 mg per day for all patients. Dose modifications were based on the Summary of Product Characteristics [20]. Adverse events were assessed following the Common Terminology Criteria for Adverse Events (CTCAE) v5.0 [21]. Patients were duly informed of all potential AEs and were actively encouraged to provide details regarding any changes associated with their treatment. Subsequently, AEs were thoroughly assessed at follow-up appointments, which were scheduled every two weeks. Treatment persisted until either disease progression or the onset of significant toxicity, classified as Grade 4 (G4). Any necessary adjustments to the dosage were carefully deliberated in collaboration with the patient, following a comprehensive benefit–risk assessment. A comprehensive record detailing all AEs that manifested during the course of treatment is provided in Table 4.

Table 4. Adverse events observed in patients and the need for dose reduction.

| Variable | Values Observed in mRCC Patients ($n = 71$) |
|---|---|
| any adverse event, $n$ (%) | 65 (92) |
| hypothyroidism, $n$ (%) | 35 (49) |
| hand–foot syndrome, $n$ (%) | 33 (46) |
| hypertension, $n$ (%) | 28 (39) |
| diarrhea, $n$ (%) | 28 (39) |
| asthenia, $n$ (%) | 24 (34) |
| liver toxicity, $n$ (%) | 11 (15) |
| >1 reported adverse event, $n$ (%) | 39 (55) |
| median number of adverse events (Q1, Q3) | 2 (1–4) |
| dose reduction | 35 (49) |

*2.4. Statistical Analysis*

Categorical variables were summarized with the number and percentage of the respective group. Quantitative variables were summarized with mean and standard deviation (SD; normally distributed) or median, first, and third quartile (Q1; Q3; non-normally distributed), as specified in the Results Section. Progression-free survival (PFS) times were calculated from the date of initiation of cabozantinib (i.e., the start of the study) until the date of diagnosis of progressive disease (PD), death, or were censored on the date of loss to follow-up or the end of the study (5 February 2022). Overall survival (OS) times were calculated from the date of initiation of cabozantinib (i.e., the start of the study) until the date of death or censored on the date of the end of the study (5 February 2022). Survival times were estimated with the Kaplan–Meier method and compared between the groups using log-rank tests. Cox proportional hazard regression was used to verify the associations between patients' baseline characteristics, laboratory results, adverse events of ponatinib treatment, and survival (PFS and OS). The multiple Cox models were calculated with a backward stepwise method using the predictors significant in a simple analysis. All the statistical tests were two-tailed, and the results were interpreted as significant at $p < 0.05$. Statistica software (version 13; Tibco, Tulsa, OK, USA) was used for computations.

## 3. Results

The study included patients ranging in age between 42 and 80 years, between 4 months and 19 years (237 months) from RCC diagnosis (median 52 months), who were treated between the 30 January 2017 and the 23 June 2021. Thirty (42%) of them were receiving cabozantinib as a second-line treatment (2L), thirty-six (50%) as a third-line treatment, and only five (7%) as a fourth- or fifth-line treatment.

Observation time (from the start of the initiation of treatment with cabozantinib until death or the end of the study on 5 February 2022) was between 1 and 61 months; median (Q1; Q3): 15 months (95%CI: 9; 31). Progression was observed in fifty-five (77%) patients, forty-seven (66%) passed away before the end of the study, and sixteen (23%) patients who did not progress continued cabozantinib at/to the end of the study.

The main histological subtype was clear cell RCC (n = 69; 97%). According to International Metastatic Renal Cell Carcinoma Database Consortium (IMDC) criteria, 16 (23%) patients were in the favorable risk group, 45 (63%) were in the intermediate group, and 10 (14%) were in the poor prognosis group. Full characterization of the enrolled patients is shown in Table 1.

Adverse events occurred in almost every patient, with 65 (92%) of them experiencing at least one. The most common AE was hypothyroidism (n = 35; 49%), followed by hand–foot syndrome (n = 33; 46%), hypertension (n = 28; 39%), diarrhea (n = 28; 39%), asthenia (n = 24; 34%), and liver toxicity (n = 11; 15%). Thirty-nine (55%) patients experienced two or more AEs. Dose reduction was necessary in 35 (49%) cases due to toxicity.

During the course of treatment, the presence of hypothyroidism displayed a statistically significant association with prolonged overall survival (OS) and progression-free survival (PFS) (HR: 0.31; $p < 0.001$, and HR:0.34; $p < 0.001$, respectively), as determined through multiple Cox regression analyses. Likewise, the occurrence of hand–foot syndrome exhibited a noteworthy association with improved OS (HR: 0.46, $p = 0.021$) using the multiple Cox regression analysis model. Furthermore, the presence of diarrhea or hand–foot syndrome (HFS) was correlated with enhanced OS and PFS (HR: 0.53; $p = 0.039$ and HR: 0.49; $p = 0.02$, respectively) using a simple Cox regression analysis model. Patients experiencing multiple adverse events also demonstrated superior OS and PFS compared to those with only one or no adverse events (HR: 0.36; $p < 0.001$ and HR: 0.30; $p < 0.001$, respectively). However, it is noteworthy that hypertension, asthenia, and liver toxicity did not exhibit any significant correlation with improved OS or PFS. All the analyses carried out can be found in Tables 5 and 6, while a graphical representation of the correlations is shown in Figures 1 and 2.

Table 5. Predictors of OS in simple and multiple Cox regression.

| Variable | Simple Analysis | | Multiple Model | |
|---|---|---|---|---|
| | HR (95% CI) | $p$ | HR (95% CI) | $p$ |
| cabozantinib in 3rd line or further (vs. 2nd) | 0.50 (0.28–0.89) | 0.019 | 0.49 (0.24–0.97) | 0.041 |
| time from RCC diagnosis, per 1 year | 0.91 (0.85–0.99) | 0.031 | not included | |
| IMDC (score 3 or 4) | 2.99 (1.41–6.35) | 0.004 | 2.23 (1.00–5.02) | 0.51 |
| hypothyroidism | 0.35 (0.19–0.65) | <0.001 | 0.31 (0.15–0.62) | 0.001 |
| hand–foot syndrome | 0.49 (0.27–0.90) | 0.020 | 0.46 (0.24–0.89) | 0.021 |
| diarrhea | 0.53 (0.29–0.97) | 0.039 | not included | |
| number of adverse events, per 1 event | 0.71 (0.57–0.88) | 0.002 | not included | |
| multiple adverse events | 0.36 (0.19–0.66) | 0.001 | not included | |
| hemoglobin, per 1 g/dL | 0.81 (0.70–0.93) | 0.003 | not included | |
| neutrophils, per 1 G/L | 1.20 (1.03–1.40) | 0.017 | not included | |
| platelets, per 100 G/L | 1.45 (1.12–1.87) | 0.005 | not included | |
| NLR | 1.19 (1.05–1.35) | 0.007 | 1.29 (1.12–1.48) | <0.001 |
| PLR | 1.005 (1.003–1.008) | <0.001 | not included | |

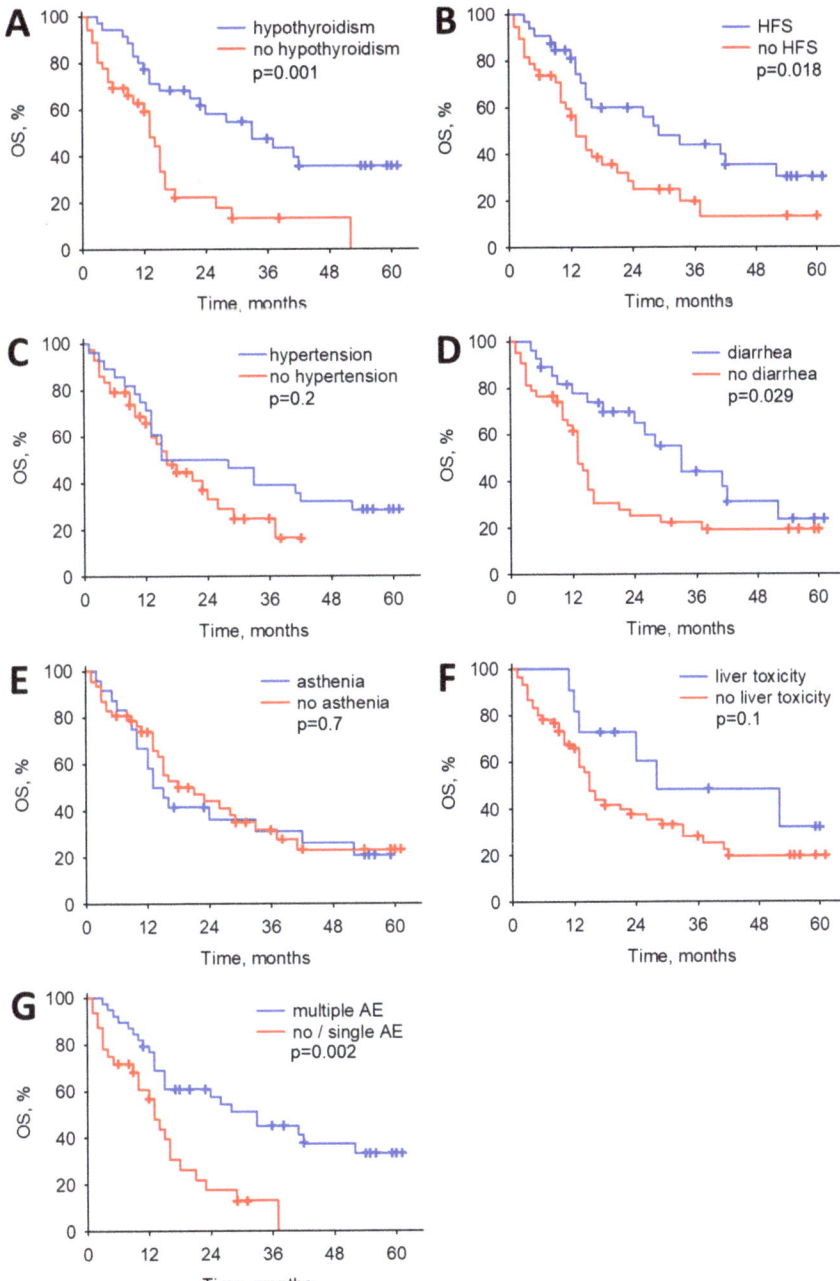

**Figure 1.** The associations between adverse events (AE) of cabozantinib and overall survival (OS). (**A**) The associations between hypothyroidism and OS. (**B**) The associations between HFS and OS. (**C**) The associations between hypertension and OS. (**D**) The associations between diarrhea and OS. (**E**) The associations between asthenia and OS. (**F**) The associations between liver toxicity and OS. (**G**) The associations between multiple AE and OS. Occurrence of hypothyroidism, HFS, diarrhea and multiple significantly prolongs OS.

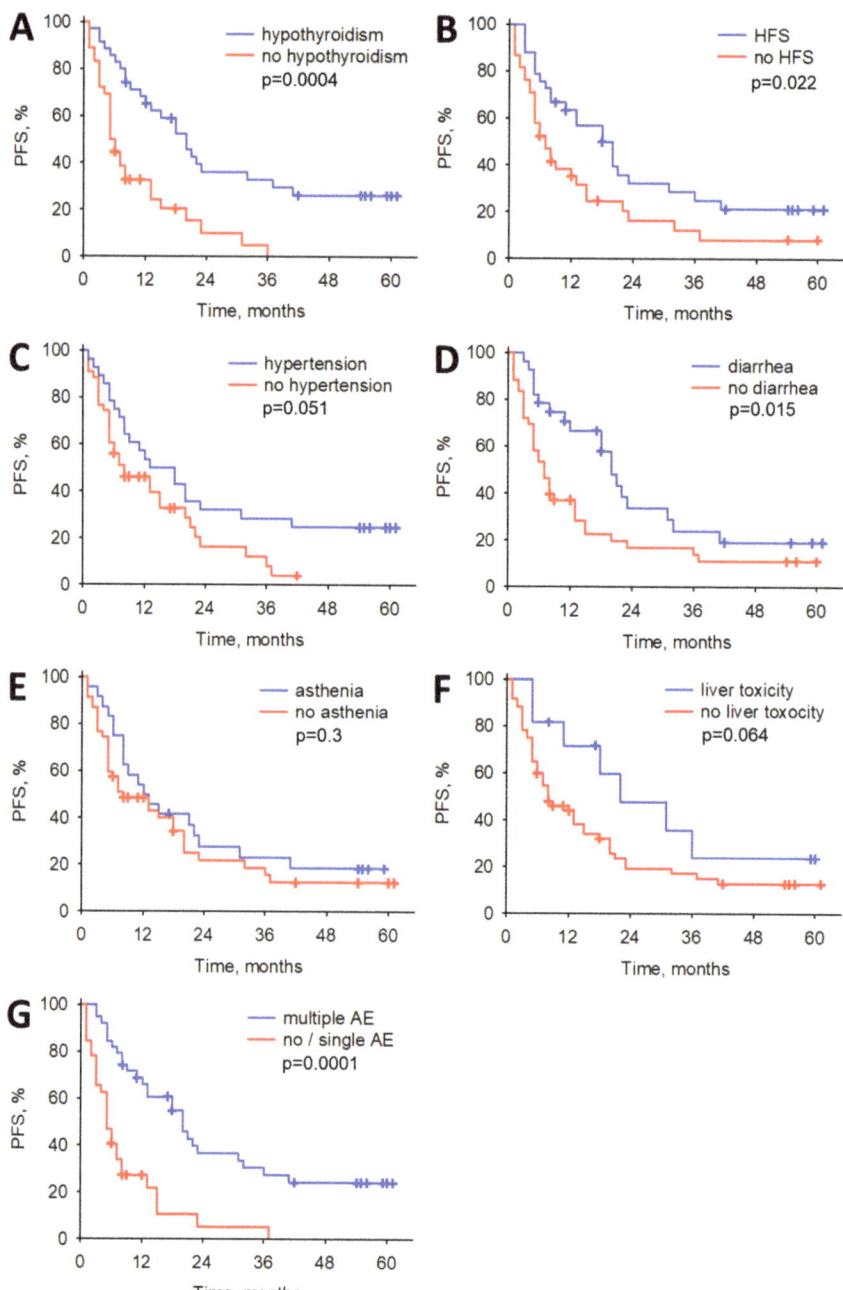

**Figure 2.** The associations between adverse events of cabozantinib and progression-free survival (PFS). (**A**) The associations between hypothyroidism and PFS. (**B**) The associations between HFS and PFS. (**C**) The associations between hypertension and PFS. (**D**) The associations between diarrhea and PFS. (**E**) The associations between asthenia and PFS. (**F**) The associations between liver toxicity and PFS. (**G**) The associations between multiple AE and PFS. Occurrence of hypothyroidism, HFS, diarrhea and multiple significantly prolongs PFS.

Table 6. Predictors of PFS in simple and multiple Cox regression.

| Variable | Simple Analysis | | Multiple Model | |
|---|---|---|---|---|
| | HR (95% CI) | p | HR (95% CI) | p |
| cabozantinib in 3rd line or further (vs. 2nd) | 0.34 (0.20–0.59) | <0.001 | 0.29 (0.16–0.53) | <0.001 |
| IMDC–poor risk (score 3 or 4) | 2.13 (1.03–4.41) | 0.042 | 1.58 (0.73–3.41) | 0.2 |
| hypothyroidism | 0.35 (0.20–0.62) | <0.001 | 0.34 (0.18–0.65) | <0.001 |
| hand–foot syndrome | 0.54 (0.31–0.93) | 0.026 | not included | |
| diarrhea | 0.52 (0.30–0.92) | 0.024 | not included | |
| number of adverse events, per 1 event | 0.68 (0.55–0.83) | <0.001 | not included | |
| multiple adverse events | 0.30 (0.17–0.53) | <0.001 | not included | |
| hemoglobin, per 1 g/dL | 0.80 (0.70–0.91) | <0.001 | 0.82 (0.70–0.97) | 0.017 |
| platelets, per 100 G/L | 1.26 (1.001–1.58) | 0.049 | not included | |
| PLR | 1.004 (1.002–1.007) | <0.001 | 1.004 (1.001–1.007) | 0.016 |

## 4. Discussion

In this single-center retrospective cohort study, we present real-world data illuminating the prognostic significance of adverse events occurring during cabozantinib treatment among patients with advanced RCC or mRCC who had previously experienced disease progression on the previous line. Our findings indicate that cabozantinib was generally well-tolerated, with no new safety concerns or treatment-related fatalities identified. The comprehensive analysis of adverse events in our study underscores that treatment with cabozantinib consistently leads to the occurrence of at least one such event. The overall incidence of adverse events, irrespective of type and grade, stood at 92%. This observation aligns with findings from the METEOR study, where the incidence rate was 100%, and from the CABOSUN study, where it was 99% [22,23]. More than one AE occurred in 55% of patients. The necessity for dose reduction, observed in 49% of our patients in this study, closely parallels findings from the METEOR and CABOSUN trials, where dose reductions were required in 62% and 46% of patients, respectively. In another real-world experience study conducted by Bodnar et al., the incidence of all AEs was reported at 100% [24], while a study conducted by Iinuma et al. reported an incidence of 79% [25].

An exposure–response (ER) analysis of cabozantinib within the CheckMate 9ER study [26] showed no significant correlation between the extent of exposure to cabozantinib during treatment and progression-free survival (PFS) or risk of death [26]. However, it did unveil a statistically significant association between cabozantinib exposure and the incidence of hand–foot syndrome (HFS) at Grade 1 or higher, as well as severe diarrhea at Grade 3 or higher. Notably, the ER analysis conducted for the METEOR study yielded different results, suggesting a positive correlation between the average concentration of cabozantinib and improved PFS. These differing conclusions can likely be attributed to variations in study designs. Specifically, in the METEOR study, the exposure-response analysis involved simulating cabozantinib concentrations in patients receiving doses lower than 60 mg, whereas the CheckMate 9ER analysis was based on individual average plasma concentrations of the drug. Additionally, it is important to consider that patients in the METEOR study received cabozantinib as monotherapy, while those in the CheckMate 9ER trial were administered a combination of nivolumab and cabozantinib. Furthermore, it is worth noting that in the CheckMate 9ER trial, the median time elapsed before the first-level dose reduction was significantly longer, at 106 days, compared to the METEOR study, where it occurred at 55 days [22].

In other real-world studies with cabozantinib, researchers did not delve into how the occurrence of AEs might affect PFS or OS. However, similar analyses have been conducted with other TKIs, such as sorafenib or sunitinib, which have demonstrated an enhancement in both OS and PFS when AEs like palmar–plantar erythrodysesthesia, hypothyroidism, and hypertension occurred [17,27–32].

In this study, approximately 46% of the patients experienced HFS—a common symptom associated with systemic treatment using classical cytostatic agents [33] or targeted tyrosine kinase inhibitors [17,34,35]. The development of HFS is closely tied to the impact of TKIs on endothelial and fibroblastic cells [30]. The inhibition of VEGF-R can impair wound healing, particularly in areas subjected to high pressure and repeated trauma, making them more susceptible to HFS [36,37]. Notably, in this study, HFS was linked to a 50% reduction in the risk of both PFS and overall OS, consistent with findings from similar studies assessing other TKIs [17,38,39].

Numerous theories surround the topic of TKI-induced hypothyroidism; however, the precise mechanism remains a subject of ongoing investigation and is not yet fully understood [40]. It appears to be closely associated with the inhibition of VEGF-R as it is responsible for proper blood flow, which is crucial for the functioning of the thyroid gland. VEGF-R inhibition can also lead to tissue ischemia potentially resulting in thyroid dysfunction [41,42]. In this study, hypothyroidism occurred in 35 patients (55%), making it the most prevalent adverse event. Interestingly, the occurrence of this side effect was associated with a reduction in the risk of PFS and OS by nearly 70%. Some studies have shown statistical significance only for PFS, failing to demonstrate the same significance for OS [43–45]. However, several studies have confirmed statistical significance for OS [27,46,47], and Schmidinger et al. established a correlation between hypothyroidism and overall response rate (ORR) [48]. While these aforementioned studies primarily focus on sunitinib and sorafenib, similar associations can also be observed in cabozantinib therapy.

It is important to acknowledge the fact that most patients undergoing treatment with cabozantinib have previously received some form of radical treatment. The resulting reduction in the number of active nephrons makes these patients more susceptible to chronic kidney disease and acute kidney injury (AKI). AKI, characterized by a considerable mortality rate, substantially restricts therapeutic options [49]. Timely management of side effects is crucial, underscoring the importance of the study by Allinovi et al., which describes biomarkers that may be useful in detecting patients at high risk of AKI and in limiting the progression of renal failure [50]. Notably, assignment to a risk group can be made at the stage of radical treatment, and the method is non-invasive. These risk stratification possibilities are particularly valuable due to the potential of cabozantinib to cause rhabdomyolysis, which in turn may contribute to the development of AKI, putting the patient's life at risk [51]. While a comprehensive examination remains crucial, these biomarkers offer valuable insights, especially in the early stages of emerging renal complications.

Interestingly, in the context of this study, we identified a notable pattern where the presence of multiple AEs emerged as a favorable predictive factor. This intriguing observation presents a dual challenge for both patients and clinicians. Hence, the swift and effective management of AEs becomes imperative, enhancing patients' ability to endure the therapy successfully [52]. Clearance of cabozantinib varies across the population [26], necessitating dose adjustments for individuals with lower clearance due to their increased susceptibility to developing multiple or severe AEs. Importantly, it has been reported that there is no significant disparity in terms of PFS or OS between patients who underwent a dose reduction to 20 mg and those who maintained the standard 40 mg dose.

Some limitations of this study include the small size of the subgroups, the use of descriptive statistics, and the retrospective nature of the research. Further studies should be conducted to assess the other correlations between adverse events and PFS, OS, or ORR. Uncovering and reporting these correlations can contribute to the development of novel prognostic factors and ultimately provide more informed and personalized patient care. Our findings, therefore, serve as a valuable reference point for future real-world studies focusing on metastatic renal cell carcinoma (mRCC).

**Author Contributions:** All authors contributed to the study conception and design. Material preparation, data collection, and analysis were performed by P.D. (Piotr Domański), M.P., B.K., J.J., A.M., T.D., W.K., M.D. and B.S.-K. [P.D. (Paulina Dumnicka)—statistical analysis] and [J.K.—senior supervisor]. The first draft of the manuscript was written by P.D. (Piotr Domański) and M.P. All authors have read and agreed to the published version of the manuscript.

**Funding:** This research received no external funding.

**Institutional Review Board Statement:** The study was conducted in accordance with the Declaration of Helsinki, and approved by the Institutional Ethics Committee the Maria Sklodowska-Curie National Research Institute of Oncology (permission number 38/2018).

**Informed Consent Statement:** Informed consent was obtained from all individual participants included in the study.

**Data Availability Statement:** The data presented in this study are available on request from the corresponding author (accurately indicate status).

**Conflicts of Interest:** Honoraria: Angelini, Astellas, Astra Zeneca, Bayer, Bristol Myers Squibb, IPSEN, Janssen, Merck MSD, Novartis, Pfizer, Research Funding: Novartis. All unrelated to the present paper.

# References

1. Libertino, J.; Gee, J. *Renal Cancer Contemporary Management: Contemporary Management*; Springer International Publishing: Berlin/Heidelberg, Germany, 2020.
2. Sharma, R.; Kadife, E.; Myers, M.; Kannourakis, G.; Prithviraj, P.; Ahmed, N. Determinants of Resistance to Vegf-Tki and Immune Checkpoint Inhibitors in Metastatic Renal Cell Carcinoma. *J. Exp. Clin. Cancer Res.* **2021**, *40*, 186. [CrossRef]
3. Swiatek, M.; Jancewicz, I.; Kluebsoongnoen, J.; Zub, R.; Maassen, A.; Kubala, S.; Udomkit, A.; Siedlecki, J.A.; Sarnowski, T.J.; Sarnowska, E. Various Forms of Hif-1α Protein Characterize the Clear Cell Renal Cell Carcinoma Cell Lines. *IUBMB Life* **2020**, *72*, 1220–1232. [CrossRef]
4. Choueiri, T.K.; Escudier, B.; Powles, T.; Mainwaring, P.N.; Rini, B.I.; Donskov, F.; Hammers, H.; Hutson, T.E.; Lee, J.L.; Peltola, K.; et al. Cabozantinib Versus Everolimus in Advanced Renal-Cell Carcinoma. *N. Engl. J. Med.* **2015**, *373*, 1814–1823. [CrossRef]
5. Ott, P.A.; Hodi, F.S.; Buchbinder, E.I. Inhibition of Immune Checkpoints and Vascular Endothelial Growth Factor as Combination Therapy for Metastatic Melanoma: An Overview of Rationale, Preclinical Evidence, and Initial Clinical Data. *Front. Oncol.* **2015**, *5*, 202. [CrossRef]
6. Voron, T.; Marcheteau, E.; Pernot, S.; Colussi, O.; Tartour, E.; Taieb, J.; Terme, M. Control of the Immune Response by Pro-Angiogenic Factors. *Front. Oncol.* **2014**, *4*, 70. [CrossRef]
7. Apolo, A.B.; Nadal, R.; Tomita, Y.; Davarpanah, N.N.; Cordes, L.M.; Steinberg, S.M.; Cao, L.; Parnes, H.L.; Costello, R.; Merino, M.J.; et al. Cabozantinib in Patients with Platinum-Refractory Metastatic Urothelial Carcinoma: An Open-Label, Single-Centre, Phase 2 Trial. *Lancet Oncol.* **2020**, *21*, 1099–1109. [CrossRef]
8. Kwilas, A.R.; Ardiani, A.; Donahue, R.N.; Aftab, D.T.; Hodge, J.W. Dual Effects of a Targeted Small-Molecule Inhibitor (Cabozantinib) on Immune-Mediated Killing of Tumor Cells and Immune Tumor Microenvironment Permissiveness When Combined with a Cancer Vaccine. *J. Transl. Med.* **2014**, *12*, 294. [CrossRef]
9. Choueiri, T.K.; Powles, T.; Burotto, M.; Escudier, B.; Bourlon, M.T.; Zurawski, B.; Oyervides Juárez, V.M.; Hsieh, J.J.; Basso, U.; Shah, A.Y.; et al. Nivolumab Plus Cabozantinib Versus Sunitinib for Advanced Renal-Cell Carcinoma. *N. Engl. J. Med.* **2021**, *384*, 829–841. [CrossRef] [PubMed]
10. Heng, D.Y.; Xie, W.; Regan, M.M.; Warren, M.A.; Golshayan, A.R.; Sahi, C.; Eigl, B.J.; Ruether, J.D.; Cheng, T.; North, S.; et al. Prognostic Factors for Overall Survival in Patients with Metastatic Renal Cell Carcinoma Treated with Vascular Endothelial Growth Factor-Targeted Agents: Results from a Large, Multicenter Study. *J. Clin. Oncol.* **2009**, *27*, 5794–5799. [CrossRef] [PubMed]
11. Powles, T.; Motzer, R.J.; Escudier, B.; Pal, S.; Kollmannsberger, C.; Pikiel, J.; Gurney, H.; Rha, S.Y.; Park, S.H.; Geertsen, P.F.; et al. Outcomes Based on Prior Therapy in the Phase 3 Meteor Trial of Cabozantinib Versus Everolimus in Advanced Renal Cell Carcinoma. *Br. J. Cancer* **2018**, *119*, 663–669. [CrossRef] [PubMed]
12. McGregor, B.A.; Lalani, A.A.; Xie, W.; Steinharter, J.A.; Bakouny, Z.E.; Martini, D.J.; Fleischer, J.H.; Abou-Alaiwi, S.; Nassar, A.; Nuzzo, P.V.; et al. Activity of Cabozantinib after Immune Checkpoint Blockade in Metastatic Clear-Cell Renal Cell Carcinoma. *Eur. J. Cancer* **2020**, *135*, 203–210. [CrossRef]
13. Navani, V.; Wells, J.C.; Boyne, D.J.; Cheung, W.Y.; Brenner, D.M.; McGregor, B.A.; Labaki, C.; Schmidt, A.L.; McKay, R.R.; Meza, L.; et al. Caboseq: The Effectiveness of Cabozantinib in Patients with Treatment Refractory Advanced Renal Cell Carcinoma:

Results from the International Metastatic Renal Cell Carcinoma Database Consortium (Imdc). *Clin. Genitourin. Cancer* **2023**, *21*, 106.e1–106.e8. [CrossRef]
14. Shah, A.Y.; Kotecha, R.R.; Lemke, E.A.; Chandramohan, A.; Chaim, J.L.; Msaouel, P.; Xiao, L.; Gao, J.; Campbell, M.T.; Zurita, A.J.; et al. Outcomes of Patients with Metastatic Clear-Cell Renal Cell Carcinoma Treated with Second-Line Vegfr-Tki after First-Line Immune Checkpoint Inhibitors. *Eur. J. Cancer* **2019**, *114*, 67–75. [CrossRef] [PubMed]
15. Bedke, J.; Albiges, L.; Capitanio, U.; Giles, R.H.; Hora, M.; Lam, T.B.; Ljungberg, B.; Marconi, L.; Klatte, T.; Volpe, A.; et al. Updated European Association of Urology Guidelines on Renal Cell Carcinoma: Nivolumab Plus Cabozantinib Joins Immune Checkpoint Inhibition Combination Therapies for Treatment-Naïve Metastatic Clear-Cell Renal Cell Carcinoma. *Eur. Urol.* **2021**, *79*, 339–342. [CrossRef] [PubMed]
16. Rathmell, W.K.; Rumble, R.B.; Van Veldhuizen, P.J.; Al-Ahmadie, H.; Emamekhoo, H.; Hauke, R.J.; Louie, A.V.; Milowsky, M.I.; Molina, A.M.; Rose, T.L.; et al. Management of Metastatic Clear Cell Renal Cell Carcinoma: Asco Guideline. *J. Clin. Oncol.* **2022**, *40*, 2957–2995. [CrossRef] [PubMed]
17. Kucharz, J.; Budnik, M.; Dumnicka, P.; Pastuszczak, M.; Kuśnierz-Cabala, B.; Demkow, T.; Popko, K.; Wiechno, P. Hand-Foot Syndrome and Progression-Free Survival in Patients Treated with Sunitinib for Metastatic Clear Cell Renal Cell Carcinoma. *Adv. Exp. Med. Biol.* **2019**, *1133*, 35–40. [CrossRef] [PubMed]
18. Wolfe, J.D.; Wolfe, N.K.; Rich, M.W. Perioperative Care of the Geriatric Patient for Noncardiac Surgery. *Clin. Cardiol.* **2020**, *43*, 127–136. [CrossRef] [PubMed]
19. Anderson, S.; Brenner, B.M. The Aging Kidney: Structure, Function, Mechanisms, and Therapeutic Implications. *J. Am. Geriatr. Soc.* **1987**, *35*, 590–593. [CrossRef]
20. European Medicines Agency. Summmary of Product Characteristics Cabozantinib. 2021. Available online: https://Www.Ema.Europa.Eu/En/Documents/Product-Information/Cabometyx-Epar-Product-Information_En.Pdf (accessed on 11 November 2023).
21. U.S. Department of Health and Human Services. Common Terminology Criteria for Adverse Events (Ctcae) Version 5.0. 2017. Available online: https://ctep.cancer.gov/protocoldevelopment/electronic_applications/docs/ctcae_v5_quick_reference_5x7.pdf (accessed on 20 December 2023).
22. Choueiri, T.K.; Escudier, B.; Powles, T.; Tannir, N.M.; Mainwaring, P.N.; Rini, B.I.; Hammers, H.J.; Donskov, F.; Roth, B.J.; Peltola, K.; et al. Cabozantinib Versus Everolimus in Advanced Renal Cell Carcinoma (Meteor): Final Results from a Randomised, Open-Label, Phase 3 Trial. *Lancet Oncol.* **2016**, *17*, 917–927. [CrossRef]
23. Choueiri, T.K.; Halabi, S.; Sanford, B.L.; Hahn, O.; Michaelson, M.D.; Walsh, M.K.; Feldman, D.R.; Olencki, T.; Picus, J.; Small, E.J.; et al. Cabozantinib Versus Sunitinib as Initial Targeted Therapy for Patients with Metastatic Renal Cell Carcinoma of Poor or Intermediate Risk: The Alliance A031203 Cabosun Trial. *J. Clin. Oncol.* **2017**, *35*, 591–597. [CrossRef]
24. Bodnar, L.; Kopczyńska, A.; Żołnierek, J.; Wieczorek-Rutkowska, M.; Chrom, P.; Tomczak, P. Real-World Experience of Cabozantinib as Second- or Subsequent Line Treatment in Patients with Metastatic Renal Cell Carcinoma: Data from the Polish Managed Access Program. *Clin. Genitourin. Cancer* **2019**, *17*, e556–e564. [CrossRef]
25. Iinuma, K.; Tomioka-Inagawa, R.; Kameyama, K.; Taniguchi, T.; Kawada, K.; Ishida, T.; Nagai, S.; Enomoto, T.; Ueda, S.; Kawase, M.; et al. Efficacy and Safety of Cabozantinib in Patients with Advanced or Metastatic Renal Cell Carcinoma: A Multicenter Retrospective Cohort Study. *Biomedicines* **2022**, *10*, 3172. [CrossRef] [PubMed]
26. Tran, B.D.; Li, J.; Ly, N.; Faggioni, R.; Roskos, L. Cabozantinib Exposure-Response Analysis for the Phase 3 Checkmate 9er Trial of Nivolumab Plus Cabozantinib Versus Sunitinib in First-Line Advanced Renal Cell Carcinoma. *Cancer Chemother. Pharmacol.* **2023**, *91*, 179–189. [CrossRef] [PubMed]
27. Buda-Nowak, A.; Kucharz, J.; Dumnicka, P.; Kuzniewski, M.; Herman, R.M.; Zygulska, A.L.; Kusnierz-Cabala, B. Sunitinib-Induced Hypothyroidism Predicts Progression-Free Survival in Metastatic Renal Cell Carcinoma Patients. *Med. Oncol.* **2017**, *34*, 68. [CrossRef] [PubMed]
28. Li, J.; Gu, J. Hand-Foot Skin Reaction with Vascular Endothelial Growth Factor Receptor Tyrosine Kinase Inhibitors in Cancer Patients: A Systematic Review and Meta-Analysis. *Crit. Rev. Oncol. Hematol.* **2017**, *119*, 50–58. [CrossRef] [PubMed]
29. Bono, P.; Rautiola, J.; Utriainen, T.; Joensuu, H. Hypertension as Predictor of Sunitinib Treatment Outcome in Metastatic Renal Cell Carcinoma. *Acta Oncol.* **2011**, *50*, 569–573. [CrossRef] [PubMed]
30. Belum, V.R.; Serna-Tamayo, C.; Wu, S.; Lacouture, M.E. Incidence and Risk of Hand-Foot Skin Reaction with Cabozantinib, a Novel Multikinase Inhibitor: A Meta-Analysis. *Clin. Exp. Dermatol.* **2016**, *41*, 8–15. [CrossRef]
31. Di Nunno, V.; Frega, G.; Gatto, L.; Brandi, G.; Massari, F. Hypothyroidism in Patients with Hepatocellular Carcinoma Receiving Cabozantinib: An Unassessed Issue. *Future Oncol.* **2019**, *15*, 563–565. [CrossRef]
32. Peverelli, G.; Raimondi, A.; Ratta, R.; Verzoni, E.; Bregni, M.; Cortesi, E.; Cartenì, G.; Fornarini, G.; Facchini, G.; Buti, S.; et al. Cabozantinib in Renal Cell Carcinoma with Brain Metastases: Safety and Efficacy in a Real-World Population. *Clin. Genitourin. Cancer* **2019**, *17*, 291–298. [CrossRef]
33. Janusch, M.; Fischer, M.; Marsch, W.; Holzhausen, H.J.; Kegel, T.; Helmbold, P. The Hand-Foot Syndrome—A Frequent Secondary Manifestation in Antineoplastic Chemotherapy. *Eur. J. Dermatol.* **2006**, *16*, 494–499.
34. Escudier, B.; Eisen, T.; Stadler, W.M.; Szczylik, C.; Oudard, S.; Siebels, M.; Negrier, S.; Chevreau, C.; Solska, E.; Desai, A.A.; et al. Sorafenib in Advanced Clear-Cell Renal-Cell Carcinoma. *N. Engl. J. Med.* **2007**, *356*, 125–134. [CrossRef]

35. Motzer, R.J.; Hutson, T.E.; Tomczak, P.; Michaelson, M.D.; Bukowski, R.M.; Rixe, O.; Oudard, S.; Negrier, S.; Szczylik, C.; Kim, S.T.; et al. Sunitinib Versus Interferon Alfa in Metastatic Renal-Cell Carcinoma. *N. Engl. J. Med.* **2007**, *356*, 115–124. [CrossRef]
36. Pożarowska, D.; Pożarowski, P. The Era of Anti-Vascular Endothelial Growth Factor (Vegf) Drugs in Ophthalmology, Vegf and Anti-Vegf Therapy. *Cent. Eur. J. Immunol.* **2016**, *41*, 311–316. [CrossRef] [PubMed]
37. Lipworth, A.D.; Robert, C.; Zhu, A.X. Hand-Foot Syndrome (Hand-Foot Skin Reaction, Palmar-Plantar Erythrodysesthesia): Focus on Sorafenib and Sunitinib. *Oncology* **2009**, *77*, 257–271. [CrossRef] [PubMed]
38. Michaelson, M.D.; Cohen, D.P.; Li, S.; Motzer, R.; Escudier, B.J.; Barrios, C.H.; Burnett, P.; Puzanov, I. Hand-Foot Syndrome (Hfs) as a Potential Biomarker of Efficacy in Patients (Pts) with Metastatic Renal Cell Carcinoma (Mrcc) Treated with Sunitinib (Su). *J. Clin. Oncol. Off. J. Am. Soc. Clin. Oncol.* **2011**, *29* (Suppl. S7), 320. [CrossRef]
39. Poprach, A.; Pavlik, T.; Melichar, B.; Puzanov, I.; Dusek, L.; Bortlicek, Z.; Vyzula, R.; Abrahamova, J.; Buchler, T. Skin Toxicity and Efficacy of Sunitinib and Sorafenib in Metastatic Renal Cell Carcinoma: A National Registry-Based Study. *Ann. Oncol.* **2012**, *23*, 3137–3143. [CrossRef] [PubMed]
40. Wu, J.; Huang, H. Acquired Hypothyroidism in Patients with Metastatic Renal Cell Carcinoma Treated with Tyrosine Kinase Inhibitors. *Drug Des. Dev. Ther.* **2020**, *14*, 3977–3982. [CrossRef] [PubMed]
41. Makita, N.; Iiri, T. Tyrosine Kinase Inhibitor-Induced Thyroid Disorders: A Review and Hypothesis. *Thyroid* **2013**, *23*, 151–159. [CrossRef]
42. Makita, N.; Miyakawa, M.; Fujita, T.; Iiri, T. Sunitinib Induces Hypothyroidism with a Markedly Reduced Vascularity. *Thyroid Off. J. Am. Thyroid Assoc.* **2010**, *20*, 323–326. [CrossRef]
43. Wolter, P.; Stefan, C.; Decallonne, B.; Dumez, H.; Fieuws, S.; Wildiers, H.; Clement, P.; Debaere, D.; Van Oosterom, A.; Schöffski, P. Evaluation of Thyroid Dysfunction as a Candidate Surrogate Marker for Efficacy of Sunitinib in Patients (Pts) with Advanced Renal Cell Cancer (Rcc). *J. Clin. Oncol.* **2008**, *26*, 5126. [CrossRef]
44. Kust, D.; Prpić, M.; Murgić, J.; Jazvić, M.; Jakšić, B.; Krilić, D.; Bolanča, A.; Kusić, Z. Hypothyroidism as a Predictive Clinical Marker of Better Treatment Response to Sunitinib Therapy. *Anticancer Res.* **2014**, *34*, 3177–3184.
45. Kucharz, J.; Dumnicka, P.; Kusnierz-Cabala, B.; Demkow, T.; Wiechno, P. The Correlation between the Incidence of Adverse Events and Progression-Free Survival in Patients Treated with Cabozantinib for Metastatic Renal Cell Carcinoma (Mrcc). *Med. Oncol.* **2019**, *36*, 19. [CrossRef]
46. Riesenbeck, L.M.; Bierer, S.; Hoffmeister, I.; Köpke, T.; Papavassilis, P.; Hertle, L.; Thielen, B.; Herrmann, E. Hypothyroidism Correlates with a Better Prognosis in Metastatic Renal Cancer Patients Treated with Sorafenib or Sunitinib. *World J. Urol.* **2011**, *29*, 807–813. [CrossRef]
47. Pinto, F.A.I.; Pereira, A.A.R.; Formiga, M.N.; Fanelli, M.F.; Chinen, L.T.D.; Lima, V.C.; De Melo Gagliato, D.; Santos, E.S.; Dettino, A.A.; Sousa, C.E.P.; et al. Association of Hypothyroidism with Improved Outcomes in First-Line Treatment of Renal Cell Carcinoma with Sunitinib. *J. Clin. Oncol.* **2012**, *30*, 466. [CrossRef]
48. Schmidinger, M.; Vogl, U.M.; Bojic, M.; Lamm, W.; Heinzl, H.; Haitel, A.; Clodi, M.; Kramer, G.; Zielinski, C.C. Hypothyroidism in Patients with Renal Cell Carcinoma: Blessing or Curse? *Cancer* **2011**, *117*, 534–544. [CrossRef]
49. Wang, H.E.; Muntner, P.; Chertow, G.M.; Warnock, D.G. Acute Kidney Injury and Mortality in Hospitalized Patients. *Am. J. Nephrol.* **2012**, *35*, 349–355. [CrossRef] [PubMed]
50. Allinovi, M.; Sessa, F.; Villa, G.; Cocci, A.; Innocenti, S.; Zanazzi, M.; Tofani, L.; Paparella, L.; Curi, D.; Cirami, C.L.; et al. Novel Biomarkers for Early Detection of Acute Kidney Injury and Prediction of Long-Term Kidney Function Decline after Partial Nephrectomy. *Biomedicines* **2023**, *11*, 1046. [CrossRef] [PubMed]
51. Yamanaka, T.; Takemura, K.; Hayashida, M.; Suyama, K.; Urakami, S.; Miura, Y. Cabozantinib-Induced Serum Creatine Kinase Elevation and Rhabdomyolysis: A Retrospective Case Series. *Cancer Chemother. Pharmacol.* **2023**, *92*, 235–240. [CrossRef] [PubMed]
52. Schmidinger, M.; Danesi, R. Management of Adverse Events Associated with Cabozantinib Therapy in Renal Cell Carcinoma. *Oncologist* **2018**, *23*, 306–315. [CrossRef] [PubMed]

**Disclaimer/Publisher's Note:** The statements, opinions and data contained in all publications are solely those of the individual author(s) and contributor(s) and not of MDPI and/or the editor(s). MDPI and/or the editor(s) disclaim responsibility for any injury to people or property resulting from any ideas, methods, instructions or products referred to in the content.

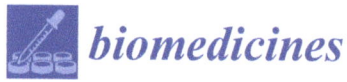 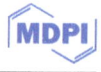

Article

# Expression of Basal Compartment and Superficial Markers in Upper Tract Urothelial Carcinoma Associated with Balkan Endemic Nephropathy, a Worldwide Disease

Ljubinka Jankovic Velickovic [1,2,*], Ana Ristic Petrovic [1,2,*], Zana Dolicanin [3], Slavica Stojnev [1,2], Filip Velickovic [4] and Dragoslav Basic [5]

1. Center for Pathology, University Clinical Center Nis, 18000 Nis, Serbia; slavicastojnev@gmail.com
2. Department of Pathology, Faculty of Medicine, University of Nis, 18000 Nis, Serbia
3. Department of Biomedical Sciences, State University of Novi Pazar, 36300 Novi Pazar, Serbia; dolicanin_z@yahoo.com
4. Department of Nuclear Medicine, Faculty of Medicine, University of Nis, 18000 Nis, Serbia; velickovicfilip@yahoo.com
5. Department of Urology, Faculty of Medicine, University of Nis, 18000 Nis, Serbia; basicdr@gmail.com
* Correspondence: ljubinkavelickovic60@gmail.com (L.J.V.); ana.v.ristic.petrovic@gmail.com (A.R.P.); Tel.: +381-64-2284789 (L.J.V.)

**Abstract:** The aim of this study was to determine the association of basal compartment and superficial markers, comprising CK5/6, CD44, CK20, and the pathological characteristics of upper tract urothelial carcinoma (UTUC) associated with Balkan endemic nephropathy (BEN). Comparing the expression of the investigated markers in 54 tumors from the BEN region and 73 control UTUC, no significant difference between them was detected. In regression analysis, CK20 expression was not determined with expression of CK5/6, CD44, and the phenotypic characteristics of BEN and control UTUC. Parameters with predictive influence on the expression of CD44 in BEN UTUC included growth pattern ($p = 0.010$), necrosis ($p = 0.019$); differentiation ($p = 0.001$), and lymphovascular invasion ($p = 0.021$) in control UTUC. Divergent squamous differentiation in BEN tumors ($p = 0.026$) and stage in control tumors ($p = 0.049$) had a predictive influence on the expression of CK5/6. This investigation detected a predictive influence of the phenotypic characteristics of UTUC on the expression of basal compartment and superficial markers, with a significant influence of necrosis in BEN tumors ($p = 0.006$) and differentiation in control UTUC ($p = 0.036$).

**Keywords:** upper tract urothelial cancer; Balkan endemic nephropathy; morphology; CKs; CD44

**Citation:** Jankovic Velickovic, L.; Ristic Petrovic, A.; Dolicanin, Z.; Stojnev, S.; Velickovic, F.; Basic, D. Expression of Basal Compartment and Superficial Markers in Upper Tract Urothelial Carcinoma Associated with Balkan Endemic Nephropathy, a Worldwide Disease. *Biomedicines* **2024**, *12*, 95. https://doi.org/10.3390/biomedicines12010095

**Academic Editors:** Łukasz Zapała and Paweł Rajwa

Received: 31 October 2023
Revised: 30 November 2023
Accepted: 14 December 2023
Published: 1 January 2024

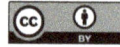

**Copyright:** © 2024 by the authors. Licensee MDPI, Basel, Switzerland. This article is an open access article distributed under the terms and conditions of the Creative Commons Attribution (CC BY) license (https://creativecommons.org/licenses/by/4.0/).

## 1. Introduction

Upper tract urothelial carcinoma (UTUC) constitutes only 5–6% of all epithelial tumors of the urinary tract, but in some regions of the world, the incidence of urothelial neoplasms of the renal pelvis and ureter is quite high [1–3]. Balkan endemic nephropathy (BEN) is a chronic, slowly progressive tubulointerstitial disease, and in the area of BEN, UTUC may occur alone or in combination with BEN [4].

UTUC is more invasive and worse differentiated than bladder cancer; thus, it requires as precise as possible an assessment of disease progression and tumor invasiveness for every individual case. Factors such as age, tumor grade, stage, sessile tumor growth, lymphovascular invasion (LVI), lymph node involvement, necrosis, and tumor location have been reported in the literature to be associated with the prognosis of patients with UTUC [1–4].

Some investigations have suggested that differentiation in the majority of urothelial carcinomas mirrors normal urothelial differentiation [5]. CK20 is a marker of cellular differentiation and is considered a useful and reliable marker of neoplastic change in urothelial cells. In normal urothelium, CK20 expression is confined to umbrella cells and occasional intermediate cells [6–8]. On the other hand, CD44 and CK5/6 are markers of basal compartment in the urothelium [9]. Chan et al. [10] have described a tumor-initiating cell subpopulation in primary human bladder cancer based on the expression of markers similar to those of normal bladder basal cells (lineage CD44 + CK5 + CK20−).

CD44 is a transmembrane glycoprotein involved in all essential cellular processes, like survival, differentiation, proliferation, migration, angiogenesis, and cellular signaling, through the presentation of cytokines and growth factors to the corresponding receptors. CD44 expression is associated with bladder cancer aggressiveness and resistance to chemo and radio treatment, and the ratio in urothelial cancer tissue and urinary exfoliated cells showed a significant correlation in the same patients; therefore, it was proposed as a prognostic predictor [9,11,12].

The aims of this study were to determine the association of basal compartment and superficial markers (CK5/6, CK20, and CD44) with the pathological characteristics of UTUC in BEN and a control population and to estimate the predictive impact of these markers in UTUC.

## 2. Patients and Methods

### 2.1. Patient's Population

We studied 127 patients with UTUC who had undergone nephroureterectomy with bladder cuff removal and extended lymphadenectomy. All cases of UTUC were diagnosed at the Center for Pathology, University Clinical Center Nis. The study included 93 pelvic and 34 ureteral urothelial. Patients were divided into two groups: 54 patients were from villages along the South Morava River basin, which are endemic settlements for BEN (BEN tumors); and 73 were residents of areas that are free of BEN (control subjects).

### 2.2. Histologic Analysis

The histological sections were processed from tissue fixed in 10% formalin and stained with hematoxylin and eosin (H&E). Obtained H&E slides were used to estimate histological variant, divergent differentiation, growth pattern (papillary/solid), tumor grade (low/high grade), and the presence of necrosis and lymphovascular invasion (LVI), as well as to determine pathologic stage (pT) [13]. The authors compared low-stage non-muscle invasive tumors (pTa and pT1) and high-stage muscle invasive (pT2-pT4) tumors [3]. The tumor necrosis was based on macroscopic and microscopic examination of the tumor, and the cut-off was the presence of 10% macroscopic necrosis confirmed microscopically [14]. The squamous differentiation was defined as the presence of intercellular bridges or keratinization [15].

### 2.3. Immunohistochemical Scoring

Monoclonal antibodies against CK 20, CK 5/6, and CD44 (Dako, Glostrup, Denmark) at dilution 1:50, 1:50, and 1:50, respectively, with a standard En Vision system were used. Slides were reviewed independently by three researchers (LJV, ARP, SS), and areas with greater positivity were selected. Cytoplasmic (CK20, CK5/6) and membranous (CD44) expression was recorded for the investigated antibodies.

Based on personal observations and findings derived from the previously reported literature, immunohistochemical expression of CK20, CK5/6, CD44 in UTUC was defined as normal or altered as follows.

CK20 immunoreactivity was classified as normal (N) group (expression in superficial cells or absent staining) and altered (A) group (focal pattern or diffuse pattern, in which more than 10% of tumor cells were positive) [11]. CK5/6 was classified as normal (N) group (no staining or staining only in basal/parabasal cells) and altered (A) group (moderate to strong staining usually through the full thickness of the urothelium) [7]. The CD44 normal (N) group included strong expression on the plasma membranes of basal cells or the immunoreactivity of CD44 in basal, suprabasal, and intermediate cells, but not in the superficial cells (accentuated pattern). The altered (A) group included tumors which displayed a focal or total loss of basal CD44 expression or a focal loss of staining in an otherwise-accentuated pattern [11].

According to the investigated antigens, all tumors were classified into four groups based on normal (N) or altered (A) expression of CK5/6/CD44/CK20. Altered expression of all three markers was detected in only 4/127 (3.14%) UTUC (two in BEN and two in control UTUC). Therefore, groups 1, 2, and 3 contain tumors with either normal or altered CK5/6 expression. Group 1 comprised tumors with altered CK20 ($n = 26/127$ (20.5%)), group 2 included tumors with alteration of both CK20 and CD44 ($n = 39/127$ (30.7%)), group 3 contained tumors with altered expression of CD44 ($n = 32/127$ (25.2%)), and group 4 comprised tumors with normal expression of all three markers ($n = 26/127$ (20.47%)).

### 2.4. Statistical Analysis

For the purposes of analysis, pathological tumor stage (low vs. high), grade (low vs. high), growth pattern (papillary vs. solid), LVI (no vs. yes), necrosis (no vs. yes), squamous differentiation (no vs. yes), and clinical parameters, i.e., sex (M vs. F) and localization (pelvis vs. ureter), were evaluated as dichotomized variables. The $\chi^2$ (Fisher's exact) test was used to estimate the expression of CK20, CK5/6, and CD44 in regard to pathological parameters (stage, grade, growth pattern, LVI, necrosis, squamous differentiation of tumors). Logistic regression analysis was used to detect the influence of every morphological characteristic, respectively, and each separately to the expression of CK5/6, CD44, and CK20. PLUM (Polytomous Universal Model) regression analysis was used to detect the predictive influence of the investigated pathological characteristics on the expression of basal compartment and superficial markers.

The result was considered statistically significant if $p < 0.05$. All analyses were performed with the Statistical Package for Social Sciences (version 24.0 statistical software (SPSS, Chicago, IL, USA).

## 3. Results

### 3.1. Clinical Features in UTUC

The age of the 127 patients with UTUC ranged from 22 to 85 years, with a mean age of 64.74 ± 8.31 years for tumors in BEN regions and 63.89 ± 10.7 years for control tumors. There were 25 male (46%) and 29 female (54%) patients in the BEN-associated UTUC group with ratio M:F = 1.2:1; while in the control group, there were 39 men (53%) and 34 women (47%) with ratio M:F = 1.1:1. With respect of localization, tumors were more frequent localized on the left side in both BEN and control UTUC, albeit without a statistical difference between these two groups (32/22 versus 46/27).

### 3.2. Immunohistochemical Evaluation of CKs and CD44 and the Association with Pathological Characteristics in BEN and Control UTUC

The investigated markers—CK20, CK5/6, and CD44—were altered in 65 (51.2%), 14 (11%), and 71 (55.9%) UTUC, respectively (Figure 1).

Through investigation of the relationships between conventional pathological parameters and the altered immunohistochemical staining of CK20, CK5/6, and CD44 in UTUC, BEN tumors showed that altered expression of CK20 was significantly associated with grade (high 22/10 (68.8%) versus low 9/13 (40.9%), $\chi^2 = 4.06$, $p < 0.05$); and CD44 was significantly linked to tumor grade, stage, growth, and presence of necrosis (high-grade 24/8 (75%) versus low grade 7/15 (31.8%), $\chi^2 = 9.76$, $p < 0.005$; high-stage 22/9 (71%) versus low-stage 9/14 (39.1%), $\chi^2 = 5.37$, $p < 0.05$; solid growth 28/8 (77.8%) versus papillary 3/15 (16,7%), $\chi^2 = 17.99$, $p < 0.00005$; necrosis (yes 20/2 (90.9%) versus no 11/21 (34.4%), $\chi^2 = 16.73$, $p < 0.00005$)) (Table 1).

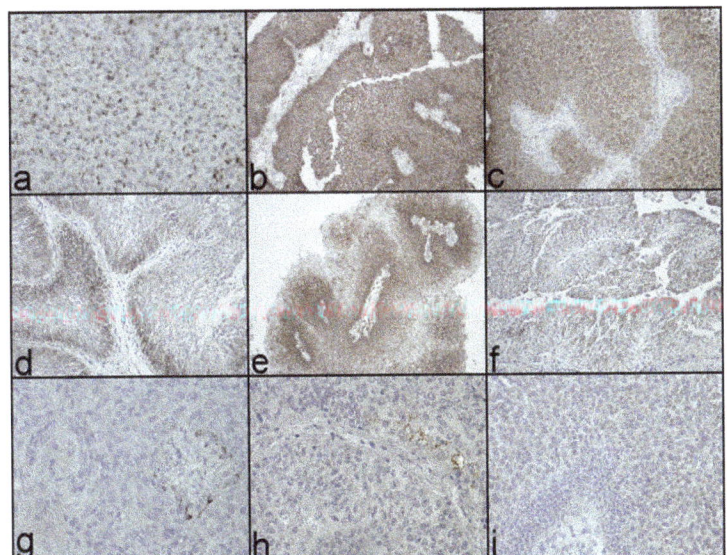

**Figure 1.** The representative altered and normal immunohistochemical expression of basal compartment and superficial markers (CK5/6 (**a,d,g**), CD44 (**b,e,h**), and CK20 (**c,f,i**)) in BEN-associated upper tract urothelial carcinoma with coexpression patterns (**a,b,c**) (original magnification: ×400).

**Table 1.** Association of CK20, CK5/6, and CD44 expression with pathological characteristics of BEN and control tumors.

| UTUC | BEN N54 | CK20 | CK5/6 | CD44 | Control N73 | CK20 | CK5/6 | CD44 |
|---|---|---|---|---|---|---|---|---|
| Grade | | | | | | | | |
| Low | 22 | 9 | 1 | 7 | 25 | 8 | 3 | 6 |
| High | 32 | 22 | 4 | 24 | 48 | 25 | 6 | 34 |
| p< | | 0.05 | NS * | 0.005 | | NS * | NS * | 0.0005 |
| Stage | | | | | | | | |
| Low | 23 | 11 | 1 | 9 | 23 | 8 | 6 | 8 |
| High | 31 | 20 | 4 | 22 | 50 | 26 | 3 | 32 |
| p< | | NS * | NS * | 0.05 | | NS * | NS * | 0.05 |
| Growth | | | | | | | | |
| Papillary | 18 | 7 | 1 | 3 | 27 | 9 | 3 | 9 |
| Solid | 36 | 24 | 4 | 28 | 46 | 25 | 6 | 31 |
| p< | | NS * | NS * | 0.00005 | | NS * | NS * | 0.005 |
| LVI | | | | | | | | |
| no | 42 | 23 | 4 | 28 | 50 | 19 | 7 | 21 |
| yes | 12 | 8 | 1 | 9 | 23 | 15 | 2 | 19 |
| p< | | NS * | NS * | NS * | | 0.05 | NS * | 0.005 |
| Necrosis | | | | | | | | |
| no | 32 | 18 | 1 | 11 | 40 | 17 | 5 | 19 |
| yes | 22 | 13 | 4 | 20 | 33 | 17 | 4 | 21 |
| p< | | NS * | NS * | 0.00005 | | NS * | NS * | NS * |
| Divergent dif. | | | | | | | | |
| no | 40 | 23 | 1 | 22 | 53 | 24 | 4 | 27 |
| yes | 14 | 8 | 4 | 9 | 20 | 10 | 5 | 13 |
| p< | | NS * | NS * | NS * | | NS * | NS * | NS * |

* NS: not significant.

Control tumors displayed a statistically significant association between altered expression of CK20 and LVI (LVI yes 15/8 (65.2%) versus LVI no 19/31 (38%), $\chi^2 = 4.63$, $p < 0.05$); CD44 was in statistically significant association with grade, stage, growth, and LVI (high-grade 34/14 (70.8%) versus low-grade 6/19 (24%), $\chi^2 = 14.36$, $p < 0.0005$; high-stage 32/18 (64%) versus low-stage 8/15 (34.8%), $\chi^2 = 5.35$, $p < 0.05$; solid growth 31/15 (67.4%) versus papillary 9/18 (33.3%), $\chi^2 = 7.86$, $p < 0.005$; LVI yes 19/4 (82.6%) versus LVI no 21/29 (42%), $\chi^2 = 10.34$, $p < 0.005$). A significant association was not detected between the phenotypic characteristics of BEN and control UTUC and altered expression of CK5/6 (Table 1).

Comparing the expression of CK20, CK5/6, and CD44 and group, a significant difference was not detected between BEN and control tumors. However, BEN tumors with necrosis had a significant difference in altered expression of CD44 compared to control tumors with the same morphological findings (20/2 (90.9%) versus 21/12 (63.6%), $\chi^2 = 5.08$, $p < 0.05$).

### 3.3. Influence of Expression of Basal Compartment and Superficial Markers-CKs and CD44 on Pathological Characteristics of BEN and Control UTUC

BEN tumors contain 11/54 (20.37%) UTUC from group 1; 20/54 (37.03%) from group 2; 11/54 (20.37%) from group 3; and 12/54 (22.2%) from group 4 UTUC. Group 2 is significantly differentiated from group 4 in grade, stage, growth, and necrosis (high-grade, $\chi^2 = 12.92$, $p < 0.0005$; high-stage, $\chi^2 = 5.91$, $p < 0.05$; solid growth, $\chi^2 = 16.67$, $p < 0.00005$; and presence of necrosis, $\chi^2 = 9.74$, $p < 0.005$, respectively). Group 2 UTUC is very similar to that of group 1 and differentiated in terms of growth ($\chi^2 = 4.94$, $p < 0.05$), and no significant difference was detected between groups 2 and 3. Also, tumors from group 3 are significantly differentiated from UTUC group 4 in terms of grade, stage, growth, and necrosis ($\chi^2 = 12.06$, $p < 0.001$; $\chi^2 = 5.01$, $p < 0.05$; $\chi^2 = 12.13$, $p < 0.0005$; and $\chi^2 = 15.43$, $p < 0.0001$, respectively). Group 1 UTUC, with alteration of superficial marker CK20, has a significant difference in grade compared with group 4 ($\chi^2 = 7.40$, $p < 0.001$) (Table 2).

Table 2. Expression of basal compartment and superficial markers in BEN and control UTUC.

| UTUC | BEN N 54 | | | | | | Control N73 | | | | | |
|---|---|---|---|---|---|---|---|---|---|---|---|---|
| | 1:2 | 1:3 | 1:4 | 2:3 | 2:4 | 3:4 | 1:2 | 1:3 | 1:4 | 2:3 | 2:4 | 3:4 |
| Grade | 4/7 | 4/7 | 4/7 | 5/15 | 5/15 | 2/9 | 7/8 | 7/8 | 7/8 | 1/18 | 1/18 | 3/18 |
|  | 5/15 | 2/9 | 11/1 | 2/9 | 11/1 | 11/1 | 1/18 | 3/18 | 12/2 | 3/18 | 12/2 | 12/2 |
| $p<$ | NS * | NS * | 0.01 | NS * | 0.0005 | 0.001 | 0.001 | 0.05 | 0.05 | NS * | 0.000005 | 0.00005 |
| Stage | 5/6 | 5/6 | 5/6 | 6/14 | 6/14 | 3/8 | 6/9 | 6/9 | 6/9 | 2/17 | 2/17 | 6/15 |
|  | 6/14 | 3/8 | 9/3 | 3/8 | 9/3 | 9/3 | 2/17 | 6/15 | 6/8 | 6/15 | 6/8 | 6/8 |
| $p<$ | NS * | NS * | NS * | NS * | 0.05 | 0.05 | 0.05 | NS * | NS * | NS * | 0.05 | NS * |
| Growth | 5/6 | 5/6 | 5/6 | 2/18 | 2/18 | 1/10 | 6/9 | 6/9 | 6/9 | 3/16 | 3/16 | 6/15 |
|  | 2/18 | 1/10 | 10/2 | 1/10 | 10/2 | 10/2 | 3/16 | 6/15 | 11/3 | 6/15 | 11/3 | 11/3 |
| $p<$ | 0.05 | NS * | NS * | NS * | 0.00005 | 0.0005 | NS * | NS * | 0.05 | NS * | 0.0005 | 0.005 |
| LVI | 10/1 | 10/1 | 10/1 | 13/7 | 13/7 | 9/2 | 13/2 | 13/2 | 13/2 | 6/13 | 6/13 | 15/6 |
|  | 13/7 | 9/2 | 10/2 | 9/2 | 10/2 | 10/2 | 6/13 | 15/6 | 13/1 | 15/6 | 13/1 | 13/1 |
| $p<$ | NS * | NS * | NS * | NS * | NS * | NS * | 0.005 | NS * | NS * | 0.05 | 0.001 | NS * |
| Necrosis | 9/2 | 9/2 | 9/2 | 9/11 | 9/11 | 2/9 | 8/7 | 8/7 | 8/7 | 9/10 | 9/10 | 10/11 |
|  | 9/11 | 2/9 | 12/0 | 2/9 | 12/0 | 12/0 | 9/10 | 10/11 | 10/4 | 10/11 | 10/4 | 10/4 |
| $p<$ | NS * | 0.005 | 0.005 | NS * | NS * | 0.005 | 0.0001 | NS * | NS * | NS * | NS * | NS * |
| Squamous differentiation | 8/3 | 8/3 | 8/3 | 15/5 | 15/5 | 7/4 | 11/4 | 11/4 | 11/4 | 13/6 | 13/6 | 14/7 |
|  | 15/5 | 7/2 | 10/2 | 7/4 | 10/2 | 10/2 | 13/6 | 13/6 | 14/7 | 14/7 | 13/1 | 13/1 |
| $p<$ | NS * | NS * | NS * | NS * | NS * | NS * | NS * | NS * | NS * | NS * | NS * | NS * |

1. CK5/6 N and A, CD44 N, CK20 A; 2. CK5/6 N and A, CD44 A, CK20 A; 3. CK5/6 N and A, CD44 A, CK20 N; 4. CK5/6 N, CD44 N, CK20 N. * NS: not significant.

Control tumors account for 15/73 (20.54%) UTUC from group 1; 19/73 (26.02%) from group 2; 21/73 (28.76%) from group 3; and 14/73 (19.17%) from group 4 UTUC. In group 2 of control UTUC, compared to group 4, there was a significant difference in grade, stage, growth, and LVI was detected ($\chi^2 = 21.19$, $p < 0.000005$; $\chi^2 = 4.45$, $p < 0.005$; $\chi^2 = 12.61$, $p < 0.0005$; $\chi^2 = 12.02$, $p < 0.0015$, respectively). Group 2 is very similar to group 3 (difference only in LVI, $\chi^2 = 6.19$, $p < 0.05$), but the difference was evident between this group and group 1 in terms of grade, stage, and LVI (high-grade, $\chi^2 = 7.75$, $p < 0.01$; high-stage, $\chi^2 = 3.93$, $p < 0.05$, and presence of LVI, $\chi^2 = 10.01$, $p < 0.005$). UTUC with alteration of CD44 (group 3) differed significantly from group 1 in grade (high grade, ($\chi^2 = 4.45$, $p < 0.05$), and differed from group 4 in grade and growth (high grade, $\chi^2 = 17.00$, $p < 0.00005$; solid growth, $\chi^2 = 8.17$, $p < 0.005$, respectively) (Table 2).

In addition, the multistep logistic regression model, which included investigated basal and superficial markers (CK5/6, CD44, CK20), as well as group, localization, and pathological characteristics, showed that alteration of CK20 was not determined by expression of CD44 and CK5/6 and the phenotypic characteristics of UTUC and the groups (BEN and control UTUC). Differentiation and LVI had a prominent influence on the expression of CD44 in control UTUC (Wald = 10.464 $p = 0.001$; Wald = 5.316 $p = 0.021$). Growth pattern and necrosis had the prominent influence on the expression of CD44 in BEN UTUC (Wald = 6.654 $p = 0.010$; Wald = 5.460 $p = 0.019$). Squamous divergent differentiation in BEN UTUC had a notable influence on the expression of CK5/6 (Wald = 4.974 $p = 0.026$), and stage in the control UTUC determined the expression of CK5/6 (Wald = 3.890 $p = 0.049$) (Table 3).

**Table 3.** Logistic regression analysis of basal compartment and superficial markers, CK5/6, CD44, and CK20, and morphological characteristics in UTUC.

| Dependent Variable | Variable | Basal Compartment and Superficial Markers | | | | | | |
|---|---|---|---|---|---|---|---|---|
| | | B | S.E. | Wald | Sig. | Exp(B) | 95.0% C.I. for EXP(B) | Dependent Variable |
| CK20 | CD44 | −0.344 | 0.359 | 0.917 | 0.338 | 0.709 | 0.350 | 1.434 |
| | CK5/6 | 0.384 | 0.574 | 0.447 | 0.504 | 1.468 | 0.476 | 4.522 |
| | | Morphological characteristics: BEN UTUC | | | | | | |
| CK20 | All entered variables ** | | | | NS *** | | | |
| CD44 | GROWTH | −3.364 | 1.304 | 6.654 | 0.010 | 0.035 | 0.003 | 0.446 |
| | NECROSIS | −2.530 | 1.083 | 5.460 | 0.019 | 0.080 | 0.010 | 0.665 |
| | All others | | | | NS *** | | | |
| CK5/6 | DIFF | −2.973 | 1.333 | 4.974 | 0.026 | 0.051 | 0.004 | 0.698 |
| | All others | −3.364 | 1.304 | 6.654 | 0.010 | 0.035 | 0.003 | 0.446 |
| | | Morphological characteristics: CONTROL UTUC | | | | | | |
| CK20 | All entered variables ** | | | | N.S. | | | |
| CD44 | LG/HG | −3.795 | 1.173 | 10.464 | 0.001 | 0.022 | 0.002 | 0.224 |
| | LVI | −1.879 | 0.815 | 5.316 | 0.021 | 0.153 | 0.031 | 0.754 |
| | All others | | | | NS *** | | | |
| CK5/6 | STAGE | 2.365 | 1.199 | 3.890 | 0.049 | 10.639 | 1.015 | 111.527 |
| | All others * | | | | NS *** | | | |

\* All entered variables: group, localization (pyelon/ureter), LG/HG, stage, growth, LVI, necrosis, divergent differentiation. ** All entered variables: P/U, LG/HG, stage, growth, LVI, necrosis, divergent differentiation. *** NS: not significant.

PLUM regression analysis of expression CK5/6, CD44, and CK20 in control UTUC showed that differentiation had a predictive influence on expression of the basal compartment and superficial markers (Wald = 4.404, $p = 0.036$) and on necrosis in BEN tumors (Wald = 7.707, $p = 0.006$) (Table 4).

Table 4. PLUM regression analysis of expression of basal compartment and superficial markers, CK5/6, CD44, and CK20, and morphological characteristics in UTUC.

|  |  | Estimate | Std. Error | Wald | Sig. | 95% Confidence Interval Lower Bound | Upper Bound |
|---|---|---|---|---|---|---|---|
|  |  | BEN UTUC |  |  |  |  |  |
| Threshold | [Group = 1–2] | −2.651 | 1.675 | 2.506 | 0.113 | −5.934 | 0.631 |
|  | [Group = 2–3] | 0.763 | 1.655 | 0.213 | 0.645 | −2.481 | 4.007 |
| Location | NECROSIS | 2.278 | 0.821 | 7.707 | 0.006 | 0.670 | 3.886 |
|  | All others * |  |  |  | NS ** |  |  |
|  |  | CONTROL UTUC |  |  |  |  |  |
| Threshold | [Group = 1–2] | −0.349 | 1.195 | 0.085 | 0.770 | −2.690 | 1.993 |
|  | [Group = 2–3] | 2.062 | 1.228 | 2.816 | 0.093 | −0.346 | 4.469 |
| Location | DIF | 1.523 | 0.726 | 4.404 | 0.036 | 0.101 | 2.946 |
|  | All others * |  |  |  | NS ** |  |  |

* All entered variables: P/U, dif., stage, growth (pap/sol), LVI (no/yes), necrosis (no/yes), divergent diff (no/yes).
** NS: not significant.

## 4. Discussion

In the urothelium, the transition from basal to terminally differentiated superficial cells is reflected in the different protein synthesis for each layer, which leads to the various morphological and antigenic characteristics [11,16]. CD44 is a cell adhesion molecule involved in tumor growth and biological behavior. CD44 realizes its functions through Fas inhibition, activating the mitogen-activated protein kinase (MAPK), and signaling and regulating the matrix metalloproteinases (MMPs) [17–20]. Recent data suggested that CD44 and p53 are important markers for the differential diagnosis of CIS from reactive/normal urothelium [11]. Inactivation of p53 results in overexpression of CD44, which may act as a tumor-promoting agent. However, the complexity of the problem stems from the poorly explained dualistic nature of CD44, which was found to be implicated in both tumor suppression and tumor promotion [21].

Our study showed that the dominant pattern of CD44 expression was altered, i.e., through the loss of CD44, in 55.9% of UTUC. The loss of CD44 expression is significantly connected with the morphological characteristics of aggressiveness in both control and BEN UTUC, which is reflected in high-grade, muscle-invasive disease, and the solid architecture pattern, as well as the presence of LVI in control tumors and necrosis in BEN UTUC.

Parameters with predictable influence on the expression of CD44 in BEN UTUC included architectural pattern and necrosis. Our previous comparative morphological study of BEN-associated tumors identified the sessile tumor architecture as a particular characteristic of these tumors [4], and this investigation detected that the solid growth of BEN tumors determined the loss of CD44 antigen. A predictable influence on the expression of CD44 in control UTUC was had by WHO grade and LVI. Similar findings related to the correlation of CD44 immunoreactivity and WHO grade, differentiation and LVI, have been reported by others [22,23].

CK5/6 is identified in squamous epithelium, the basal cells of the prostate, myoepithelial cells, and in different epithelial neoplasms [24]. In our study, parameters that had predictable influence on the expression of CK5/6 were squamous differentiation in BEN UTUC and stage of the control tumor, which has been shown in regression analysis [25]. Our previous morphological study of BEN tumors detected a higher frequency of divergent changes in BEN UTUC than in control tumors [4]. Additionally, urothelial lesions with squamous features showed higher CK5/6 expression. The CK 5/6 staining pattern varied between well-differentiated and poorly differentiated urothelial carcinoma. In low-grade papillary urothelial neoplasms, the CK 5/6-positive cells were observed at the basal cells; whereas in high-grade urothelial carcinoma, tumor cells were diffusely positive for CK 5/6 [24,26,27].

High expression of superficial marker CK20 was significantly associated with high grade in BEN tumors and the presence of LVI in control UTUC, but in regression analysis, the morphology of UTUC did not have a predictive influence on the expression of CK20, or the expression of CK5/6 and CD44.

BEN and control tumors have a similar presentation of basal compartment and superficial antigen. On the other hand, the absence of these antigens in BEN tumors is reflected in a significant presence of necrosis in regard to tumors with coexpression and heterogenous expression of the investigated antigens; moreover, the loss of coexpression in control tumors is associated with high grade in regard to other antigens profiles. In regression analysis, we detected that necrosis in BEN tumors and differentiation in control UTUC had a significant predictive influence on the change in the antigenic profile, from coexpression to the loss of coexpression, of basal compartment and superficial antigens.

This investigation showed that BEN and control tumors have a similar antigen presentation of basal compartment and superficial layer. Our findings indicate a predictive influence of the phenotypic characteristics of UTUC on the expression of basal compartment and superficial markers, with a significant influence of necrosis in BEN tumors and differentiation in control UTUC.

**Author Contributions:** Conceptualization, L.J.V.; Methodology, L.J.V., A.R.P., Z.D., S.S. and D.B.; Software, L.J.V., A.R.P. and F.V.; Validation, L.J.V., A.R.P. and S.S.; Formal analysis, L.J.V., A.R.P. and S.S.; Investigation, L.J.V., A.R.P., Z.D., S.S. and F.V.; Resources, L.J.V. and F.V.; Data curation, L.J.V. and D.B.; Writing—original draft, L.J.V.; Writing—review & editing, L.J.V., A.R.P., Z.D., S.S., F.V. and D.B. All authors have read and agreed to the published version of the manuscript.

**Funding:** This work was supported by Grant no. 175092 from the Ministry of Education and Science of Serbia.

**Institutional Review Board Statement:** The study was conducted in accordance with the Declaration of Helsinki, and approved by the Ethical Committee of the Medical Faculty, University of Nis (12-15637-2/6; 17 July 2019).

**Informed Consent Statement:** Informed consent was obtained from all subjects involved in the study.

**Data Availability Statement:** Data are contained within the article.

**Conflicts of Interest:** The authors declare no conflict of interest.

## References

1. Colin, P.; Koenig, P.; Ouzzane, A.; Berthon, N.; Villers, A.; Biserte, J.; Rouprêt, M. Environmental factors involved in carcinogenesis of urothelial cell carcinomas of the upper urinary tract. *BJU Int.* **2009**, *104*, 1436–1440. [CrossRef] [PubMed]
2. Tufano, A.; Perdonà, S.; Viscuso, P.; Frisenda, M.; Canale, V.; Rossi, A.; Del Prete, P.; Passaro, F.; Calarco, A. The Impact of Ethnicity and Age on Distribution of Metastases in Patients with Upper Tract Urothelial Carcinoma: Analysis of SEER Data. *Biomedicines* **2023**, *11*, 1943. [CrossRef] [PubMed]
3. Soualhi, A.; Rammant, E.; George, G.; Russell, B.; Enting, D.; Nair, R.; Hemelrijck, M.; Bosco, C. The incidence and prevalence of upper tract urothelial carcinoma: A systematic review. *BMC Urol.* **2021**, *21*, 110. [CrossRef] [PubMed]
4. Jankovic Velickovic, L.; Hattori, T.; Dolicanin, Z.; Visnjic, M.; Krstic, M.; Ilic, I.; Cukuranovic, R.; Rajic, M.; Stefanovic, V. Upper urothelial carcinoma in Balkan endemic nephropathy and non-endemic regions: A comparative study of pathological features. *Pathol. Res. Pract.* **2009**, *205*, 89–96. [CrossRef] [PubMed]
5. He, X.; Marchionni, L.; Hansel, E.D.; Yu, W.; Sood, A.; Yang, J.; Parmigiani, G.; Matsui, W.; Berman, D.M. Differentiation of a highly tumorigenic basal cell compartment in urothelial carcinoma. *Stem Cells* **2009**, *27*, 1487–1495. [CrossRef]
6. Arville, B.; O'Rourke, E.; Chung, F.; Amin, M.; Bose, S. Evaluation of a triple combination of cytokeratin 20, p53 and CD44 for improving detection of urothelial carcinoma in urine cytology specimens. *CytoJournal* **2013**, *10*, 25. [CrossRef] [PubMed]
7. Jung, S.; Wu, C.; Eslami, Z.; Tanguay, S.; Aprikian, A.; Kassouf, W.; Brimo, F. The role of immunohistochemistry in the diagnosis of flat urothelial lesions: A study using CK20, CK5/6, P53, Cd138, and Her2/Neu. *Ann. Diagn. Pathol.* **2014**, *18*, 27–32. [CrossRef]
8. Jung, M.; Kim, B.; Moon, K.C. Immunohistochemistry of cytokeratin (CK) 5/6, CD44 and CK20 as prognostic biomarkers of non-muscle-invasive papillary upper tract urothelial carcinoma. *Histopathology* **2019**, *74*, 483–493. [CrossRef]
9. Dimov, I.; Visnjic, M.; Stefanovic, V. Urothelial cancer stem cells. *Sci. World J.* **2010**, *10*, 1400–1415. [CrossRef]
10. Chan, K.S.; Espinosa, I.; Chao, M.; Wong, D.; Ailles, L.; Diehn, M.; Gill, H.; Presti, J., Jr.; Chang, H.Y.; van de Rijn, M.; et al. Identification, molecular characterization, clinical prognosis, and therapeutic targeting of human bladder tumor-initiating cells. *Proc. Natl. Acad. Sci. USA* **2009**, *106*, 14016–14021. [CrossRef]

11. Yoo, D.; Min, K.-W.; Pyo, J.-S.; Kim, N.Y. Diagnostic Roles of Immunohistochemical Markers CK20, CD44, AMACR, and p53 in Urothelial Carcinoma In Situ. *Medicina* **2023**, *59*, 1609. [CrossRef] [PubMed]
12. Erdogan, G.; Küçükosmanoğlu, I.; Akkaya, B.; Köksal, T.; Karpuzoğlu, G. CD44 and MMP-2 expression in urothelial carcinoma. *Turk. J. Pathol.* **2008**, *24*, 147–152.
13. Rouprêt, M.; Seisen, T.; Birtle, A.J.; Capoun, O.; Compérat, E.M.; Dominguez-Escrig, J.L.; Andersson, I.G.; Liedberg, F.; Mariappan, P.; Mostafid, A.H.; et al. European Association of Urology Guidelines on Upper Urinary Tract Urothelial Carcinoma: 2023 Update. *Eur. Urol.* **2023**, *84*, 49–64. [CrossRef] [PubMed]
14. Lee, S.E.; Hong, S.K.; Han, B.K.; Yu, J.H.; Han, J.H.; Jeong, S.J.; Byun, S.S.; Park, Y.H.; Choe, G. Prognostic significance of tumor necrosis in primary transitional cell carcinoma of upper urinary tract. *Jpn. J. Clin. Oncol.* **2007**, *37*, 49–55. [CrossRef] [PubMed]
15. Mirsya, W.S.; Dharma, K.D.; Putra, S.G.; Ali, H. The difference between cytokeratin 20 expression in high- and low-grade urothelial bladder carcinomas: A cross-sectional study. *Urol. Ann.* **2023**, *15*, 383–387.
16. Yeh, B.-W.; Yu, L.-E.; Li, C.-C.; Yang, J.-C.; Li, W.-M.; Wu, Y.-C.; Wei, Y.-C.; Lee, H.-T.; Kung, M.-L.; Wu, W.-J. The protoapigenone analog WYC0209 targets CD133+ cells: A potential adjuvant agent against cancer stem cells in urothelial cancer therapy. *Toxicol. Appl. Pharmacol.* **2020**, *402*, 115129. [CrossRef] [PubMed]
17. Marhaba, R.; Bourouba, M.; Zoller, M. CD44v6 promotes proliferation by persisting activation of MAP kinases. *Cell. Signal.* **2005**, *17*, 961–973. [CrossRef]
18. Kudelski, J.; Tokarzewicz, A.; Gudowska-Sawczuk, M.; Mroczko, B.; Chłosta, P.; Bruczko-Goralewska, M.; Mitura, P.; Młynarczyk, G. The Significance of Matrix Metalloproteinase 9 (MMP-9) and Metalloproteinase 2 (MMP-2) in Urinary Bladder Cancer. *Biomedicines* **2023**, *11*, 956. [CrossRef]
19. Wang, H.; Tan, M.; Zhang, S.; Li, X.; Gao, J.; Zhang, D.; Hao, Y.; Gao, S.; Liu, J.; Lin, B. Expression and significance of CD44, CD47 and c-met in ovarian clear cell carcinoma. *Int. J. Mol. Sci.* **2015**, *16*, 3391–3404. [CrossRef]
20. Godar, S.; Ince, T.A.; Bell, G.W.; Feldser, D.; Donaher, J.L.; Bergh, J.; Liu, A.; Miu, K.; Watnick, R.S.; Reinhardt, F.; et al. Growth-inhibitory and tumor-suppressive functions of p53 depend on its repression of CD44 expression. *Cell* **2008**, *134*, 62–73. [CrossRef]
21. Louderbough, J.M.; Schroeder, J.A. Understanding the dual nature of CD44 in breast cancer progression. *Mol. Cancer Res.* **2011**, *9*, 1573–1586. [CrossRef] [PubMed]
22. Hu, Y.; Zhang, Y.; Gao, J.; Lian, X.; Wang, Y. The clinicopathological and prognostic value of CD44 expression in bladder cancer: A study based on meta-analysis and TCGA data. *Bioengineered* **2020**, *11*, 572–581. [CrossRef] [PubMed]
23. Apollo, A.; Ortenzi, V.; Scatena, C.; Zavaglia, K.; Aretini, P.; Lessi, F.; Franceschi, S.; Tomei, S.; Sepich, C.A.; Viacava, P.; et al. Molecular characterization of low grade and high grade bladder cancer. *PLoS ONE* **2019**, *14*, e0210635. [CrossRef] [PubMed]
24. Akhtar, M.; Rashid, S.; Gashir, M.B.; Taha, N.M.; Al Bozom, I. CK20 and CK5/6 Immunohistochemical staining of urothelial neoplasms: A perspective. *Adv. Urol.* **2020**, *2020*, 4920236. [CrossRef]
25. Chu, P.G.; Weiss, L.M. Expression of cytokeratin 5/6 in epithelial neoplasms: An immunohistochemical study of 509 cases. *Mod. Pathol.* **2002**, *15*, 6–10. [CrossRef]
26. Jankovic Velickovic, L.; Dolicanin, Z.; Hattori, T.; Pesic, I.; Djordjevic, B.; Stojanovic, M.; Stankovic, J.; Visnic, M.; Stefanovic, V. Divergent squamous differentiation in upper urothelial carcinoma-comparative clinicopathological and molecular study. *Pathol. Oncol. Res.* **2011**, *17*, 535–539. [CrossRef]
27. Edgecombe, A.; Nguyen, B.N.; Djordjevic, B.; Belanger, E.C.; Mai, K.T. Utility of cytokeratin 5/6, cytokeratin 20, and p16 in the diagnosis of reactive urothelial atypia and noninvasive component of urothelial neoplasia. *Appl. Immunohistochem. Mol. Morphol.* **2012**, *20*, 264–271. [CrossRef]

**Disclaimer/Publisher's Note:** The statements, opinions and data contained in all publications are solely those of the individual author(s) and contributor(s) and not of MDPI and/or the editor(s). MDPI and/or the editor(s) disclaim responsibility for any injury to people or property resulting from any ideas, methods, instructions or products referred to in the content.

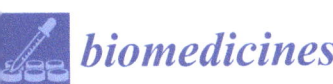 

*Article*

# Basement Membrane-Associated lncRNA Risk Model Predicts Prognosis and Guides Clinical Treatment in Clear Cell Renal Cell Carcinoma

Xinxin Li [1,†], Qihui Kuang [1,†], Min Peng [2,\*], Kang Yang [3] and Pengcheng Luo [1,\*]

1. Department of Urology, Wuhan Third Hospital (Tongren Hospital of Wuhan University), Wuhan 430060, China; xinxinli0408@whu.edu.cn (X.L.); 2021283030166@whu.edu.cn (Q.K.)
2. Department of Oncology, Renmin Hospital of Wuhan University, Wuhan 430060, China
3. Department of Urology, Renmin Hospital of Wuhan University, Wuhan 430060, China; kangyang@whu.edu.cn
\* Correspondence: mpeng320@whu.edu.cn (M.P.); pluo@whu.edu.cn (P.L.)
† These authors contributed equally to this work.

**Abstract:** The basement membrane (BM) affects the invasion and growth of malignant tumors. The role and mechanism of BM-associated lncRNAs in clear cell renal cell carcinoma (ccRCC) are unknown. In this study, we identified biomarkers of ccRCC and developed a risk model to assess patient prognosis. We downloaded transcripts and clinical data from the Cancer Genome Atlas (TCGA). Differential analysis, co-expression analysis, Cox regression analysis, and lasso regression were used to identify BM-associated prognostic lncRNAs and create a risk prediction model. We evaluated and validated the accuracy of the model using multiple methods and constructed a nomogram to predict the prognosis of ccRCC. GO, KEGG, and immunity analyses were used to explore differences in biological function. We constructed a risk model containing six BM-associated lncRNAs (LINC02154, IGFL2-AS1, NFE4, AC112715.1, AC092535.5, and AC105105.3). The risk model has higher diagnostic efficiency compared to clinical characteristics and can be used to forecast patient prognoses. We used renal cancer cells and tissue microarrays to verify the expression of lncRNAs in the risk model. We found that knocking down LINC02154 and AC112715.1 could inhibit the invasion ability of renal cancer cells. The risk model based on BM-associated lncRNAs can well predict ccRCC and guide clinical treatment.

**Keywords:** basement membrane; diagnostic; renal cancer; lncRNA; prognostic model; biomarker; immunotherapy

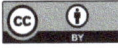

## 1. Introduction

As the most prevalent form of kidney cancer, ccRCC is highly aggressive and metastatic [1]. Approximately 80% of all renal cell carcinomas are clear cell renal cell carcinomas (ccRCCs) [2], which are the second most frequent kind of urinary system cancer, behind bladder cancer. Approximately one third of ccRCC patients may have metastases at the time of their first diagnosis, and one fourth of individuals with localized cancer may experience disease recurrence after a complete surgical excision [3]. A significant death rate is often linked with metastatic ccRCC [4,5]. Even with surgery, chemotherapy, radiation therapy, targeted therapy, and the newly suggested immunotherapy, ccRCC remains one of urology's greatest clinical difficulties [6]. A late diagnosis and a high risk of metastases are the primary causes [7]. Given the significant mortality and morbidity associated with ccRCC, it is essential to identify effective therapeutic targets, develop more accurate prognostic models, and identify relevant biomarkers for ccRCC patients.

The basement membrane (BM) is a thin, dense extracellular matrix (ECM) layer that is essential for the formation and function of normal tissues [8]. The BM contains an abundance of biochemical and mechanical signals and is necessary for cell signaling, structural integrity, and barrier protection against cells and macromolecules. Cancer is linked to changes in the mechanical and chemical properties of the BM [9]. As a protective structural barrier that impedes the invasion, migration, and extravasation of cancer cells, the BM plays an essential function in epithelial carcinomas and carcinomas. To metastasize, cells must enter through the basement membrane, which is a physical barrier preventing cancer cells from invading the surrounding stromal tissue. The endothelial BM impedes the invasion (intraluminal) and outflow (extravasation) of blood and lymphatic vessels by cancer cells during metastasis, which is associated with 90% of cancer deaths [10]. The growth of metastases or malignancies is a significant obstacle for cancer therapy and is a key factor contributing to higher mortality. The 5-year survival rate reduces considerably after cells enter the surrounding region via the BMS [11]; BM integrity is a crucial prognostic indication for patients. A thorough understanding of BM structure and processes, as well as cancer cell invasion of the BM, may lead to the development of innovative techniques for inhibiting cancer growth and metastasis.

RNAs longer than 200 base pairs (bps) are called long non-coding RNA (lncRNA), which do not have protein-coding activity and have an essential role in the regulation of the immune response. It is associated with immune cell infiltration, tumor elimination, antigen recognition, and exposure [12]. According to recent research, lncRNAs are involved in various tumor development pathways, encompassing carcinogenesis, proliferation, migration, invasion, and metastasis, as well as angiogenesis [13,14]. Liu demonstrated that lncRNAs participate in tumor autophagy [15]. Numerous studies have revealed that lncRNAs may influence target gene expression by competing with target genes [12,16,17]. LncRNAs are also associated with tumor therapy resistance [18]. However, the functions of basement membrane-associated lncRNAs in the prognosis of ccRCC and tumor immunotherapy remain unknown. This work aimed to build a prognostic risk model of basement membrane-associated lncRNAs to assess prognosis and guide clinical treatment in clear cell renal cell carcinoma.

## 2. Materials and Methods

*2.1. Collect and Identify lncRNAs Connected with Basement Membranes*

From the TCGA database, we collected clinical and transcriptome information for 541 ccRCC patients (https://portal.gdc.cancer.gov/repository (accessed on 1 December 2022)). Patients with inadequate clinical data were eliminated from the study. By doing a literature search, genes associated with basement membranes were found [19]. We screened for basement membrane genes and lncRNAs with differential expression between normal and renal clear cell carcinoma tissues using a $p$-value of 0.05 and $|\log2FC| > 1.5$ as cutoff values. We then identified lncRNAs linked with differentially expressed basement membrane genes using Pearson correlation analysis (|correlation coefficient| > 0.60, $p < 0.001$).

*2.2. Construction and Verification of a Basement Membrane-Associated lncRNA Risk Model*

The ccRCC patient data were assigned randomly to either the training set or the testing set in a ratio of 1:1. The training set was used to construct a risk model for basement membrane-associated lncRNAs, whereas the testing set and the overall set were utilized to verify the risk model. Basement membrane-associated lncRNAs linked with kidney carcinoma prognosis were identified using univariate Cox regression analysis. A prognostic risk model based on the optimal lncRNA was developed by utilizing the LASSO Cox regression technique and multivariate Cox regression analysis. Using this risk model, a risk score was assigned to every individual. This is how the risk score is computed: risk score = $\sum i = \ln\text{Coef}(i) \times \text{Expr}(i)$. In the equation, Coef (i) represents the regression coefficient of each lncRNA, and Expr (i) represents the normalized expression level of each lncRNA. Using the median risk score, the training set was divided into low- and high-risk groups. We applied Kaplan–Meier curves to explore if the two risk groups differed in terms of overall survival. We drew receiver operating characteristic (ROC) curves for clinical characteristics and prognostic models, evaluated the area under the curve (AUC), and used the concordance index (C-index) to evaluate the risk model's accuracy.

*2.3. Creating and Validating Predicted Nomograms and Evaluating the Relationship between the Prognostic Signatures and Clinicopathological Features*

To predict OS in ccRCC patients at 1, 3, and 5 years, we built nomograms using the rms R package (R 4.2.1) based on clinical parameters and risk scores. According to the nomogram scoring technique, each variable is given a score, and the total score for each sample is calculated by summing the scores of every variable. The prediction ability of an existing nomogram model was evaluated using a nomogram calibration plot. The connection between basement membrane-associated lncRNAs and clinicopathological characteristics was studied using logistic regression and heat maps.

*2.4. PCA, Functional Enrichment, Tumor Immunity, Drug Sensitivity, and Mortality Analysis*

Principal component analysis (PCA) was used to investigate the geographical distribution of two risk groups across four expression profiles (total gene expression profile, basement membrane gene expression profile, basement membrane-associated lncRNA expression profile, and six basement membrane-associated lncRNA expression profiles in the risk model). We evaluated enrichment pathways and biological processes for genes that were expressed differently in two risk groups using GO and KEGG. The enrichment of biological processes and pathways was highly significant only when $p < 0.05$ and FDR $<0.05$.

The dataset of tumor immune cells was obtained using TIMER 2.0 (http://timer.cistrom.org (accessed on 5 December 2022)). We used seven algorithms to simultaneously compare differences in the immune infiltration profile between the two risk groups (TIMER, CIBERSORT, CIBERSORT-ABS, QUANTISEQ, MCPCOUNTER, XCELL, and EPIC). We employed heatmaps to illustrate variations in immune infiltration status under varied algorithmic conditions. Additionally, single-sample GSEA (ssGSEA) was performed to evaluate immune-related functions of ccRCC, and a heat map was shown. We collated previous studies to identify potential immune checkpoints and assess expression differences between the two risk groups [20]. These stages used the R packages limma, pHeatmap, ggpubr, GSEABase, reshape2, and ggplot2. We obtained the tumor immune dysfunction and exclusion (TIDE) scoring result of every ccRCC patient from the TIDE database (http://tide.dfci.harvard.edu (accessed on 10 December 2022)).

We used the "ggpubr" tool to compare the immune checkpoint blockade (ICB) responses of the two risk populations. Subsequently, we used the pRRophetic program to predict the medicines that may be used to treat ccRCC and to estimate the IC50 values of the pharmaceuticals in the two patient groups. We assessed the relationship between patient mortality and risk score by calculating the proportion of patients who died in the two risk groups and the risk score for dead and surviving patients. In addition, we also compared whether there was a significant difference in progression-free survival (PFS) between the two risk groups of patients.

*2.5. Validation of Basement Membrane-Associated lncRNA Expression in Renal Cancer Cells*

Bena Culture Collection (BNCC, Beijing, China) provided the normal kidney cell line (HK-2, RRID: CVCL_0302) and the renal cancer cell lines (ACHN, RRID: CVCL_1067; 769-P, RRID: CVCL_1050; and CAKI-1, RRID: CVCL_0234). All experimental cells were free of mycoplasma contamination via the assay (Service-bio, #G1900-50T, Wuhan, China). The cells were grown in a 10% fetal bovine serum-containing DMEM/F-12 mixture. All cells were cultivated at 37 °C and 5% $CO_2$ in the incubator. We used the TRIzol reagent to extract total RNA from cells and tissues (Servicebio, #G3013, Wuhan, China). Finally, cDNA was treated to qRT-PCR using SYBR Green qPCR Master Mix (Servicebio, #G3320-01, Wuhan, China). GAPDH served as the internal benchmark. We used GraphPad Prism 8 (San Diego, CA, USA) for statistical analysis, and various group means were compared using one-way ANOVA. Below are the primer sequences we used: LINC02154-F: ACCAATGA-

GACAATGCCACTGAACC; LINC02154-R: TGACCC CTGATTGTGCCTGAAAG; IGFL2-AS1-F: TGGTCTAGCGGTAGCGTCAGTG, IGFL2-AS1-R: ACAAGAGGTGGTGGAGC AGAGTC; NFE4-F: GGGGTGGGCATGTGTTGACTT, NFE4-R: GCTGGAGTGTGG ATG-GTG GAAAC; AC112715.1-F: GCTGCTGTGCTGACCAGTCTG, AC112715.1-R: CTTGGTG-GAATG GCAGGAAGAGC; AC092535.5-F: GCCACACTTGCCTTCCTGCTG, AC092535.5-R: CCTG TCC ACTTGCCTGTTGCC; and AC105105.3-F: TGGCACTCCTGGAGCACTCTG, AC105105.3-R: TGTA GGACGCTATGGCTGGGAAG.

*2.6. RNA Fish*

Clear cell renal cell carcinoma tissue chips were purchased from Shanghai Outdo Biotech Co., Ltd., Shanghai, China, (#HKid-CRCC060PG-01). The tissue chips were deparaffinized, fixed with 4% paraformaldehyde, and permeabilized. Design RNA probes are complementary to the target RNA sequence (lncRNA LINC02154: TTAGTGGCTTCTCCC-CACAGTGAAC, AAAGCCACGACACAATCAAAACCTC, TTGACCCACTGATTGTGC-CTGAAAG; lncRNA AC112715.1: ACTGAAACTTCCGTGGTAGGTGGCT, CAAAACGG GACTC CACCTTGACATC, AAGAACCAGGCAATCCTTTGTCTCC, TTAGCAATGAA GTC TCGGATGGCAT; lncRNA AC092535.5: AACCACCACCTCATCAACGACTTCA, TGTCT GCCT GTGTTCTCTTCCTCCC, GACCAGTCCGTTTGACACTGAGTGG, TGTG-GAAGAGAATGGCAGAGACAGA; and lncRNA AC105105.3: AGGAAACTCTGTAGC-CACGAAGGTG, GCAAACGATGCCAAGACATTTATCG, GCTGGGAAGAAA CAGTGA-GAGGTGA, GAGGGAAGGATTGCCTAGCAGTAGC). The probe was labeled with Cy3 fluorescent dye. Labeled RNA probes were prepared in formamide hybridization buffer to maintain probe stability and facilitate hybridization. Fixed and permeabilized tissue was also incubated in hybridization buffer. The sample was washed multiple times with wash buffer to remove the unbound probe and reduce the background signal. Samples were coated with appropriate mounting medium and coverslips, and images of labeled RNA molecules were captured using a fluorescence microscope (BX41; Olympus, Tokyo, Japan).

*2.7. Invasion Assay*

We transferred small interfering RNA and negative control RNA of two risk model lncRNAs (AC112715.1 and LINC02154) into ACHN and 769P cell lines. After twenty-four hours in serum-free medium, $1 \times 10^5$ cells were grown in a 24-well transwell plate with Matrigel for the invasion assay. The transwell plate was placed in a 37 °C, 5% $CO_2$ cell culture incubator for 24 h. All cells were treated with 4% paraformaldehyde and crystal violet after twenty-four hours incubation. A random selection of five fields from each slide was randomly utilized for statistical analysis.

## 3. Results

*3.1. Construction of a Basement Membrane-Associated lncRNA Signature*

We analyzed normal and cancer tissues for 68 basement membrane-related genes with differential expression (Figure 1A) and 2573 lncRNAs with differential expression (Figure 1B). Correlation analysis revealed 784 differential (Pearson $R > 0.60$, $p < 0.001$) basement membrane-associated lncRNAs (Figure 1C). We discovered 38 basement membrane-related lncRNAs linked with patient prognosis using univariate Cox regression (Figure 1D). Next, we performed LASSO-Cox regression on the training set to reduce multicollinearity and found 13 lncRNAs (Figure 1E,F). Subsequent multivariate Cox analysis revealed a risk model comprising six basement membrane-associated lncRNAs (LINC02154, IGFL2-AS1, NFE4, AC112715.1, AC092535.5, and AC105105.3). Next, we explain how the expression levels of basement membrane-associated lncRNAs may be utilized to generate a risk score. The risk score for each patient is as follows: risk score = (LINC02154*0.2227 + IGFL2-AS1*0.3000 + NFE4*0.4607 + AC112715.1*0.5587 + AC092535.5*0.2509 + AC105105.3*0.7305).

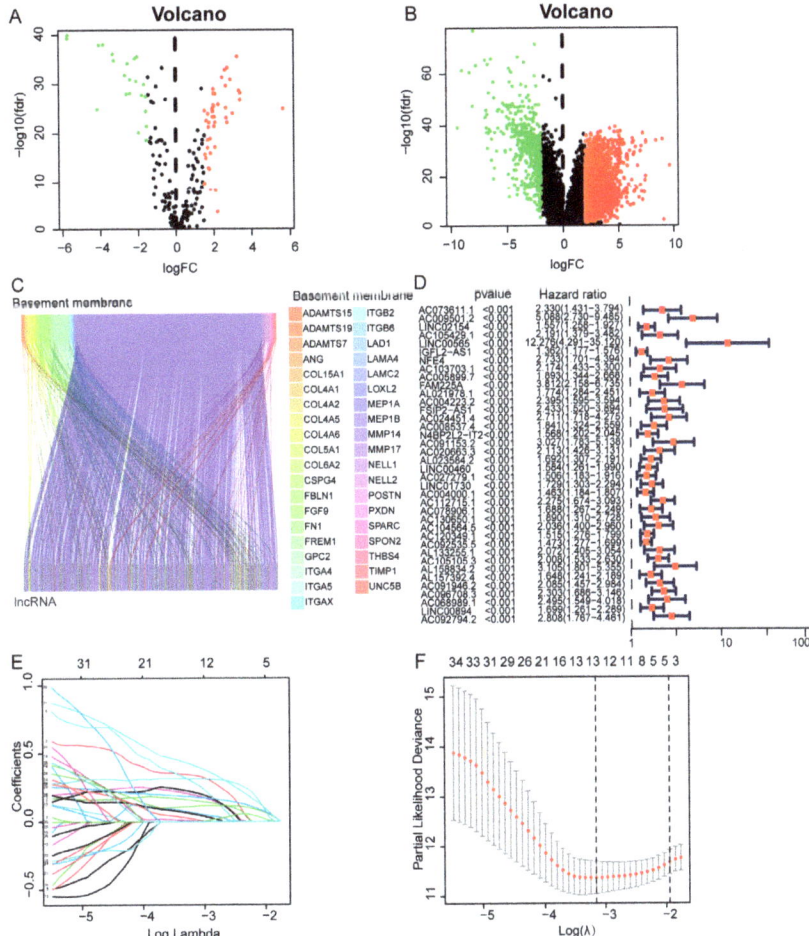

**Figure 1.** Identification of basement membrane-associated ccRCC prognostic lncRNAs. (**A**) Differential expression of basement membrane genes in ccRCC. (**B**) Differential expression of lncRNAs in ccRCC. (**C**) Sankey relationship diagram of basement membrane genes and basement membrane-associated lncRNAs. (**D**) Basement membrane-associated ccRCC prognostic lncRNAs. (**E**) The least absolute shrinkage and selection operator (LASSO) algorithm's 10-fold cross-validation of variable selection. (**F**) Distribution of LASSO coefficients of basement membrane-associated lncRNAs.

*3.2. Expression and Survival Analysis of Prognostic Model lncRNAs*

A heat map shows how much six lncRNAs linked to the basement membrane are expressed in patients with ccRCC. All six of these lncRNAs are highly expressed in renal cancer tissues (Figure 2A). We further visualized lncRNAs using the ggalluvial R package (R 4.2.1) and Cytoscape software (3.9.1). The co-expression network included 27 lncRNA-mRNA pairings (Figure 2B, |correlation coefficient| > 0.6 and $p < 0.001$). LINC02154 was co-expressed with eight basement membrane-associated genes (COL4A5, COL4A6, COL7A1, FBN1, NID2, TIMP1, ITGA2, and TENM2), IGFL2-AS1 was co-expressed with three basement membrane-associated genes (LAMA1, MMP17, and VTN), NFE4 was co-expressed with seven basement membrane-associated genes (COL4A5, COL4A6, COL7A1, FBN1, NID2, TIMP1, and ITGA2), AC112715.1 was co-expressed with six basement membrane-associated genes (COL6A1, COL6A2, COL6A3, LOXL2, TIMP1, and ITGA2B), AC092535.5

was co-expressed with SPON2, and AC105105.3 was co-expressed with MEP1 and BMMP21. Figure 2C–H display the expression levels of six lncRNAs associated with the basement membrane in ccRCC patients. They are all highly expressed in cancer tissues, and individuals with high expression of these lncRNAs had shorter overall survival (OS) (Figure 3A–F).

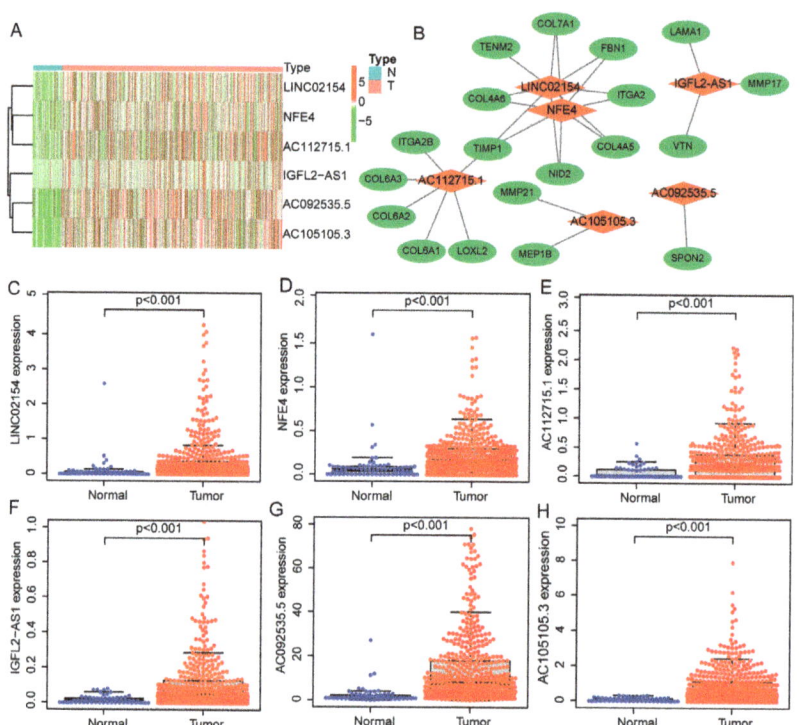

Figure 2. Expression levels and lncRNA-mRNA network of six basement membrane-associated lncRNAs. (A) A heat map of the lncRNA expression levels in the risk model. N, normal; T, tumor. (B) The co-expression network of prognostic basement membrane-associated lncRNAs. (C–H) The expression levels of six basement membrane-associated lncRNAs in tumor and normal tissues.

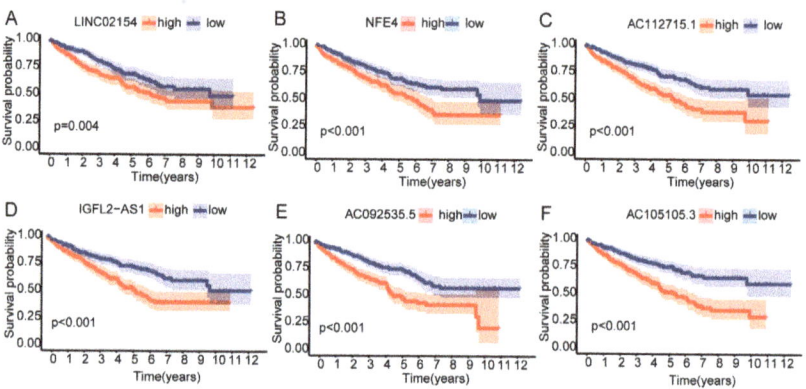

Figure 3. Overall survival of six basement membrane-associated lncRNAs. (A) LINC02154, (B) NFE4, (C) AC112715.1, (D) IGFL2-AS1, (E) AC092535.5, and (F) AC105105.3.

## 3.3. Survival Results and Multivariate Analysis

To examine the validity and reliability of the risk model, we also used the median risk score to classify patients in the testing and all sets into two risk groups. Figure 4A–C depict the expression patterns of six basement membrane-associated lncRNAs. Each of the six lncRNAs associated with the basement membrane was enriched in the high-risk population; the risk scores are depicted in Figure 4D–F, and the patient's survival status is depicted in Figure 4G–I. Clearly, the incidence of ccRCC patient fatalities increased as the risk score rose, and the low-risk category had longer survival times (Figure 4J,K).

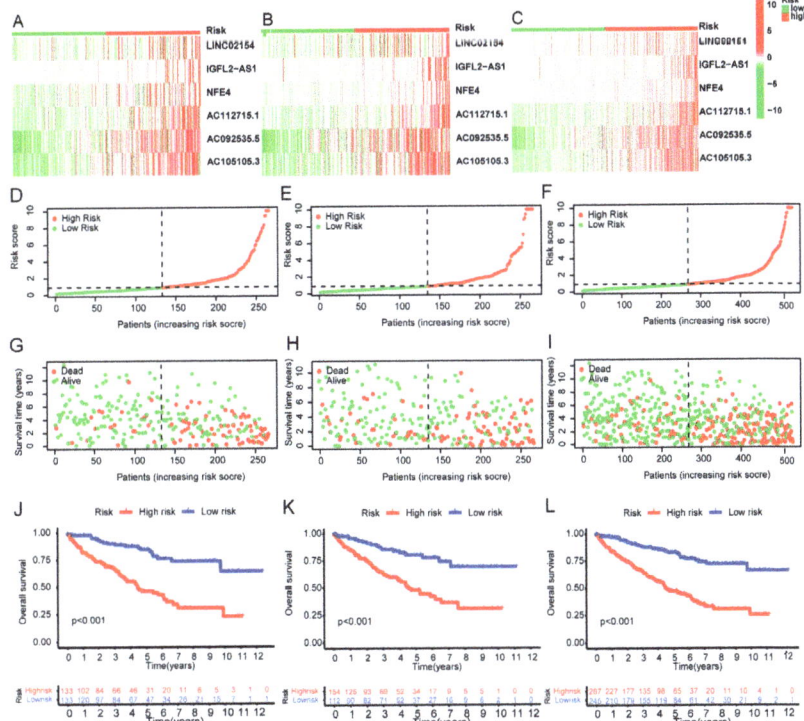

**Figure 4.** Prognostic analysis of the risk model in training, testing, and overall groups. (**A–C**) The clustering analysis heatmap depicts the six lncRNA expression levels for each patient in training, testing, and overall sets. (**D–F**) Distribution of basement membrane-associated lncRNA model-based risk score in training, testing, and overall sets. (**G–I**) Patterns of survival time and survival status were ranked by risk score in training, testing, and entire sets. (**J–L**) Kaplan–Meier survival curves of overall survival of patients in training, testing, and overall sets.

We analyzed whether there is a difference in survival between the two risk groups at various clinical stages (age, gender, grade TMN stage, T stage, and M stage). Statistically, the low-risk category had a much greater overall survival rate than the high-risk category (Figure 5A–L). The findings imply that the risk model may be applied to evaluate the survival of ccRCC patients with various clinicopathological characteristics.

## 3.4. Independent Prognostic Value of the Risk Score

The 1-, 3-, and 5-year ROCs had corresponding AUC values of 0.733, 0.729, and 0.759 (Figure 6A). In the 5-year ROC curve of the model, the AUC of the risk score was 0.759, displaying more prominent predictive power than other clinicopathological features (Figure 6B). The risk model's 10-year C-index was similarly high in all aspects (Figure 6C).

Using univariate and multivariate Cox regression analyses, age, grade, stage, and the risk model for six basement membrane-associated lncRNAs were identified as independent predictive variables for ccRCC (Figure 6D,E). These results demonstrate the excellent predictive power of the risk model.

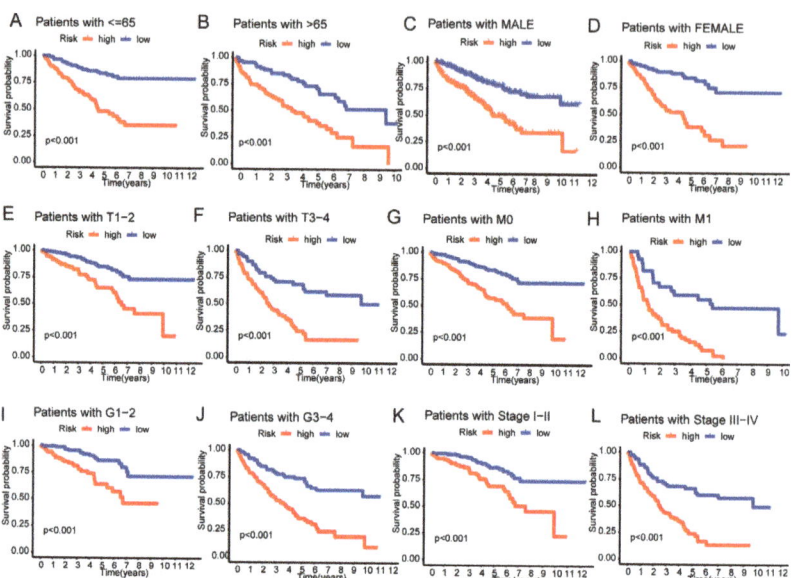

**Figure 5.** Kaplan–Meier survival curves for low- and high-risk populations according to various clinical factors. (**A**,**B**) age. (**C**,**D**) gender. (**E**,**F**) T stage. (**G**,**H**) M stage. (**I**,**J**) grade. (**K**,**L**) TMN stage.

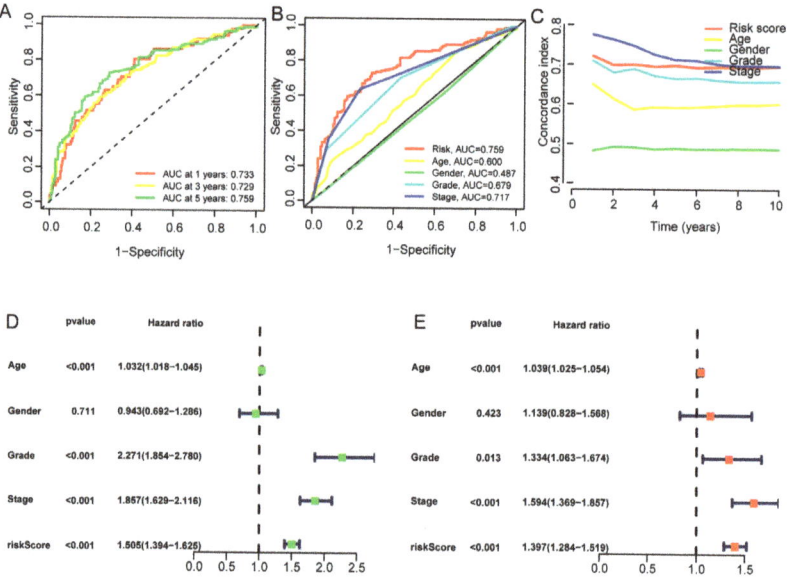

**Figure 6.** Assessment of the prognostic signature of the basement membrane-associated lncRNAs in the overall set. (**A**) The 1-year, 3-year, and 5-year ROCs of the risk model. (**B**) The 5-year ROC curve of the risk model and clinicopathological variables. (**C**) The C-index curve of the risk model. (**D**) Forest plot for univariate Cox regression analysis. (**E**) Forest plot for multivariate Cox regression analysis.

## 3.5. Nomogram and Heatmap of Clinical Factors

We evaluated the outcomes of patients with ccRCC at 1, 3, and 5 years using a nomogram comprising clinicopathological features and the risk score (Figure 7A). The calibration curve shows that the predicted result of the nomogram and the actual result are very close (Figure 7B). A heatmap depicting the relationship between the prediction signature of basement membrane-associated lncRNAs and clinicopathological characteristics was also drawn (Figure 7C). The risk score was related to T stage, M stage, TMN stage, and grade; patients with higher risk scores tended to have a higher clinical stage.

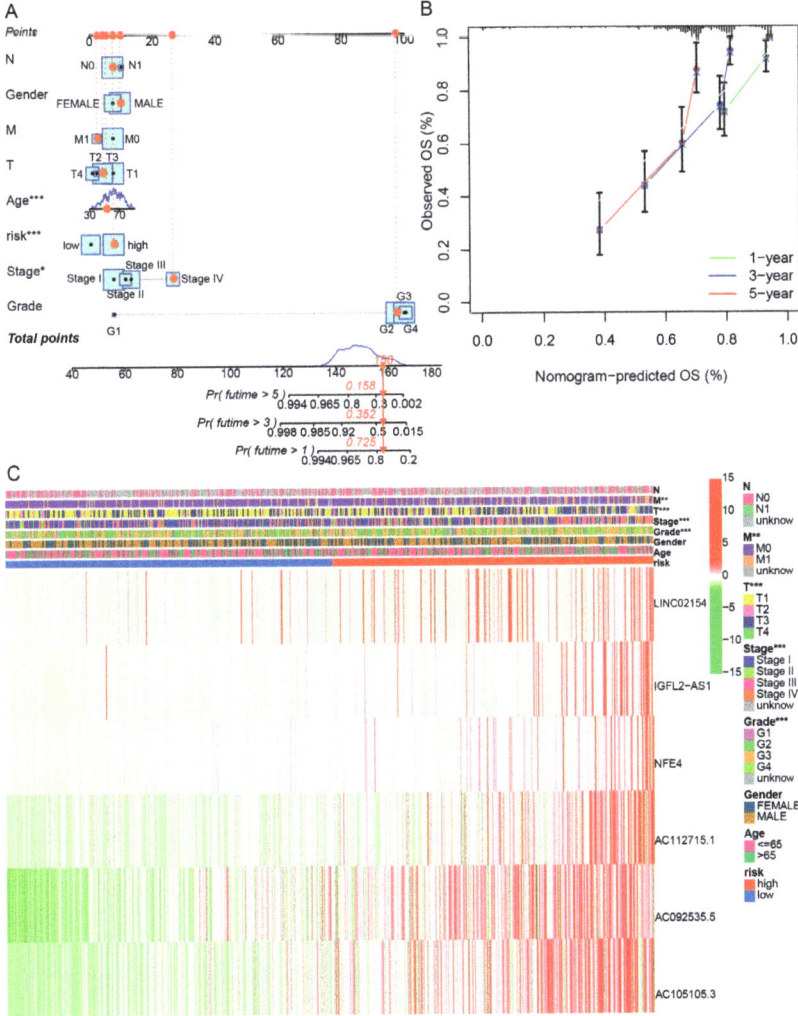

**Figure 7.** Nomograms and heatmaps of risk scores and clinicopathological features. (**A**) Nomogram of clinicopathological factors and risk scores. (**B**) Calibration curves for detecting nomogram predictions. (**C**) Heatmap for basement membrane-associated lncRNAs prognostic signature and clinicopathological variables. * $p < 0.05$; ** $p < 0.01$; *** $p < 0.001$.

## 3.6. PCA and Enrichment Analysis

We examined the spatial distribution of two risk groups across four expression profiles using PCA (total gene expression profile, basement membrane gene expression profile, basement membrane-associated lncRNA expression profile, and six basement membrane-associated expression profiles in the risk model) (Figure 8A–D). The results suggested that six basement membrane-associated lncRNAs had the greatest potential to differentiate between populations at low and high risk.

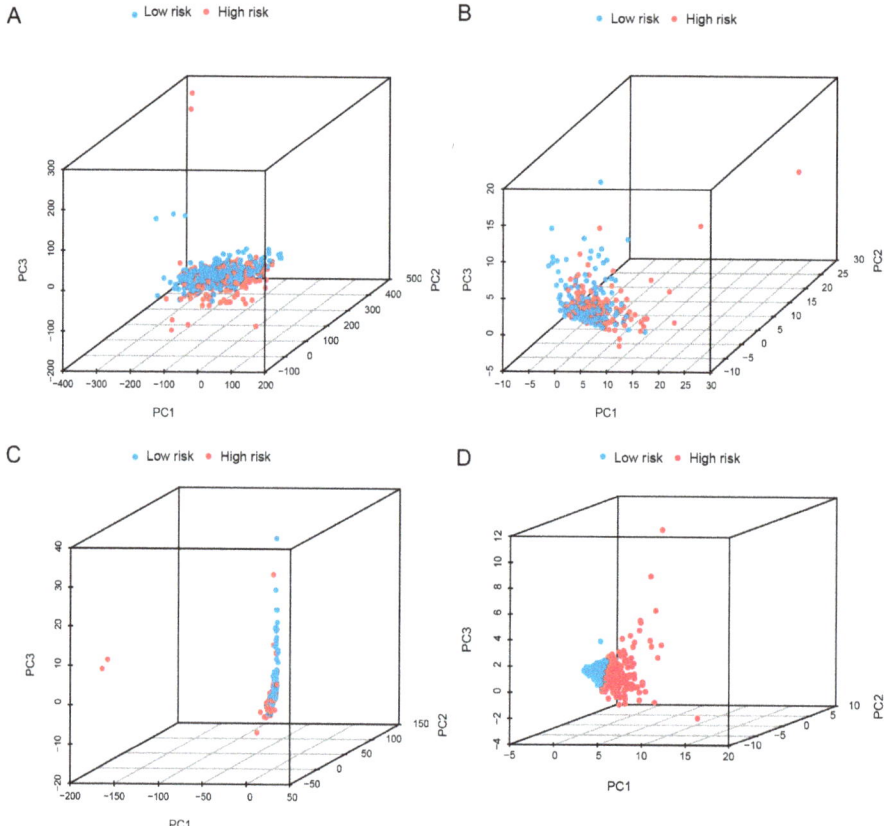

**Figure 8.** Principal component analysis between the high- and low-risk populations. (**A**) PCA of all genes. (**B**) PCA of basement membrane genes. (**C**) PCA of basement membrane-associated lncRNAs. (**D**) PCA of risk lncRNAs.

The basement membrane-associated lncRNAs were substantially connected with extracellular matrix structure and inflammatory cell motility, according to GO analysis (Figure 9A,C). The KEGG study resulted mainly in cytokine receptor and IL-17 signaling route; cancer-related signaling pathways including NF-kappa B, TGF-β, TNF, PI3K-Akt; and the viral carcinogenesis signaling pathway (Figure 9B,D). These results suggest that basement membrane-associated lncRNA plays an important role in the development of clear cell renal cell carcinoma.

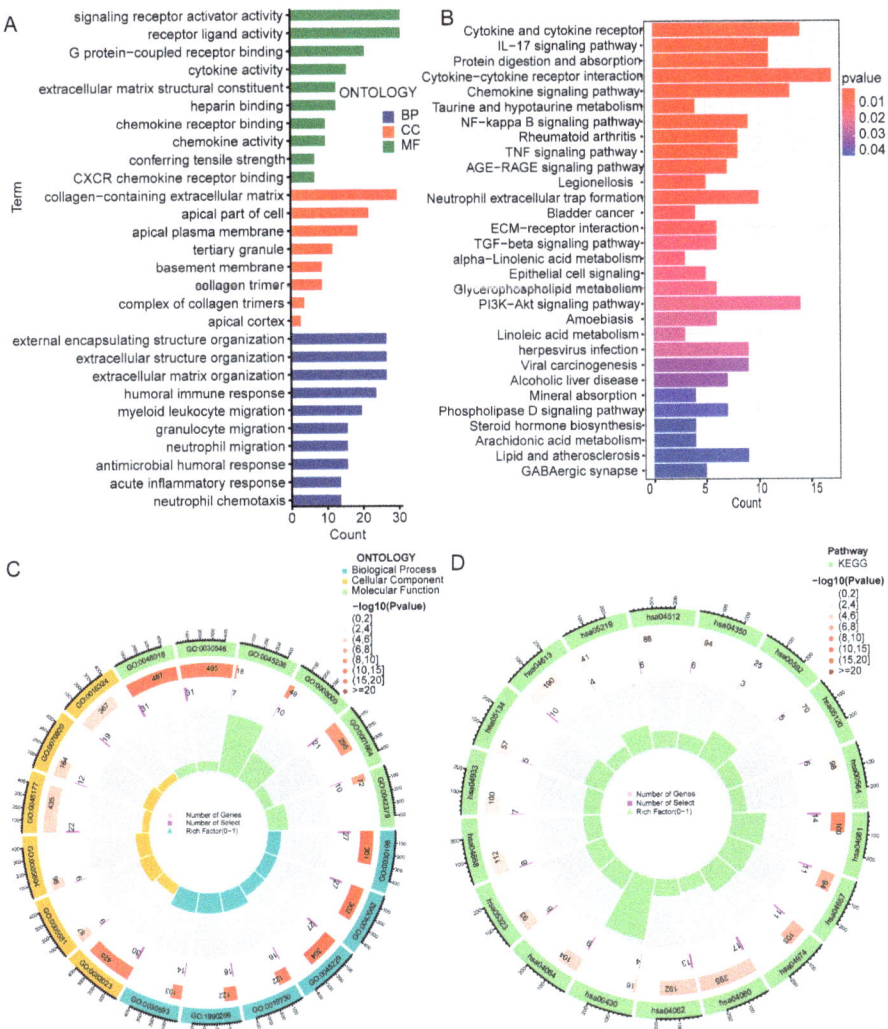

**Figure 9.** GO and KEGG analysis of DEGs in high- and low-risk groups. (**A,C**) GO analysis of DEGs. (**B,D**) KEGG analysis of DEGs. GO, gene ontology; KEGG, Kyoto Encyclopedia of Genes and Genomes; DEGs, differentially expressed genes; BP, biological process; CC, cellular component; MF, molecular function.

*3.7. Examination of Immune Characteristics Using the Basement Membrane-Related lncRNA Signature*

The heatmap in Figure 10A displays immune cell infiltration based on seven algorithms. We examined the association between risk score and immune-related response. The data show that type II IFN response, type I IFN response, T cell co-inhibition, checkpoints, T cell co-stimulation, and inflammatory promotion are differently active across two risk groups (Figure 10B). Moreover, we compared immune checkpoint alterations between the two risk groups (Figure 10C). The majority of immunological checkpoints were expressed at higher levels in the high-risk group, which may explain patients' shorter survival time. The high-risk population had higher TIDE scores, suggesting reduced responses and shorter survival in ICI-treated patients, which may explain their poor prognoses (Figure 10D).

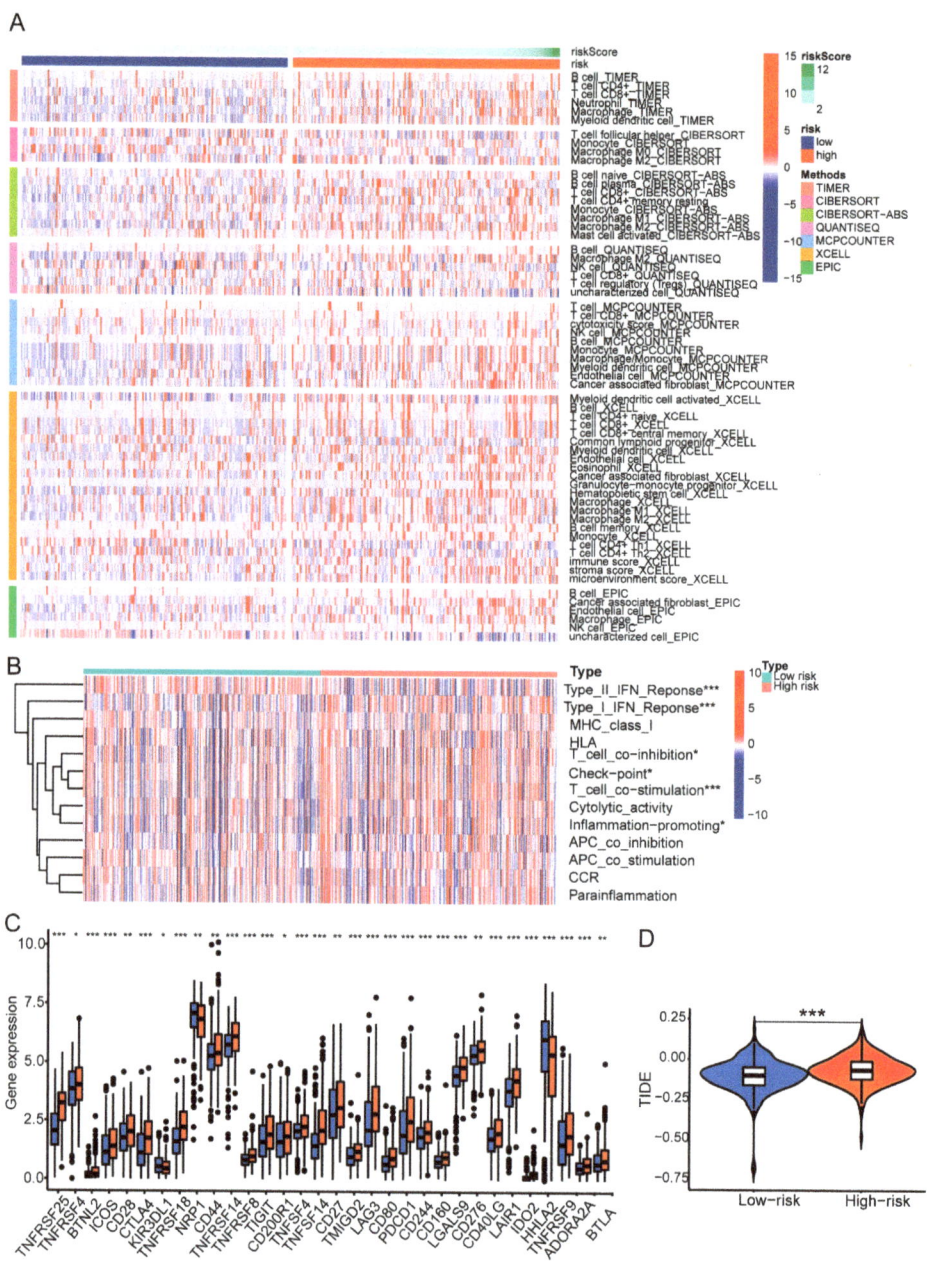

**Figure 10.** Differences in the tumor immune microenvironment between the low- and high-risk groups. (**A**) Heatmap for immune cell infiltration landscape between the two risk groups. (**B**) ssGSEA scores of immune cells and immune function in the two risk groups. (**C**) Expression of immune checkpoints between high- and low-risk groups. (**D**) TIDE scores between the two groups. * $p < 0.05$; ** $p < 0.01$; *** $p < 0.001$.

## 3.8. Therapeutic Drug Sensitivity and Mortality Rate

We discovered considerable disparities in IC50 values for various medicines between the two patient groups by evaluating their drug susceptibilities. Cyclopamine, imatinib, and rapamycin were more efficient in low-risk populations (Figure 11A–C), whereas phenformin, pyrimethamine, and tubastatin A were more efficient in high-risk populations (Figure 11D–F). These results suggest that risk scores may be useful in guiding clinical treatment. By comparing the percentage of patients who died in the two risk categories, we determined that the high-risk group had a larger percentage of deceased patients (Figure 11G). Patients who died had a much higher risk score than survivors (Figure 11H). Moreover, we analyzed the progression-free survival (PFS) of patients in the two risk categories and found that PFS durations were shorter for the high-risk categories (Figure 11I). These results suggest that risk models can predict patient mortality.

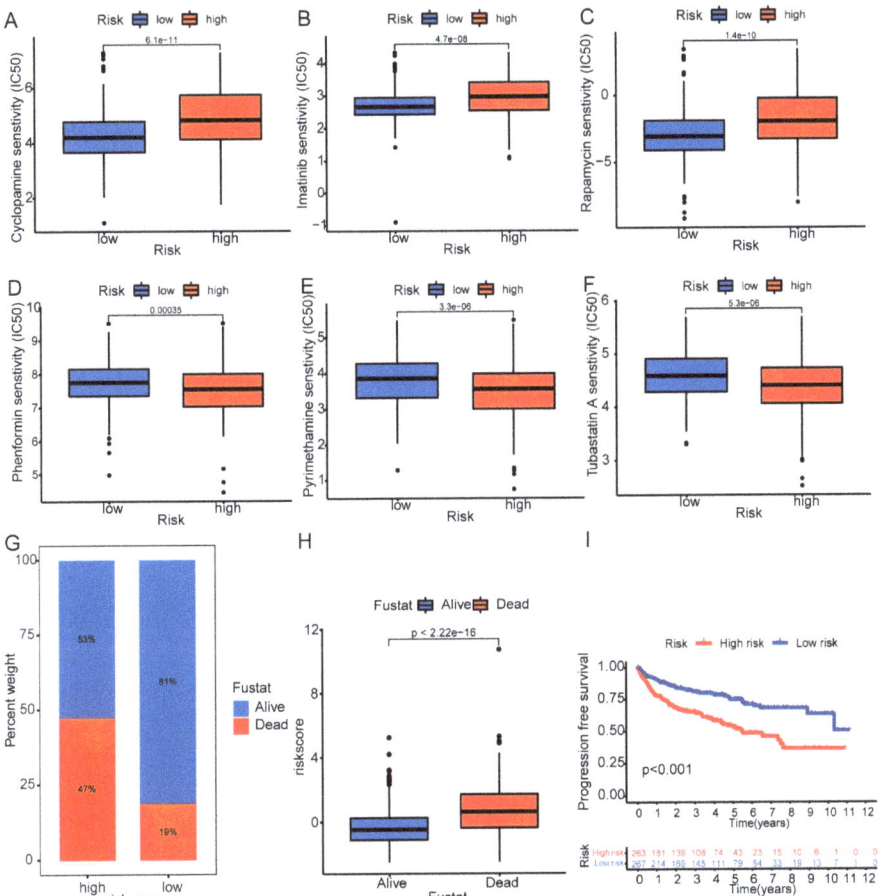

**Figure 11.** Differences in drug sensitivity and prognoses between high- and low-risk groups. Sensitive drugs in low-risk groups: (**A**) cyclopamine, (**B**) imatinib, and (**C**) rapamycin; Sensitive drugs in high-risk groups: (**D**) phenformin, (**E**) pyrimethamine and (**F**) tubastatin. (**G**) The difference in the proportion of dead patients between the two risk groups. (**H**) The differences in risk scores between dead and alive patients. (**I**) The difference in PFS of patients in the two risk groups.

## 3.9. Expression of Risk Model lncRNAs

Compared with the normal renal cell line HK-2, LINC02154, AC112715.1, AC092535.5, and AC105105.3 were significantly upregulated in the renal cancer cell lines ACHN, 769-P, and CAKI-1 (Figure 12A–D). The expression of IGFL2-AS1 was only increased in the renal carcinoma cell line 769-P (Figure 12E), while the expression of NFE4 was increased in the renal carcinoma cell lines ACHN and CAKI-1 (Figure 12F).

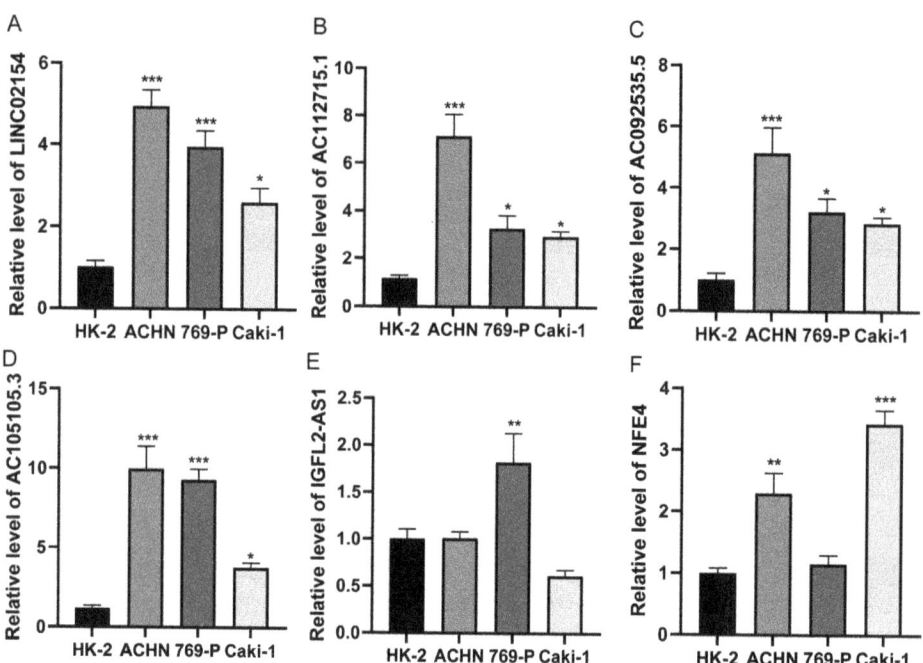

**Figure 12.** qRT-PCR for detection of lncRNA expression levels in a risk model in cancer cells (HK-2, ACHN, 769-P, and CAKI-1). (**A**) LINC02154; (**B**) AC112715.1; (**C**) AC092535.5; (**D**) AC105105.3; (**E**) IGFL2-AS1; (**F**) NFE4 in HK-2, ACHN, 769-P, and CAKI-1. * $p < 0.05$; ** $p < 0.01$; *** $p < 0.001$.

## 3.10. Expression of Risk Model lncRNAs in Renal Cancer Tissue and Functional Verification

We used RNA FISH technology to find out where LINC02154, AC112715.1, AC092535.5, and AC105105.3 were expressed and where they were located in kidney cancer tissue chips (Figure 13A). We found that these four lncRNAs are highly expressed in renal cancer tissues. AC112715.1 is mostly found in the nucleus, while lNC02154, AC092535.5, and AC105105.3 are mostly found in the cytoplasm. We used si-LINC02154 and si-AC112715.1 to knock down the expression of LINC02154 and AC112715.1 in ACHN and 769P, respectively. Among them, si-AC112715.1-2 and si-LINC02154-3 had the best knockdown effects (Figure 13B,D). Through invasion experiments, we found that knocking down LINC02154 and AC112715.1 could inhibit the invasion ability of renal cancer cells (Figure 13C,E).

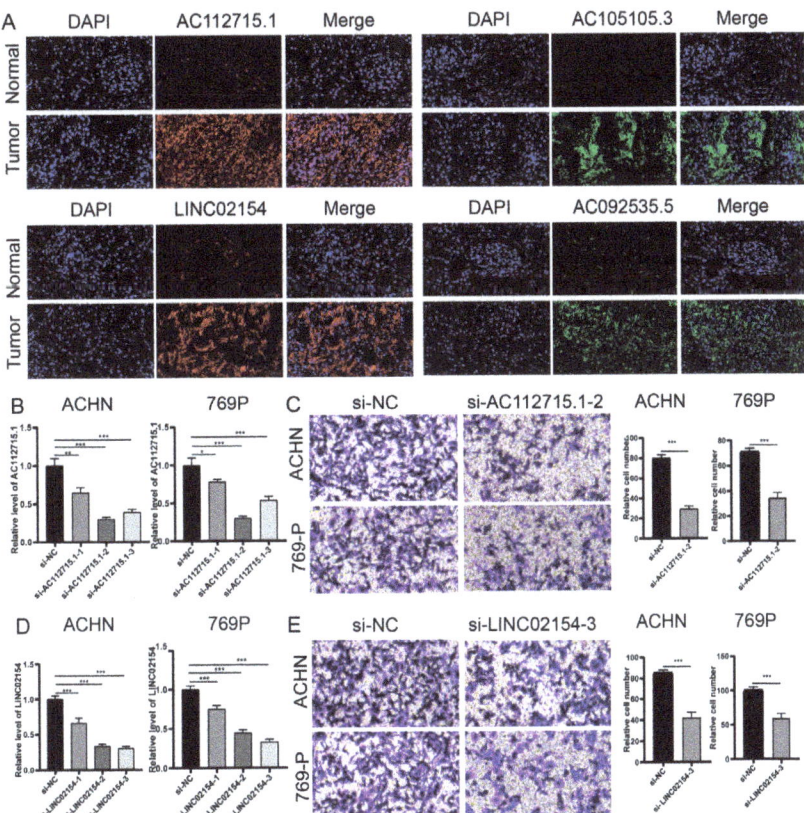

**Figure 13.** Verification of the expression of model lncRNA in renal cancer tissues and exploration of the impact on the invasion ability of renal cancer cell lines. (**A**) RNA FISH shows that AC112715.1, LINC02154, AC092535.5, and AC105105.3 are highly expressed in renal cancer tissues. (**B**) Effect of si-AC112715.1 on AC112715.1 expression in ACHN and 769P cells. (**C**) Effect of AC112715.1 knockdown on the invasion ability of ACHN and 769P cells. (**D**) Effect of si-LINC02154 on LINC021541 expression in ACHN and 769P cells. (**E**) Effect of LINC0215 knockdown on the invasion ability of ACHN and 769P cells. * $p < 0.05$; ** $p < 0.01$; *** $p < 0.001$.

## 4. Discussion

During the development of kidney cancer, cancer cells usually penetrate the renal tubular epithelial cell layer and the corresponding basement membrane and enter the deep tissue of the kidney [21]. They may then begin to spread to surrounding tissue or spread further to other sites through the blood vessels or lymphatic system. The basement membrane typically deteriorates and ruptures as a result of renal cancer cell invasion [22]. This disruption helps cancer cells penetrate the basement membrane and enter deeper tissues [23]. Therefore, studying the integrity and recovery capabilities of the basement membrane is important for understanding the development and treatment of renal cancer.

Recent research indicates that lncRNAs are involved in various tumor genesis mechanisms, including carcinogenesis, proliferation, metastasis, migration, invasion, and angiogenesis [24]. Studies have shown that SNHG6 interacts with YBX1 to enhance the translation of HIF1, ultimately promoting ccRCC development and metastasis [25]. According to research, MRCCAT1 is an important lncRNA that promotes metastasis in ccRCC by suppressing NPR3 and promoting p38-MAPK signaling [26]. Song et al. reported that elevated expression of lncRNA ATB may promote renal cell cancer via binding to DNMT1, downregulating P53 and inhibiting the proliferation and migration of apoptotic cells [27]. However, basement membrane-associated lncRNAs in ccRCC have never been studied. Our team created a signature of the lncRNAs associated with basement membranes to predict the survival of ccRCC patients and validated the expression of risk model lncRNAs at the cellular level.

We discovered 784 basement membrane lncRNAs related to prognosis via differential and co-expression studies. According to univariate, LASSO, and multivariate Cox regression analyses, we found six basement membrane-associated lncRNAs (LINC02154, IGFL2-AS1, NFE4, AC112715.1, AC092535.5, and AC105105.3) that were substantially related to survival. Using the lncRNAs outlined before, we developed a risk model of basement membrane-associated lncRNAs to estimate the survival of ccRCC patients, and these lncRNAs are significantly expressed in kidney tissue cancer. LINC02154, AC112715.1, AC092535.5, and AC105105.3 were all significantly upregulated in three renal cancer cell lines, while the expression of IGFL2-AS1 and NFE4 was elevated in some renal cancer cell lines. We used RNA FISH to confirm that LINC02154, AC112715.1, AC092535.5, and AC105105.3 are highly expressed in renal cancer tissues. This is basically consistent with their expression levels in TCGA data.

LINC02154 increases liver cancer cell growth and spread by increasing SPC24 promoter activity and modulating the PI3K-AKT signaling pathway [28]; it may also be used to estimate the prognosis of laryngeal squamous cell carcinoma [29]. Studies have shown that renal cancer patients with high expression of LINC02154 have a poor prognosis, and knocking down LINC02154 can inhibit the invasion ability of cancer cells, which is consistent with our experimental results [30,31]. IGFL2-AS1 exerts a tumor-promoting effect in TSCC through the Wnt/β-catenin pathway and enhances the development of tongue squamous cell carcinoma [32]. KLF5's proliferative and pro-survival effects are mediated by IGFL2-AS1 [33], and KLF5 promotes basal-like breast cancer by upregulating the expression of IGFL1 and cell growth and survival [34–36]. In renal cancer cells, IGFL2-AS1 contributes to the development of drug resistance in cancer cells [37,38]. According to ccRCC studies, patients who had a high level of lncRNA NEF4 expression had a shorter OS; this may be an independent prognostic factor for ccRCC [39]. Recently made available to the public are the last three lncRNAs (AC112715.1, AC092535.5, and AC105105.3). Specifically, these newly discovered basement membrane-associated lncRNAs could help us better comprehend ccRCC and explore innovative cancer therapy strategies.

Risk score prognosis accuracy was validated using the ROC and C-index. The risk score is an independent prognostic risk factor, as established via multivariate Cox analyses. The prognosis of patients with ccRCC was then predicted using a nomogram, and the calibration curve demonstrates that the actual measurements and projected values correspond well. Heatmaps of predictive and clinicopathological characteristics of basement membrane-associated lncRNAs demonstrated a correlation between risk scores and N stage, M stage, TMN stage, and grade. PCA study results show that risk model lncRNAs can better distinguish patients from two risk groups. The GO enrichment study indicates that binding activation of receptor, ligand, and cytokine signaling is tightly connected with basement membrane-associated lncRNAs. KEGG analysis revealed the cancer-related signaling pathways NF-kappa B pathway, TNF pathway, TGF-β pathway, and PI3K-Akt pathway and viral carcinogenesis were significantly active in basement membrane-associated lncRNAs. The TGF-β signaling pathway plays a crucial role in epithelial-mesenchymal transition (EMT) and cancer-associated fibroblast (CAF) production, and it has a significant influence on the progression of cancer [40]. In inflammatory-stimulated mammary epithelial cells, the long non-coding RNA NKILA may form a stable complex with NF-B/IκB and inhibit excessive activation of the NF-κB pathway [41]. Numerous studies have shown that the PI3K/Akt signaling pathway is inappropriately active in cancer and promotes tumor formation [42]. These findings indicate that basement membrane-associated lncRNAs play a crucial role in cancer formation.

Using multiple approaches to evaluate immune cell infiltration, we discovered substantial disparities between the two risk categories. Moreover, ssGSEA data demonstrated that the Type II IFN response is dormant in high-risk populations, whereas checkpoint and T cell co-inhibition is active. These findings indicate that the risk model lncRNAs may be active in the tumor immune microenvironment, working through immunological checkpoints, T cell co-inhibition, and Type II IFN response inactivation to suppress immune responses and promote ccRCC development [43].

Immune checkpoints comprise programmed death receptors and their corresponding ligands. T cells express programmed death receptors on their surfaces, while tumor cells express ligands [44]. The combination of the programmed death receptor and its ligand can exhaust T cells and render them incapable of killing tumor cells normally, allowing tumor cells to evade the host's immune surveillance [43]. Therefore, the prognosis is worse for cancer patients with active immune checkpoints. In the high-risk group, the majority of immune checkpoints are active, the patients' anti-tumor immunity is suppressed, and the patients have a dismal prognosis.

TIDE is used to evaluate the clinical response of ICI-treated patients. Higher TIDE scores represent a greater probability of immunological evasion, suggesting reduced responses and shorter survival in ICI-treated patients. High-risk individuals showed higher TIDE scores, indicating that they may respond less well to ICI therapy [45]. High-risk patients had higher mortality rates, and dead patients had a higher risk score. The high-risk category had greater rates of death, and those who passed away had higher risk scores. In addition, high-risk patients had shorter disease-free survival. We predict a number of drugs that may be therapeutically useful for kidney cancer and the susceptibility of individuals in two risk categories regarding these drugs. The prediction of patient sensitivity to drugs will help individualize chemotherapy drug selection for kidney cancer patients.

We created a basement membrane-associated lncRNA risk model in order to accurately forecast the prognosis of ccRCC patients using bioinformatics. Despite the fact that we have used a variety of techniques to improve our model, it still has a few flaws. The model is constructed based on the TCGA database. This model requires external datasets for validation and cannot avoid potential selection bias. Furthermore, to predict the prognostic value of BM-related lncRNAs, we utilized only data from public databases. We can only infer the effect of BM-related lncRNA on ccRCC based on limited clinical information, disregarding environmental and genetic variables. Lastly, we did not verify the biological functions of all risk model lncRNAs, and the mechanisms underlying their effects on ccRCC remain unknown. We will address these deficiencies in future research. We will refine and verify the role of basement membrane-associated lncRNAs in the future by collecting further clinical and experimental data.

We found that the BM-related risk model can well predict the prognosis of ccRCC patients and guide clinical treatment. The nomogram we constructed can predict the patient's 1-, 3-, and 5-year survival rates using the patient's risk score and clinical information. The BM-related risk model can divide ccRCC patients into high-risk and low-risk groups. People in the high-risk group had shorter survival times than those in the low-risk group. The risk model can be used to predict patient sensitivity to chemotherapy drugs. Based on the differences in sensitivity between high- and low-risk groups to different chemotherapy drugs, drugs can be selected according to patients' sensitivity to guide their clinical treatment. Our results may provide fresh insight on patient outcome prediction and personalized therapy.

## 5. Conclusions

Our research reveals that the basement membrane-associated lncRNA risk model may accurately assess the prognosis of individuals with ccRCC. Moreover, this research may provide insight into the development of novel therapies for ccRCC.

**Author Contributions:** Conceptualization, P.L. and K.Y.; methodology, X.L.; software, X.L.; validation, Q.K. and X.L.; formal analysis, M.P.; investigation, Q.K.; resources, X.L.; data curation, M.P.; writing—original draft preparation, X.L.; writing—review and editing, P.L.; visualization, X.L.; supervision, K.Y.; project administration, P.L.; funding acquisition, P.L. All authors have read and agreed to the published version of the manuscript.

**Funding:** This study was supported by the National Natural Science Fund of China (No. 81770688), Hubei Leading Talent Program in Medicine, and Wuhan Application Foundation and Frontier Project (No. 2020020601012209).

**Institutional Review Board Statement:** Not applicable.

**Informed Consent Statement:** Not applicable.

**Data Availability Statement:** This research examines publicly accessible datasets. This information is available here: Data accessible via TCGA (https://tcga-data.nci.nih.gov/tcga/ (accessed on 1 December 2022)) and BM-BASE (https://bmbase.manchester.ac.uk (accessed on 3 December 2022)). Further details can be obtained from the corresponding author.

**Acknowledgments:** We appreciate all participants in this study.

**Conflicts of Interest:** The authors declare no conflict of interest.

## References

1. Vuong, L.; Kotecha, R.R.; Voss, M.H.; Hakimi, A.A. Tumor Microenvironment Dynamics in Clear-Cell Renal Cell Carcinoma. *Cancer Discov.* **2019**, *9*, 1349–1357. [CrossRef] [PubMed]
2. Delman, K.A. Introducing the "Virtual Tumor Board" series in CA: A Cancer Journal for Clinicians. *CA Cancer J. Clin.* **2020**, *70*, 77. [CrossRef] [PubMed]
3. Choueiri, T.K.; Motzer, R.J. Systemic Therapy for Metastatic Renal-Cell Carcinoma. *N. Engl. J. Med.* **2017**, *376*, 354–366. [CrossRef] [PubMed]
4. Lalani, A.A.; McGregor, B.A.; Albiges, L.; Choueiri, T.K.; Motzer, R.; Powles, T.; Wood, C.; Bex, A. Systemic Treatment of Metastatic Clear Cell Renal Cell Carcinoma in 2018: Current Paradigms, Use of Immunotherapy, and Future Directions. *Eur. Urol.* **2019**, *75*, 100–110. [CrossRef]
5. Jonasch, E.; Walker, C.L.; Rathmell, W.K. Clear cell renal cell carcinoma ontogeny and mechanisms of lethality. *Nat. Rev. Nephrol.* **2021**, *17*, 245–261. [CrossRef]
6. Napolitano, L.; Manfredi, C.; Cirillo, L.; Fusco, G.M.; Passaro, F.; Abate, M.; La Rocca, R.; Mastrangelo, F.; Spirito, L.; Pandolfo, S.D.; et al. Cytoreductive Nephrectomy and Metastatic Renal Cell Carcinoma: State of the Art and Future Perspectives. *Medicina* **2023**, *59*, 767. [CrossRef]
7. Boissier, R.; Hevia, V.; Bruins, H.M.; Budde, K.; Figueiredo, A.; Lledo-Garcia, E.; Olsburgh, J.; Regele, H.; Taylor, C.F.; Zakri, R.H.; et al. The Risk of Tumour Recurrence in Patients Undergoing Renal Transplantation for End-stage Renal Disease after Previous Treatment for a Urological Cancer: A Systematic Review. *Eur. Urol.* **2018**, *73*, 94–108. [CrossRef]
8. Yurchenco, P.D. Basement membranes: Cell scaffoldings and signaling platforms. *Cold Spring Harb. Perspect. Biol.* **2011**, *3*, a004911. [CrossRef]
9. Chang, J.; Chaudhuri, O. Beyond proteases: Basement membrane mechanics and cancer invasion. *J. Cell Biol.* **2019**, *218*, 2456–2469. [CrossRef]
10. Fidler, A.L.; Darris, C.E.; Chetyrkin, S.V.; Pedchenko, V.K.; Boudko, S.P.; Brown, K.L.; Gray Jerome, W.; Hudson, J.K.; Rokas, A.; Hudson, B.G. Collagen IV and basement membrane at the evolutionary dawn of metazoan tissues. *eLife* **2017**, *6*, e24176. [CrossRef]
11. Siegel, R.L.; Miller, K.D.; Fuchs, H.E.; Jemal, A. Cancer statistics, 2022. *CA Cancer J. Clin.* **2022**, *72*, 7–33. [CrossRef] [PubMed]
12. Quinn, J.J.; Chang, H.Y. Unique features of long non-coding RNA biogenesis and function. *Nat. Rev. Genet.* **2016**, *17*, 47–62. [CrossRef] [PubMed]
13. Liu, S.J.; Dang, H.X.; Lim, D.A.; Feng, F.Y.; Maher, C.A. Long noncoding RNAs in cancer metastasis. *Nat. Rev. Cancer* **2021**, *21*, 446–460. [CrossRef] [PubMed]
14. Pandey, G.K.; Kanduri, C. Long Non-Coding RNAs: Tools for Understanding and Targeting Cancer Pathways. *Cancers* **2022**, *14*, 4760. [CrossRef] [PubMed]
15. Liu, P.F.; Farooqi, A.A.; Peng, S.Y.; Yu, T.J.; Dahms, H.U.; Lee, C.H.; Tang, J.Y.; Wang, S.C.; Shu, C.W.; Chang, H.W. Regulatory effects of noncoding RNAs on the interplay of oxidative stress and autophagy in cancer malignancy and therapy. *Semin. Cancer Biol.* **2022**, *83*, 269–282. [CrossRef]
16. Shan, G.; Huang, T.; Tang, T. Long non-coding RNA MEG8 induced by PLAG1 promotes clear cell renal cell carcinoma through the miR-495-3p/G3BP1 axis. *Pathol. Res. Pract.* **2022**, *229*, 153734. [CrossRef]
17. Zhang, Z.; Fu, X.; Gao, Y.; Nie, Z. LINC01535 Attenuates ccRCC Progression through Regulation of the miR-146b-5p/TRIM2 Axis and Inactivation of the PI3K/Akt Pathway. *J. Oncol.* **2022**, *2022*, 2153337. [CrossRef]

18. Barik, G.K.; Sahay, O.; Behera, A.; Naik, D.; Kalita, B. Keep your eyes peeled for long noncoding RNAs: Explaining their boundless role in cancer metastasis, drug resistance, and clinical application. *Biochim. Biophys Acta Rev. Cancer* **2021**, *1876*, 188612. [CrossRef]
19. Jayadev, R.; Morais, M.; Ellingford, J.M.; Srinivasan, S.; Naylor, R.W.; Lawless, C.; Li, A.S.; Ingham, J.F.; Hastie, E.; Chi, Q.; et al. A basement membrane discovery pipeline uncovers network complexity, regulators, and human disease associations. *Sci. Adv.* **2022**, *8*, eabn2265. [CrossRef]
20. Fang, C.; Liu, S.; Feng, K.; Huang, C.; Zhang, Y.; Wang, J.; Lin, H.; Wang, J.; Zhong, C. Ferroptosis-related lncRNA signature predicts the prognosis and immune microenvironment of hepatocellular carcinoma. *Sci. Rep.* **2022**, *12*, 6642. [CrossRef]
21. Morell-Quadreny, L.; Rubio, J.; Lopez-Guerrero, J.A.; Casanova, J.; Ramos, D.; Iborra, I.; Solsona, E.; Llombart-Bosch, A. Disruption of basement membrane, extracellular matrix metalloproteinases and E-cadherin in renal-cell carcinoma. *Anticancer Res.* **2003**, *23*, 5005–5010. [PubMed]
22. Majo, S.; Courtois, S.; Souleyreau, W.; Bikfalvi, A.; Auguste, P. Impact of Extracellular Matrix Components to Renal Cell Carcinoma Behavior. *Front. Oncol.* **2020**, *10*, 625. [CrossRef] [PubMed]
23. Chen, Y.; Lu, H.; Tao, D.; Fan, M.; Zhuang, Q.; Xing, Z.; Chen, Z.; He, X. Membrane type-2 matrix metalloproteinases improve the progression of renal cell cancer. *Int. J. Clin. Exp. Pathol.* **2017**, *10*, 10618–10626. [PubMed]
24. Zhou, J.; Zhang, Y.; Li, S.; Zhou, Q.; Lu, Y.; Shi, J.; Liu, J.; Wu, Q.; Zhou, S. Dendrobium nobile Lindl. alkaloids-mediated protection against CCl(4-)induced liver mitochondrial oxidative damage is dependent on the activation of Nrf2 signaling pathway. *BioMedicine* **2020**, *129*, 110351. [CrossRef]
25. Zhao, P.; Deng, Y.; Wu, Y.; Guo, Q.; Zhou, L.; Yang, X.; Wang, C. Long noncoding RNA SNHG6 promotes carcinogenesis by enhancing YBX1-mediated translation of HIF1alpha in clear cell renal cell carcinoma. *FASEB J.* **2021**, *35*, e21160. [CrossRef]
26. Li, J.K.; Chen, C.; Liu, J.Y.; Shi, J.Z.; Liu, S.P.; Liu, B.; Wu, D.S.; Fang, Z.Y.; Bao, Y.; Jiang, M.M.; et al. Long noncoding RNA MRCCAT1 promotes metastasis of clear cell renal cell carcinoma via inhibiting NPR3 and activating p38-MAPK signaling. *Mol. Cancer* **2017**, *16*, 111. [CrossRef]
27. Song, C.; Xiong, Y.; Liao, W.; Meng, L.; Yang, S. Long noncoding RNA ATB participates in the development of renal cell carcinoma by downregulating p53 via binding to DNMT1. *J. Cell. Physiol.* **2019**, *234*, 12910–12917. [CrossRef]
28. Yue, H.; Wu, K.; Liu, K.; Gou, L.; Huang, A.; Tang, H. LINC02154 promotes the proliferation and metastasis of hepatocellular carcinoma by enhancing SPC24 promoter activity and activating the PI3K-AKT signaling pathway. *Cell. Oncol.* **2022**, *45*, 447–462. [CrossRef]
29. Zhang, G.; Fan, E.; Zhong, Q.; Feng, G.; Shuai, Y.; Wu, M.; Chen, Q.; Gou, X. Identification and potential mechanisms of a 4-lncRNA signature that predicts prognosis in patients with laryngeal cancer. *Hum. Genom.* **2019**, *13*, 36. [CrossRef]
30. Liu, L.; Zhuang, M.; Tu, X.H.; Li, C.C.; Liu, H.H.; Wang, J. Bioinformatics analysis of markers based on m(6) A related to prognosis combined with immune invasion of renal clear cell carcinoma. *Cell Biol. Int.* **2023**, *47*, 260–272. [CrossRef]
31. Shen, J.; Wang, L.; Bi, J. Bioinformatics analysis and experimental validation of cuproptosis-related lncRNA LINC02154 in clear cell renal cell carcinoma. *BMC Cancer* **2023**, *23*, 160. [CrossRef]
32. Zhao, R.; Wang, S.; Tan, L.; Li, H.; Liu, J.; Zhang, S. IGFL2-AS1 facilitates tongue squamous cell carcinoma progression via Wnt/beta-catenin signaling pathway. *Oral Dis.* **2023**, *29*, 469–482. [CrossRef] [PubMed]
33. Wang, H.; Shi, Y.; Chen, C.H.; Wen, Y.; Zhou, Z.; Yang, C.; Sun, J.; Du, G.; Wu, J.; Mao, X.; et al. KLF5-induced lncRNA IGFL2-AS1 promotes basal-like breast cancer cell growth and survival by upregulating the expression of IGFL1. *Cancer Lett.* **2021**, *515*, 49–62. [CrossRef]
34. Tracy, K.M.; Tye, C.E.; Page, N.A.; Fritz, A.J.; Stein, J.L.; Lian, J.B.; Stein, G.S. Selective expression of long non-coding RNAs in a breast cancer cell progression model. *J. Cell. Physiol.* **2018**, *233*, 1291–1299. [CrossRef]
35. Ma, Y.; Liu, Y.; Pu, Y.S.; Cui, M.L.; Mao, Z.J.; Li, Z.Z.; He, L.; Wu, M.; Wang, J.H. LncRNA IGFL2-AS1 functions as a ceRNA in regulating ARPP19 through competitive binding to miR-802 in gastric cancer. *Mol. Carcinog.* **2020**, *59*, 311–322. [CrossRef] [PubMed]
36. Cen, X.; Huang, Y.; Lu, Z.; Shao, W.; Zhuo, C.; Bao, C.; Feng, S.; Wei, C.; Tang, C.; Cen, L.; et al. LncRNA IGFL2-AS1 Promotes the Proliferation, Migration, and Invasion of Colon Cancer Cells and is Associated with Patient Prognosis. *Cancer Manag. Res.* **2021**, *13*, 5957–5968. [CrossRef]
37. Cheng, B.; Xie, M.; Zhou, Y.; Li, T.; Liu, W.; Yu, W.; Jia, M.; Yu, S.; Chen, L.; Dai, R.; et al. Vascular mimicry induced by m(6)A mediated IGFL2-AS1/AR axis contributes to pazopanib resistance in clear cell renal cell carcinoma. *Cell Death Discov.* **2023**, *9*, 121. [CrossRef]
38. Pan, Y.; Lu, X.; Shu, G.; Cen, J.; Lu, J.; Zhou, M.; Huang, K.; Dong, J.; Li, J.; Lin, H.; et al. Extracellular Vesicle-Mediated Transfer of LncRNA IGFL2-AS1 Confers Sunitinib Resistance in Renal Cell Carcinoma. *Cancer Res.* **2023**, *83*, 103–116. [CrossRef] [PubMed]
39. Pan, Q.; Wang, L.; Zhang, H.; Liang, C.; Li, B. Identification of a 5-Gene Signature Predicting Progression and Prognosis of Clear Cell Renal Cell Carcinoma. *Med. Sci. Monit.* **2019**, *25*, 4401–4413. [CrossRef]
40. Peng, D.; Fu, M.; Wang, M.; Wei, Y.; Wei, X. Targeting TGF-beta signal transduction for fibrosis and cancer therapy. *Mol. Cancer* **2022**, *21*, 104. [CrossRef]
41. Liu, B.; Sun, L.; Liu, Q.; Gong, C.; Yao, Y.; Lv, X.; Lin, L.; Yao, H.; Su, F.; Li, D.; et al. A cytoplasmic NF-kappaB interacting long noncoding RNA blocks IkappaB phosphorylation and suppresses breast cancer metastasis. *Cancer Cell* **2015**, *27*, 370–381. [CrossRef] [PubMed]

42. He, Y.; Sun, M.M.; Zhang, G.G.; Yang, J.; Chen, K.S.; Xu, W.W.; Li, B. Targeting PI3K/Akt signal transduction for cancer therapy. *Signal Transduct. Target. Ther.* **2021**, *6*, 425. [CrossRef] [PubMed]
43. Kalbasi, A.; Ribas, A. Tumour-intrinsic resistance to immune checkpoint blockade. *Nat. Rev. Immunol.* **2020**, *20*, 25–39. [CrossRef] [PubMed]
44. Morad, G.; Helmink, B.A.; Sharma, P.; Wargo, J.A. Hallmarks of response, resistance, and toxicity to immune checkpoint blockade. *Cell* **2021**, *184*, 5309–5337. [CrossRef] [PubMed]
45. Jiang, P.; Gu, S.; Pan, D.; Fu, J.; Sahu, A.; Hu, X.; Li, Z.; Traugh, N.; Bu, X.; Li, B.; et al. Signatures of T cell dysfunction and exclusion predict cancer immunotherapy response. *Nat. Med.* **2018**, *24*, 1550–1558. [CrossRef]

**Disclaimer/Publisher's Note:** The statements, opinions and data contained in all publications are solely those of the individual author(s) and contributor(s) and not of MDPI and/or the editor(s). MDPI and/or the editor(s) disclaim responsibility for any injury to people or property resulting from any ideas, methods, instructions or products referred to in the content.

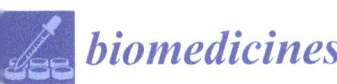 

*Article*

# A Neurosurgical Perspective on Brain Metastases from Renal Cell Carcinoma: Multi-Institutional, Retrospective Analysis

Liliana Eleonora Semenescu [1], Ligia Gabriela Tataranu [2,3,*], Anica Dricu [1], Gheorghe Vasile Ciubotaru [2], Mugurel Petrinel Radoi [4], Silvia Mara Baez Rodriguez [2] and Amira Kamel [2]

[1] Department of Biochemistry, Faculty of Medicine, University of Medicine and Pharmacy of Craiova, Str. Petru Rares nr. 2–4, 710204 Craiova, Romania; lilisicoe@yahoo.com (L.E.S.); anica.dricu@umfcv.ro (A.D.)

[2] Neurosurgical Department, Clinical Emergency Hospital "Bagdasar-Arseni", Soseaua Berceni 12, 041915 Bucharest, Romania; dr_vghciubotaru@yahoo.com (G.V.C.); mara.silvia@icloud.com (S.M.B.R.); kamel.amyra@yahoo.com (A.K.)

[3] Department of Neurosurgery, Faculty of Medicine, University of Medicine and Pharmacy "Carol Davila", 020022 Bucharest, Romania

[4] Neurosurgical Department, National Institute of Neurology and Neurovascular Diseases, Soseaua Berceni 10, 041914 Bucharest, Romania; petrinel.radoi@umfcd.ro

\* Correspondence: ligia.tataranu@umfcd.ro

**Abstract:** Background: While acknowledging the generally poor prognostic features of brain metastases from renal cell carcinoma (BM RCC), it is important to be aware of the fact that neurosurgery still plays a vital role in managing this disease, even though we have entered an era of targeted therapies. Notwithstanding their initial high effectiveness, these agents often fail, as tumors develop resistance or relapse. Methods: The authors of this study aimed to evaluate patients presenting with BM RCC and their outcomes after being treated in the Neurosurgical Department of Clinical Emergency Hospital "Bagdasar-Arseni", and the Neurosurgical Department of the National Institute of Neurology and Neurovascular Diseases, Bucharest, Romania. The study is based on a thorough appraisal of the patient's demographic and clinicopathological data and is focused on the strategic role of neurosurgery in BM RCC. Results: A total of 24 patients were identified with BM RCC, of whom 91.6% had clear-cell RCC (ccRCC) and 37.5% had a prior nephrectomy. Only 29.1% of patients harbored extracranial metastases, while 83.3% had a single BM RCC. A total of 29.1% of patients were given systemic therapy. Neurosurgical resection of the BM was performed in 23 out of 24 patients. Survival rates were prolonged in patients who underwent nephrectomy, in patients who received systemic therapy, and in patients with a single BM RCC. Furthermore, higher levels of hemoglobin were associated in our study with a higher number of BMs. Conclusion: Neurosurgery is still a cornerstone in the treatment of symptomatic BM RCC. Among the numerous advantages of neurosurgical intervention, the most important is represented by the quick reversal of neurological manifestations, which in most cases can be life-saving.

**Keywords:** brain metastases; kidney cancer; renal cell carcinoma; neurosurgery; targeted therapy

## 1. Introduction

### 1.1. A New Epidemiological Threat?

With over 15 histological subtypes identified by the World Health Organization, renal cell carcinoma (RCC) comprises 3.8% of all new cancer diagnoses. A surge in the number of new cases has been reported, with more than 70,000 new cases of RCC in 2020 and more than 14,000 deaths in the last decade in the United States [1,2]. In Europe, in 2019, the European Association of Urology (EAU) concluded that the peak incidence of RCC occurs in Western countries, leading to approximately 100,000 new RCC cases and causing more than 39,000 deaths. In some European countries, mortality rates show a rising trend, while the annual increment worldwide during the last decades exceeded 2%, with a male

**Citation:** Semenescu, L.E.; Tataranu, L.G.; Dricu, A.; Ciubotaru, G.V.; Radoi, M.P.; Rodriguez, S.M.B.; Kamel, A. A Neurosurgical Perspective on Brain Metastases from Renal Cell Carcinoma: Multi-Institutional, Retrospective Analysis. *Biomedicines* **2023**, *11*, 2485. https://doi.org/10.3390/biomedicines11092485

Academic Editors: Łukasz Zapała and Paweł Rajwa

Received: 31 July 2023
Revised: 2 September 2023
Accepted: 5 September 2023
Published: 7 September 2023

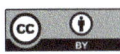

**Copyright:** © 2023 by the authors. Licensee MDPI, Basel, Switzerland. This article is an open access article distributed under the terms and conditions of the Creative Commons Attribution (CC BY) license (https://creativecommons.org/licenses/by/4.0/).

predominance. The onset age is less variable, remaining at 60–70 years of age [1–3]. In Romania, in 2018, the prevalence of RCC over the last 5 years was approximately 5400 cases, with an annual incidence of 2000 cases, while in 2020, the prevalence was 7510, with 2750 new cases [4,5].

Regarding mRCC, it has been reported to occur in approximately 25–30% of patients with RCC, while BM from RCC have a described incidence of almost 13% [6]. The incidence of BM in individuals with ccRCC has been estimated to be 8% [7], with reported cases of leptomeningeal metastases [8]. In patients with non-clear cell RCC (nccRCC), brain involvement has been reported to be 3% in papillary RCC (pRCC) and 2% in chromophobic RCC (chRCC) [7]. Multiple BM RCCs have been reported in up to 45% of patients with mRCC [9].

It is important to specify that the increasing reported number of RCC cases is also due to advancements in imaging techniques. Concerning this subject, the state of the art is represented by the use of radiomics, which is a field that combines artificial intelligence, computer science, and radiology, in order to amplify the accuracy of medical imaging [9]. In spite of various challenges, this field has demonstrated great potential for diagnostic and prognostic purposes [10]. In the current management of RCC, radiomics can distinguish between RCC and angiomyolipoma, oncocytoma, and various subtypes of RCC, as well as preoperatively predict the nuclear grade and assess the therapeutic response [11]. In mRCC patients treated with Sunitinib, diffusion-weighted imaging (DWI)-MRI and positron emission tomography/MRI radiomics analysis were used as biomarkers in order to assess treatment response [12,13]. Lately, molecular imaging has also been of interest in RCC, as it also helps differentiate between distinct subtypes [11,14]. In addition, radiogenomics, which combines radiomics features with gene expression [15], has been proven to be of great help in patients with RCC, as it can predict therapeutical responses and prognosis [16–18].

*1.2. Prognosis*

The prognostic role of RCC is decisive in determining therapeutic management. For metastatic RCC (mRCC), prognostic information is given by anatomical, histological, clinical, and molecular factors. The most important anatomical prognostic factor (PF) is represented by the tumor-node-metastasis (TNM) stage classification, but when it comes to clinical PFs, Karnofsky performance status (KPS) has persistently been the paramount determinant of survival. Regarding the histological PFs, RCC subtype, microvascular and collecting system invasion, Fuhrman nuclear grade, tumor necrosis, and sarcomatoid features are the most relevant. As for molecular PFs, worth mentioning are the expression of the Ubiquitin Carboxy-Terminal Hydrolase (BAP1) and Polybromo 1 (PBRM1) genes, chromosomal losses of regions 9p, 9q, and 14q, and CpG methylation-based assays [19–21].

*1.3. Molecular Pathogenesis*

The complexity of brain metastases from renal cell carcinoma (BM RCC) needs an understanding of this extremely heterogeneous pathology on a molecular level in an effort to address the poor prognosis. In order to succeed, treatments require adaptation to molecular susceptibilities among primary cancers and their metastases [22]. Renal cell carcinoma (RCC) is comprised of several subtypes with genetic drivers, individual histology, clinical evolution, and therapeutic responses. According to The Cancer Genome Atlas analyses of RCC, there are cardinal dissimilarities between the major histological subtypes, including metabolic pathway expression signatures and their distinct chromosomal alterations [23]. The most common subtypes of RCC are represented by the ccRCC, accounting for ~75% of cases, followed by papillary RCC (pRCC, type 1—basophilic and type 2—eosinophilic), and the chromophobic subtype (chRCC), which accounts for 5–15% of cases. The most investigated subtype is represented by the ccRCC, given the fact that it is the most frequent. The chromosome that has known relations with ccRCC is 3p. Genetic mutations in ccRCC are described in the following genes: the von Hippel–Lindau tumor suppressor gene (VHL, most frequent, up to 50%), PBMR1 (up to 40%), BAP1 (up to 15%), and other genes recounted as SET Domain Containing 2 (SET D2), Phosphatidylinositol-4,5-Bisphosphate 3-Kinase Catalytic Subunit Alpha (PIK3CA), and also TSC Complex Subunit 1 and 2 (TSC1/2) [23–26]. The last two genes are responsible for the activation and suppression of mammalian target of rapamycin (mTOR) pathways and have been defined as being involved in metabolic RCCs. The first two mentioned genes manage the regulation of hypoxia-inducible factor (HIF) protein and the encoding of BAF180 (equivalent name of PBMR1), respectively. Although the VHL gene is described in more than half of the patients with this pathology, other genetic alterations may arise progressively, worsening the prognosis. Regarding the pRCC, genetic alterations are described in the following genes: Mesenchymal Epithelial Transition (MET), Cyclin-Dependent Kinase Inhibitor 2A/B (CDKN2A/B), Telomerase reverse transcriptase (TERT), and Fumarate Hydratase (FH), the first one being the most frequent. Additionally, in the sarcomatoid subtype, mutations were described in Tumor Protein P53 (TP53), a tumor suppressor inscribing for p53, and Moesin-Ezrin-Radixin Like (MERLIN) Tumor Suppressor (NF2) [3,19,27,28].

*1.4. Therapeutic Approaches in BM RCC*

1.4.1. Hereditary versus Sporadic, and the Primary Management of RCC

The CT scan may be extremely helpful in the evaluation of RCC, with greater than 95% accuracy. A contrast-enhanced CT scan reveals an enhanced renal mass, which is a solid clue for the diagnosis of the disease. While searching for diagnostic certainty, the histopathological examination after a tissue biopsy may be essential in the diagnosis and management of RCC [29]. Subsequently, similar to CT scans, MRI and ultrasonography can be utilized to describe a specific stage before any treatment is given. Hereditary proneness to RCC is guided by the existence of many factors, of which the following are described: age younger than 50 years old, multiple enhancing lesions, and/or a family history of RCC. A thorough physical examination is required in order to assess extrarenal manifestations (e.g., ophthalmologic, neurologic, and dermatologic evaluations) [30–32]. For instance, compared to Birt–Hogg–Dubé syndrome, von Hippel–Lindau disease, and RCC, which may cause systemic damage, family ccRCC and hereditary pRCC do not reveal systemic manifestations other than renal. Genetic testing can be used to identify mutations in specific genes, as it was concluded that the von Hippel–Lindau protein has a major role in sporadic ccRCC. Monitoring and evaluation form the basis for patients with hereditary RCC to assess new renal masses, and thus, imaging studies must be carried out, sometimes with an interval difference of 6 months or more, determined by the character of the syndrome and the lesions. Finally, in the multimodal therapeutic approach, a key element is defined by the surgical treatment in selected cases (i.e., radical nephrectomy, nephron-sparing partial nephrectomy or laparoscopic nephrectomy, surgery for metastatic disease, percutaneous ablative approaches) and targeted therapy [23,32–34].

1.4.2. Multidisciplinary Opportunities in BM RCC

RCC is well known for the low rates of response to chemotherapy and radiotherapy, which gave rise to much research regarding the development and evolution of targeted therapies, including vascular endothelial growth factor (VEGF) and transforming growth factor alpha (TGF-α) pathways, mTOR inhibitors, immune checkpoint inhibitors (ICI), and more recently, combined targeted therapies. Anti-angiogenic strategies became alluring given the fact that RCC is a decidedly vascular cancer. Despite their high initial effectiveness, these agents often fail as tumors become resistant or relapse, and therefore some patients experience disease progression. Afterward, in advanced RCC, patients will frequently develop BM, and more than 80% are symptomatic at the moment of diagnosis [35–39].

Hence, despite the increased availability of targeted agents along with multimodal therapies, neurosurgery is still the main pawn when approaching BM RCC in symptomatic patients, especially with solitary BM. Among the numerous advantages of surgical intervention, the most important is represented by the quick reversal of neurological manifestations [40,41]. During neurosurgical resection, tumor tissue may be obtained for histopathological examination in favor of genetic tumor characterization. Notwithstanding its advantages, the neurosurgical approach alone is insufficient for the local control of the tumor, and the craniotomy is not risk-free, carrying a mortality rate of less than 2% and a morbidity rate between 4 and 6% [42,43]. However, accompanied by other therapies, neurosurgical treatment was proven to extend the overall survival (OS) rate.

Although RCC is appraised to be radioresistant, some studies confirm the opposite, stating that in a multimodal approach, stereotactic radiosurgery (SRS) might be a major factor in the management of the disease [44]. With the advent of minimally invasive techniques, it is now possible to decrease the disclosure of the cerebral tissue and the discomfort, maximize the safety of the central nervous system approach, reduce recovery time, and therefore increase the advantages of the method [44,45]. Some of these techniques are represented by stereotactic laser ablation (which requires the insertion of a laser catheter through the burr hole), convection-enhanced delivery (also a form of intratumoral therapy), focused ultrasound (for gaining access deep within the brain to ablate only the target tissue without harming the surrounding tissue), stereotactic laser interstitial thermal therapy (LITT, a cytoreductive neurosurgical technique), and stereotactic biopsy (most common when there is more than one lesion and with deep localization) [23,46–48].

An important part of the multimodal therapeutic approach, which can improve overall survival rates, includes cytoreductive nephrectomy (CN) [49]. CN is defined as the removal of the primary RCC tumor lesion in the presence of metastases [50]. Regarding the numerous benefits of CN, it is worth mentioning that it improves the quality of life by alleviating symptoms (e.g., hematuria, pain) [50] and removes a potential source for new metastases [51–53]. However, CN has disadvantages as well, including perioperative morbidity and mortality, as well as deferred receiving of systemic therapy [52]. Furthermore, studies like CARMENA and SURTIME highlight the paramount aspect of careful patient selection, as not every patient may benefit from CN [54,55]. Notwithstanding, patients with favorable-risk features are more likely to benefit from CN [56,57], although approximately 20% of patients with nephrectomy will still develop metastases [58]. Despite numerous studies and debates, CN remains a moving target surrounded by controversy, highlighting the need for future studies on the matter [50,59,60].

1.4.3. A Focus on Neurosurgery

The colonization of metastases in the brain is a result of tumor cells spreading throughout the blood, as well as seeding from an already existing metastasis in the body [22]. Microenvironmental interactivity, neuroinflammatory cascades, and neovascularization are the basis of developing BM [22]. Concerning the BM RCC, it is well known that this pathology has a greater tendency for vasogenic edema and hemorrhage; therefore, patients are oftentimes symptomatic [61]. Nevertheless, neuroimaging is usually recommended in symptomatic patients or at the doctor's discretion [36,61], as well as if clinically indicated [62]. However, currently, the National Comprehensive Cancer Network recommends routine neuroimaging in patients with mRCC, which is rather helpful in detecting asymptomatic BM [61]. Patients who, at the initial diagnosis, have BM usually exhibit a poor prognosis and, when left untreated, may have a median OS to the utmost of 4 months [6,63].

It is worth mentioning that several therapies can mimic intracranial disease progression, while new or incremented neuroimaging abnormalities in the course of immunotherapy or SRS may constitute pseudoprogression [64].

At present, the primary approach to BM RCC comprises neurosurgery and/or radiotherapy (RT) [65–67].

The selection of the patients is of great importance, as the decision of neurosurgical intervention must consider the advantages and disadvantages when compared to other therapeutic options. At the present time, neurosurgical resection can be considered a safe option, as it is correlated with minimal morbidity and mortality [68,69]. Nonetheless, when considering neurosurgery, several factors must be taken into account, like the status of primary cancer, Karnofsky performance status (KPS), the localization of BM in the brain areas, and patient characteristics [70]. The type of neurosurgical excision has a great impact on the clinical outcomes as well. En bloc resection and SRS are associated with better outcomes when compared to piecemeal resection, as the latter carries a higher risk of leptomeningeal dissemination in patients with single supratentorial BM [71]. In like manner, individuals with a single BM treated with neurosurgery and RT have better survival rates and quality of life in comparison to RT alone [72]. However, the therapeutic approach for patients with single BM RCC differs from patients with multiple BM RCC.

In patients with single BM, if asymptomatic and smaller than 3 cm, or if not fit for neurosurgery, SRS alone or fractioned stereotactic RT (FSRT) might be the option [73]. Individuals with lesions of 3 cm or bigger, especially if symptomatic, are candidates for neurosurgical excision. If patients are unfit for craniotomies, FSRT is preferred over single-fraction SRS [74]. It should be noted that despite general knowledge regarding the resistance of BM RCC to RT, various studies have proven otherwise [74,75]. Laser interstitial thermal therapy/ablation (LITT) might be considered in patients unfit for both neurosurgical resection and SRS [76], as in recurrent patients after SRS, LITT had similar outcomes to craniotomy [77].

In patients with multiple BMs, aggressive treatment for intracranial disease in oligometastatic cases has better outcomes when compared to whole-brain RT (WBRT) [78,79]. It has been concluded that WBRT has limited recommendations given its known relative resistance in RCC [70].

Given the fact that neurosurgery has a main role in BM RCC, our current study focuses on this exact matter in order to conclude to what extent patients with this pathology may benefit from it.

## 2. Materials and Methods

The authors of this study aimed to evaluate patients presenting with BM from RCC and their outcomes after being treated in the Neurosurgical Department of Clinical Emergency Hospital "Bagdasar-Arseni", Bucharest, Romania, and the Neurosurgical Department of the National Institute of Neurology and Neurovascular Diseases, Bucharest, Romania. We included adult patients with renal cell carcinoma as their only malignancy, and we excluded patients with more than one malignancy and patients who underwent prior neurosurgical interventions in other neurosurgical departments. In order to make the selection, registry databases from our departments, as well as the patient's physical file, were queried for all patients with histologically confirmed BM from RCC from 2012 to 2022 and evaluated retrospectively. The selected data to review were represented by the clinical notes, demographics, histology, comorbidities, BM topography, neurosurgical treatment, systemic therapy, extracranial metastases, prior nephrectomy, and outcomes. Regarding the matter of cytoreductive nephrectomy, when admitted to our departments, 37.5% of patients with BM RCC had already undergone surgery for the primary RCC lesion. Of the total of 37.5% (9 patients), 66.6% were from urban settings.

The current study is based on a thorough appraisal of the patient's demographic and clinicopathological data and is focused on the strategic role of neurosurgery in the multimodal therapy of BM from RCC.

## 3. Results

### 3.1. Statistics and Replicability

This retrospective study was carried out by reviewing the medical records from our institutional databases of 24 patients treated in our departments between January 2012 and December 2022 for BM RCC. We appraised demographic information, clinicopathological characteristics, as well as therapeutic options. Correlations between the obtained data were performed in order to draw conclusions. Statistical analyses of experimental data, figures, and tables were performed using GraphPad Prism 8.3.0 software. $p$-values less than 0.05 were considered statistically significant. The one-sample $t$-test, one-way/two-way ANOVA, and the Chi-square (and Fisher's exact) were used to assess differences in variables and correlate normally distributed data. Kaplan–Meier method was the choice for performing survival analysis. Overall survival was interpreted as the period between the histopathological diagnosis and the date of death.

*3.2. Demographic Profile, Clinicopathological Characteristics, and Correlation Analysis*

Within our institutions, 24 patients (n = 24) were admitted with BM RCC (Table 1), of whom 20.8% were women and 79.1% were men. Ten (41.6%) patients lived in urban areas, while 14 (58.3%) were living in rural settings. The median age of BM RCC diagnosis was 62.5 years (36–73), while the mean age of RCC diagnosis was 62 years. While a total of 9 (37.5%) patients underwent nephrectomy, regarding the comorbidities, 11 patients (45.8%) had a history of congestive heart failure and heart disease, and 7 (29.1%) had a history of type 2 diabetes mellitus. Seven (29.1%) patients received systemic therapy, and only two (8.3%) patients were asymptomatic at admission. The most common clinical symptoms were represented by headache (45.8%, n = 11) and limb paralysis (41.6%, n = 10), while aphasia (12.5%, n = 3), seizures (8.3%, n = 2), and pituitary dysfunction (4.1%, n = 1) were less frequent. Regarding the localization of BM RCC, the most frequent site was represented by the frontal lobe (33.3%, n = 8), followed by the cerebellum (29.1%, n = 7), and the temporal lobe (25%, n = 6). The least common sites of metastasis were represented by the parietal lobe (4.1%, n = 1), the occipital lobe (4.1%, n = 1), and the sellar region (4.1%, n = 1) (Figure 1). When comparing the distribution of lesion size by symptom status, we obtained a statistically significant result ($p$ = 0.042), showing that patients with smaller lesions were more likely to be symptomatic (Figure 2). These results may be due to the localization of BM in neurologic eloquent areas.

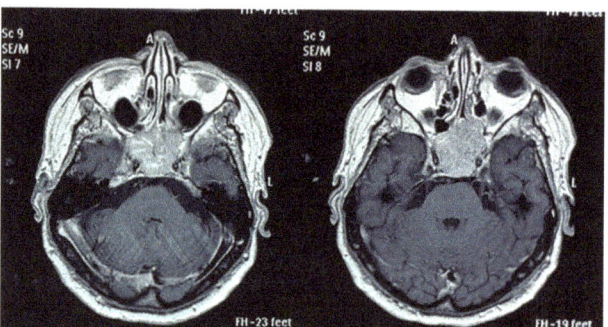

**Figure 1.** Pituitary MRI reveals a non-homogenous invasive sellar mass (BM) from RCC in a patient from our study group.

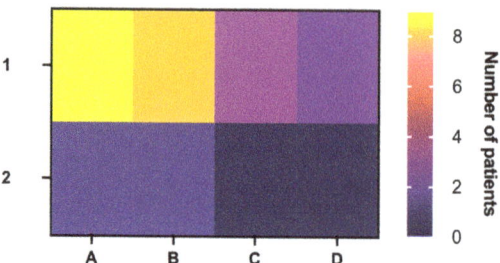

**Figure 2.** Heat map comparing the distribution of lesion size by symptom status. 1—symptomatic patients; 2—asymptomatic patients. Size of the lesion (mm): A—13–27; B—30–40; C—43–52; D—52–63.

**Table 1.** General characteristics of patients with BM from RCC in our study group.

| Characteristic | Variable | Value (total n = 24) |
|---|---|---|
| Sex | Male | 19 (79.1%) |
| | Female | 5 (20.8%) |
| Distribution area | Rural/Urban | 14 (58.3%)/10 (41.6%) |
| Age at RCC diagnosis | Median age | 62 years |
| Age at BM RCC diagnosis | Median age | 62.5 years |
| BM localization | Frontal lobe | 8 (33.3%) |
| | Temporal lobe | 6 (25%) |
| | Parietal lobe | 1 (4.1%) |
| | Occipital lobe | 1 (4.1%) |
| | Cerebellum | 7 (29.1%) |
| | Sellar region | 1 (4.1%) |
| Single or multiple BM RCC | Single BM RCC | 20 (83.3%) |
| | 2 or more BM RCC | 4 (16.6%) |
| Number of BM RCC | Mean/Median (min-max) | 1.29/1 (1–4) |
| Size of BM RCC (mm) | Mean/Median (min-max) | 32.54 mm/31 mm (13–63) |
| Symptoms at presentation | Yes | 22 (91.6%) |
| | No | 2 (8.3%) |
| Clinical symptoms/manifestations | None | 2 (8.3%) |
| | Raised intracranial Pressure syndrome | 7 (29.1%) |
| | Headache | 11 (45.8%) |
| | Cranial nerve palsies | 5 (20.8%) |
| | Pituitary dysfunction | 1 (4.1%) |
| | Limb paralysis | 10 (41.6%) |
| | Aphasia | 3 (12.5%) |
| | Seizures | 2 (8.3%) |
| Karnofsky Performance Status Scale at admission | ≥80 | 13 (54.1%) |
| | <80 | 11 (45.8%) |
| Admission to the neurosurgical department | First time | 20 (83.3%) |
| | Recurrence | 4 (16.6%) |
| Extracranial metastases [1] | Yes | 7 (29.1%) |
| | No | 17 (70.8%) |
| Systemic therapy | Yes | 7 (29.1%) |
| | No | 17 (70.8%) |
| Prior nephrectomy | Yes | 9 (37.5%) |
| | No | 15 (62.5%) |
| Stereotactic Radiosurgery (SRS) | Yes | 3 (12.5%) |
| | No | 21 (87.5%) |

[1] 7 (29.1%) of our patients had extracranial metastases (lung and intestinal metastases).

Although Romania is still a developing country with a high-income economy, in rural areas there is limited availability of healthcare resources. In our study, 9 (37.5%) patients underwent nephrectomy. From the total number (n = 9), 66.6% were from urban settings in comparison with half of that percentage (33.3%) that were from rural areas. In the group without nephrectomy (n = 15), 11 (73.3%) were from rural areas and 4 (26.6%) from urban settings; $p = 0.058$ (Figure 3).

In our study population, lesion sizes between 13 and 30 mm had a homogeneous distribution in both rural and urban settings (25% versus 25%), while the number of patients with lesion sizes between 30 and 63 mm doubled in rural areas: 33.3% in rural areas versus 16.6% in urban settings (Figure 4). However, the conclusion was not statistically significant; $p = 0.375$.

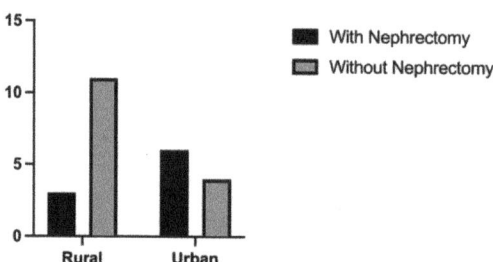

**Figure 3.** Comparison between patients from rural areas with and without nephrectomy versus patients from urban settings with and without nephrectomy ($p = 0.058$).

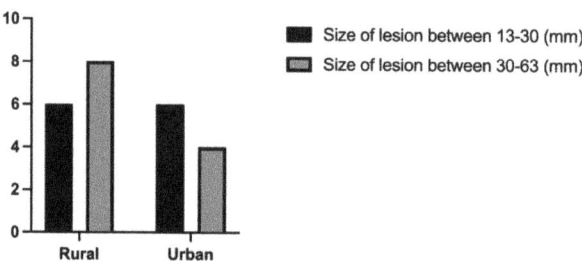

**Figure 4.** Bar graph comparing the distribution of lesion size by geographic areas ($p = 0.375$).

*3.3. Neurosurgical Results*

Out of 24 patients with BM RCC, in 23 cases a neurosurgical resection was performed, and in 1 case SRS alone was indicated. The main purposes of neurosurgical intervention were gross-total resection (which occurred in 18 patients) and relief of mass effects in order to improve neurological symptoms. Due to the infiltration and adherence of BMs, as well as their localization in eloquent brain areas, only partial resection was possible in five patients (Figure 5). In cases with multiple BMs, we approached only the symptomatic lesion.

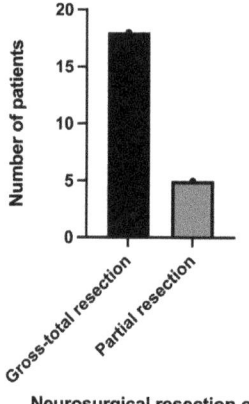

**Figure 5.** Bar graph describing the neurosurgical resection of BM RCC in our study population.

Regarding the post-surgical complications, a postoperative intracerebral hematoma has been noted in one patient, and it was operated on without further consequences. The initial KPS in patients with BM RCC was <80 in 11 (45.8%) cases (Figure 6). After neurosurgery, the score improved in 15 (62.5%) cases, remained unchanged in 8 (33.3%) cases, and worsened in 1 (4.1%) case.

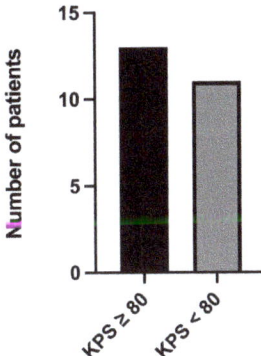

**Karnofsky Performance Status at admission**

**Figure 6.** Bar graph describing KPS at admission in our departments, in patients with BM RCC.

Seven (29.1%) of our patients had intracranial metastases: six cases of lung metastases and one case of intestinal metastasis. The remaining 17 individuals did not have extracranial metastases.

Three (12.5%) patients in our study population were treated with SRS for BM RCC. One patient with a small BM (13 mm) was treated with SRS alone, while two patients were treated with SRS and neurosurgical resection.

### 3.4. Histopathological Features

The final diagnosis based on histopathology of the neurosurgical specimen was ccRCC in 91.6% of the patients (Figure 7) and pRCC in 8.3% of the patients.

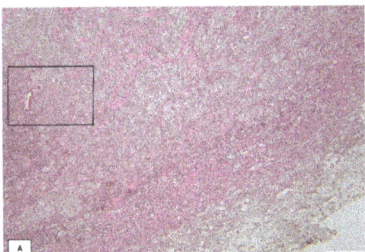
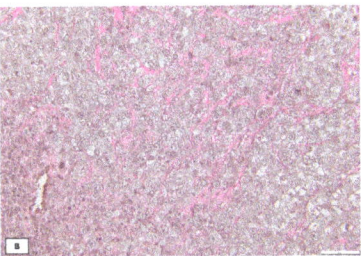

**Figure 7.** Photomicrograph of BM RCC exhibiting clear cell morphology and a prominent network of thin-walled vessels by Van Gieson staining. Magnification: (**A**)—20×, (**B**)—40×. Contributed by Laurențiu-Cătălin Cocoșilă, M.D.

### 3.5. Survival Analysis

The probability of survival was higher in patients who underwent nephrectomy than in those who did not. Overall survival was also extended in those who underwent nephrectomy (log-rank [Mantel–Cox] test). The median survival rate in patients with nephrectomy was 12 months (hazard ratio [HR] = 0.36, 95% CI 0.16–0.83), while in patients without nephrectomy, it was 7 months (HR = 2.72, 95% CI 1.19–6.21); $p = 0.004$ (Figure 8).

The probability of survival was higher for patients treated with systemic therapy. The median survival rate in patients treated with systemic therapy was 13 months (HR = 0.41; 95% CI 0.18–0.91), while in patients without systemic therapy it was 12 months (HR = 2.42; 95% CI 1.09–5.40), $p = 0.033$ (Figure 9).

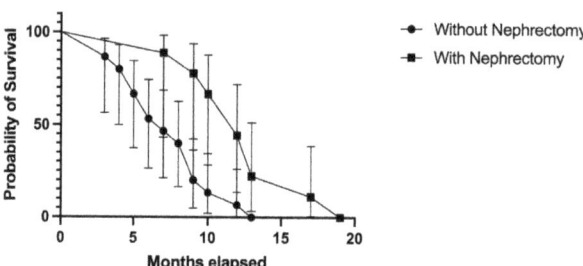

**Figure 8.** Kaplan–Meier plot describing the survival proportion in patients with and without nephrectomy.

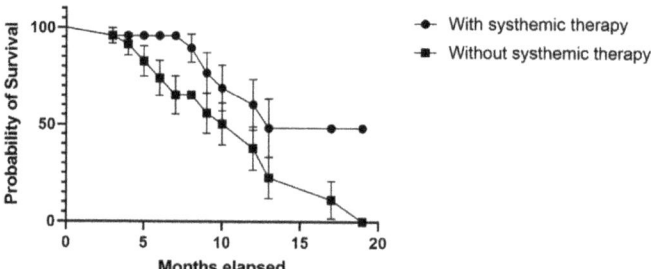

**Figure 9.** Kaplan–Meier plot describing the comparison of survival rates between neurosurgical patients treated with systemic therapy and patients who did not receive systemic therapy.

In the study population, 4 (16.6%) patients had multiple BM RCC, and 20 (83.3%) had a single BM. Compared to patients with more than one BM, those with a single BM were observed to have better survival rates: Median survival in patients with one BM was 9.5 months (HR = 2.11, 95% CI 0.72–6.17) vs. 4.5 months (HR = 0.47, 95% CI 0.16–1.38) in patients with more than one BM; $p = 0.0005$ (Figure 10).

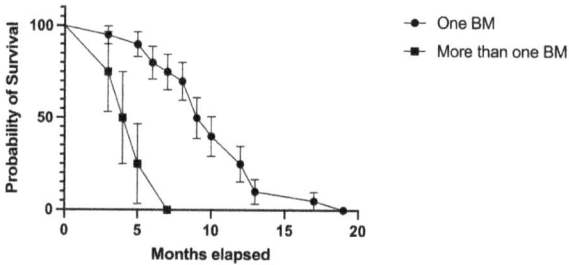

**Figure 10.** Kaplan–Meier plot describing the comparison between survival rates in patients with one BM RCC versus patients with two or more BM RCC.

In order to provide the best therapeutic options and to predict survival rates, patients with RCC were classified according to the International Metastatic Renal Cell Carcinoma Database Consortium (IMDC) risk subgroup, which currently represents the gold standard [63,64] (Table 2).

In our study, the majority of the population was in the intermediate IMDC risk subgroup (66.6%). We calculated the survival rates in each of the three subgroups (Figure 11). The favorable-risk subgroup had the longest median survival, 13 months, followed by the intermediate-risk subgroup, with a 9-month median survival. The shortest median survival rate has been registered in the poor-risk subgroup, with a median survival rate of 4 months; $p < 0.0001$.

**Table 2.** IMDC risk subgroups in our study population.

| IMDC Risk | Patients N (%) |
| --- | --- |
| Favorable-risk group | 5 (20.8%) |
| Intermediate-risk group | 16 (66.6%) |
| Poor-risk group | 3 (12.5%) |

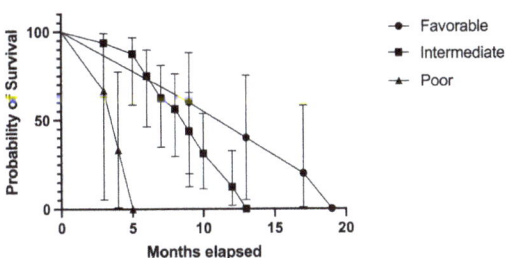

**Figure 11.** Kaplan–Meier plot describing the comparison between IMDC risk subgroups in patients with BM RCC in our study.

*3.6. The Metabolism of Ferrous Iron: A Soft Spot in the Modulation of Cancer and Metastasis?*

Back in 2005, Herbert T. Cohen and Francis J. McGovern stated in an article regarding medical progress in RCC that, among others, a low hemoglobin level predicts a poor prognosis [80]. However, in 2022, Honglin Jiang et al. found that oncogenic KRAS signaling induced ferrous iron accumulation and that elevated iron concentrations in some types of cancer are correlated with a lower survival rate. They were looking forward to exploring their ferrous iron-activatable drug conjugate (FeADC) technology, which is in effect a converted FDA-approved MEK inhibitor, in order to achieve MAPK blockade in cancerous cells [81]. However, Richard E. Gray et al. stated in an article about the diagnosis and management of RCC that a major indicator of poor prognosis is, among others, a low hemoglobin level [35,82,83]. In our study, the median value of hemoglobin was 13.7 g/dL. The normal levels of hemoglobin established by our laboratory were 12–15 g/dL for female patients and 13–17 g/dL for male patients; levels below were considered indicators of anemia, while levels above were considered elevated. The lowest value for hemoglobin in the study group was 8.8 g/dL, while the highest was 18.4 g/dL (Figure 12a). Anemia was described in 20.8% of the male population, 8.3% of the female population, and 29.1% of the total. However, higher levels of hemoglobin were associated in our study with a higher number of BM, and it was statistically significant; $p < 0.001$ (Figure 12b).

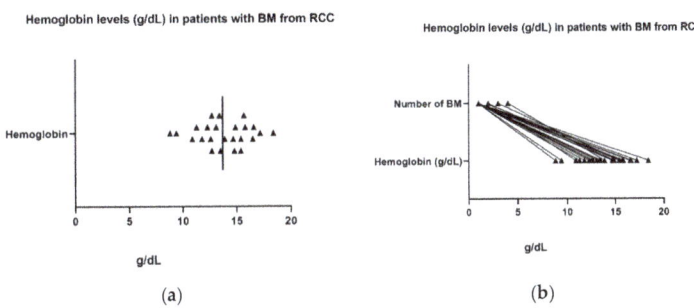

**Figure 12.** (a) Hemoglobin levels in patients with BM RCC in our study population. The median hemoglobin level was 13.7 g/dL, with the highest level of 18.4 g/dL and the lowest of 8.8 g/dL; (b) hemoglobin levels were associated with the number of BM in patients with RCC in our study population ($p < 0.001$; mean difference = 1.29, 95% CI 0.97–1.61).

The median survival in patients with normal levels of hemoglobin was 9 months, which was the same as in low hemoglobin cases, while individuals with elevated levels of hemoglobin had a lower median survival rate (median survival of 8 months; Figure 13). However, the comparison was not statistically significant ($p = 0.583$).

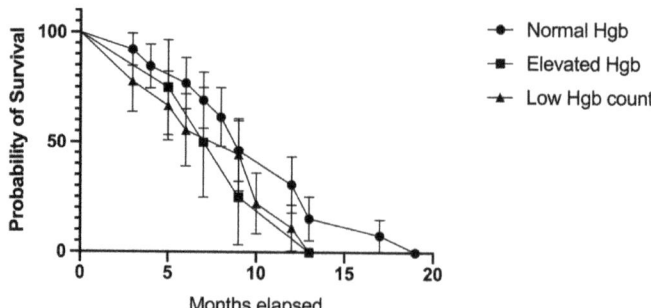

**Figure 13.** Kaplan–Meier plot describing the comparison between the survival rate in patients with normal, elevated, and low hemoglobin levels; $p = 0.210$.

## 4. Discussion

Despite the newly increased availability of multimodal therapies, BM RCC have generally poor prognostic features with dismal outcomes [69]. Notwithstanding these classically considered results, our study group experienced durable long-term survival, as patients appear to benefit from the multimodal therapeutic approach. The longest survival rate, of 19 months, has been achieved in a 63-year-old patient from a rural area with a single 24 mm cerebellar BM RCC who was admitted for cerebellar syndrome. The patient also had a pulmonary metastasis, underwent nephrectomy before neurosurgery, and did not receive systemic therapy. The shortest survival rate, of 3 months, was registered in two patients aged 70 and 73, respectively. One of them received systemic therapy, while the other did not.

Although not every patient with RCC will benefit from nephrectomy, some individuals will experience OS benefits, especially in the context of immune therapy [70–72]. In our study, 37.5% of patients with BM RCC had a prior nephrectomy (before being admitted to our departments). In this group, longer survival rates were registered, with a median survival rate of 12 months (HR = 0.36, 95% CI 0.16–0.83), in comparison to 7 months (HR = 2.72, 95% CI 1.19–6.21) in patients without nephrectomy ($p = 0.004$). When comparing this treatment with the geographic region of origin of our patients, we found that 73.3% of the patients without nephrectomy were from rural areas in comparison to only 26.6% from urban settings ($p = 0.058$). This statement is specifically significant because in Romania, there is limited availability of healthcare resources in most of the rural areas. Similarly, regarding the multimodal approach of BM RCC, in our study group, a total of 7 (29.1%) patients received systemic therapy in comparison to 17 (70.8%) who did not. Our study demonstrates that the median survival rate in patients treated with systemic therapy was longer than in those without systemic therapy: 13 months versus 12 months.

Likewise, when focusing on the number of BM RCC at the diagnosis, compared to patients with more than one BM, those with a single BM were observed to have better survival rates. Median survival in patients with one BM was 9.5 months (HR = 2.11, 95% CI 0.72–6.17), in comparison to 4.5 months (HR = 0.47, 95% CI 0.16–1.38) in patients with more than one BM; $p = 0.0005$. It is worth mentioning that only four patients from the study group had multiple metastases, while the rest of the population had a single BM RCC. Four patients (16.6%) experienced local recurrence, of whom one had a single BM RCC, while the other three patients had two or more than two BM RCC.

When comparing the distribution of lesion size by symptom status, we found that patients with smaller lesions were more likely to be symptomatic ($p = 0.042$). Nine symptomatic patients (37.5%) had lesions of sizes between 13 and 27 mm, eight symptomatic patients (33.3%) had lesions of sizes between 30 and 40 mm, three symptomatic patients (12.5%) had lesions between 43 and 52 mm, and two symptomatic patients (8.3%) had lesions between 52 and 63 mm. One asymptomatic patient (4.1%) fell into the category of the 13–27 mm lesion size group, and one asymptomatic patient fell into the category of the 30–40 mm lesion size group. A possible explanation of this result could be the fact that the localization of the tumors, regardless of their small size, was in areas of the brain with important neurological and/or neuroendocrinological functions (i.e., frontal lobe, temporal lobe, pituitary region). Even if it was not statistically significant, it is worth mentioning that in our study group, the number of patients with lesion sizes between 30 and 63 mm has doubled in rural areas (33.3% in rural areas versus 16.6% in urban settings, $p = 0.375$).

In our study population, in 23 patients, a neurosurgical resection of BM RCC was performed, with 18 gross-total resections and 5 partial resections. The partial resections were justified by tumoral infiltration and adherence, as well as localization in eloquent brain areas. One patient had a postoperative intracerebral hematoma. An emergency surgery was performed for evacuation, and the postoperative outcome was not affected by this event. No other postoperative complications have been noted.

KPS at admission in our departments was lower than 80 in 11 (45.8%) cases and higher in 13 (54.1%). After the neurosurgical intervention, the score improved in 15 (62.5%) cases, which represents more than half of the patients.

The mainstay of treatment for symptomatic patients with BM RCC is still the classical neurosurgical approach, which first and foremost offers a quick reversal of neurological manifestations. However, neurosurgery alone is insufficient, but along with other therapies, it offers long-lasting local control and may extend the OS rate [41,84].

Even though RCC is considered radioresistant, it has been proven that SRS may improve the initial poor prognosis in a multimodal approach [45,85–87]. However, unfortunately, our study consisted of only three patients who underwent SRS, so we consider this one of the study's limitations. Only one patient was treated by SRS alone, while the other two were treated with SRS and neurosurgical resection. Given the very small group of patients treated with SRS, we did not conclude a significant comparison between groups and did not include statistical analysis in this article. However, it is worth mentioning that one patient treated with SRS and neurosurgical resection had a survival of 19 months, the other one of 13 months, and the patient treated with SRS alone had a survival of 13 months. In the latter case, the patient had a single 13 mm BM, no comorbidities, minimal symptoms at a first-time admission, a prior nephrectomy, and no systemic therapy received.

In order to predict survival rates and provide the best therapeutic options for patients with RCC, the IMDC risk-scoring system has been designed [88,89]. In our study population, 5 patients were in the favorable-risk group, 16 in the intermediate-risk group, and 3 in the poor-risk group. When comparing survival rates, the first group had the longest median survival rate (13 months), followed by the intermediate-risk subgroup (9 months). The shortest survival was concluded in the poor-risk subgroup, and it was statistically significant ($p < 0.0001$).

A recent study by Honglin Jiang et al. discovered that in some categories of cancer, elevated iron concentrations are correlated with a lower survival rate [81]. The authors stated that an increased level of $Fe^{2+}$ is also linked to drug tolerance in cancer cells, but the mechanism is still undetermined. Moreover, the authors concluded that intracellular $Fe^{2+}$ is elevated by mutant RAS signaling [81]. Even though these statements represented just the basis of the study, starting from this point and inspired by other previous studies [90–93], we sought to evaluate this perspective. In our study, normal levels of hemoglobin established by our laboratory were 12–15 g/dL for female patients and 13–17 g/dL for male patients, while the levels below were considered indicators of anemia. Twelve (50%) patients had modified hemoglobin levels, and 12 were in the normal range. The median hemoglobin level in the study group was 13.7 g/dL, with the highest level of 18.4 g/dL and the lowest of 8.8 g/dL. Anemia was described in 29.1% of the study population. Interestingly, it turned out that higher levels of hemoglobin were associated with a higher number of BM, and higher numbers of BM were associated with lower survival rates.

It has been known for a long time that some cases of RCC have a hereditary constituent, and the most common examples encompass von Hippel–Lindau syndrome and the familial pRCC syndrome [94,95]. However, in our series of BM RCCs, none of the patients have been diagnosed with hereditary RCCs.

Many of the patients in our study had comorbidities that may place them at a higher risk for chronic kidney disease or even end-stage renal disease. More precisely, as many as 45.8% of patients had a history of congestive heart failure or heart disease, and 29.1% had a history of diabetes. In one of their articles, Tyler Clemmensen et al. suggested that partial nephrectomy is especially important in this category of patients as a nephron-sparing approach [1].

Overall, consistent with prior studies, the authors of this article established that neurosurgical patients with BM RCC may benefit from multimodal therapeutic approaches. Notwithstanding that neurosurgery is the gold standard for symptomatic patients with BM RCC, it alone does not suffice and, in addition to other therapies, may increase survival rates.

One of the main limitations of the current study is represented by the small sample size, which may have resulted in insufficient statistical power to permit the detection of significance for some variables (i.e., the Chi-square test is not accurate in small samples). Furthermore, the study was also limited by the small group of patients who were treated with radiation therapy (SRS). Among the limitations, we also consider the exclusion criteria regarding patients with BM RCC initially treated in other neurosurgical departments. In the current study, we solely included patients neurosurgically treated in our departments from the beginning for a better follow-up and evolution assessment. However, we are looking forward to including in future studies patients with possible recurrences initially treated in other neurosurgical departments.

To our knowledge, this is the first study focused on BM RCC patients in Romania that involves a multicentric approach, and for a better understanding of the topic, we encourage other studies regarding the matter.

## 5. Conclusions

Although the expectancy of life's duration is rather short in patients with BM RCC, neurosurgical approaches combined with other therapeutical options can offer long-lasting local control and can increase survival rates. Moreover, histopathological examination of tumoral tissue can be obtained in order to establish the best targeted therapeutic agents. Among the numerous advantages of neurosurgical intervention, the most important is represented by the quick reversal of neurological manifestations, which in most cases can be life-saving. Despite the increased availability of targeted agents along with multimodal therapies, neurosurgery is still a cornerstone in the treatment of BM RCC in symptomatic patients.

**Author Contributions:** Conceptualization, L.G.T., A.K., and M.P.R.; Resources, G.V.C. and A.D.; Supervision, L.G.T. and A.D.; Methodology, G.V.C., M.P.R., and L.G.T.; Visualization, A.K., L.G.T., and S.M.B.R.; Writing—original draft preparation, A.K.; Writing—review and editing, L.E.S., L.G.T., A.K., and A.D. All authors have read and agreed to the published version of the manuscript.

**Funding:** This research was funded by Grant PN-III-P4-ID-PCE-2020-1649, UEFISCDI, Romania.

**Institutional Review Board Statement:** The study did not require ethical approval.

**Informed Consent Statement:** Informed consent was obtained from all subjects involved in the study.

**Data Availability Statement:** Datasets analyzed or generated during the study are unavailable due to privacy and ethical restrictions.

**Conflicts of Interest:** The authors declare no conflict of interest.

## References

1. Clemmensen, T.; Matoso, A.; Graham, T.; Lai, W.S.; Rais-Bahrami, S.; Gordetsky, J. Pathologic and clinical characteristics of early onset renal cell carcinoma. *Hum. Pathol.* **2018**, *74*, 25–31. [CrossRef] [PubMed]
2. Padala, S.A.; Barsouk, A.; Thandra, K.C.; Saginala, K.; Mohammed, A.; Vakiti, A.; Rawla, P.; Barsouk, A. Epidemiology of Renal Cell Carcinoma. *World J. Oncol.* **2020**, *11*, 79–87. [CrossRef] [PubMed]
3. D'Avella, C.; Abbosh, P.; Pal, S.K.; Geynisman, D.M. Mutations in renal cell carcinoma. *Urol. Oncol.* **2020**, *38*, 763–773. [CrossRef]
4. Liviu Preda, A.; Galieta Mincă, D. Cost-Effectiveness Analysis of Treatment for Metastatic Renal Carcinoma in Romania. *J. Med. Life* **2018**, *11*, 306–311. [CrossRef] [PubMed]
5. World Health Organization. Cancer Today. 2023. Available online: https://gco.iarc.fr/today/data/factsheets/populations/642-romania-fact-sheets.pdf (accessed on 25 July 2023).
6. Kattan, J.; Rassy, E.E.; Assi, T.; Bakouny, Z.; Pavlidis, N. A comprehensive review of the role of immune checkpoint inhibitors in brain metastasis of renal cell carcinoma origin. *Crit. Rev. Oncol. Hematol.* **2018**, *130*, 60–69. [CrossRef]
7. Incorvaia, L.; Madonia, G.; Corsini, L.R.; Cucinella, A.; Brando, C.; Gagliardo, C.; Santoni, M.; Fanale, D.; Inno, A.; Fazio, I.; et al. Challenges and advances for the treatment of renal cancer patients with brain metastases: From immunological background to upcoming clinical evidence on immune-checkpoint inhibitors. *Crit. Rev. Oncol. Hematol.* **2021**, *163*, 103390. [CrossRef]
8. Dridi, M.; Bouleftour, W.; Rivoirard, R.; Dal Col, P.; Langrand-Escure, J.; Vassal, C.; Guillot, A. Leptomeningeal Metastases in Renal Cell Carcinoma at Initial Diagnosis: 2 Case Reports and Literature Review. *Cancer Investig.* **2019**, *37*, 501–505. [CrossRef] [PubMed]
9. Hasanov, E.; Yeboa, D.N.; Tucker, M.D.; Swanson, T.A.; Beckham, T.H.; Rini, B.; Ene, C.I.; Hasanov, M.; Derks, S.; Smits, M.; et al. An interdisciplinary consensus on the management of brain metastases in patients with renal cell carcinoma. *CA Cancer J. Clin.* **2022**, *72*, 454–489. [CrossRef]
10. Roshkovan, L. Chapter 11—Radiologic assessment of tumor response to immunotherapy and its complications. In *NK Cells in Cancer Immunotherapy: Successes and Challenges*; Academic Press: Cambridge, MA, USA, 2023; pp. 239–261.
11. Van Timmeren, J.E.; Cester, D.; Tanadini-Lang, S.; Alkadhi, H.; Baessler, B. Radiomics in medical imaging-"how-to" guide and critical reflection. *Insights Imaging* **2020**, *11*, 91. [CrossRef]
12. Ferro, M.; Musi, G.; Marchioni, M.; Maggi, M.; Veccia, A.; Del Giudice, F.; Barone, B.; Crocetto, F.; Lasorsa, F.; Antonelli, A.; et al. Radiogenomics in Renal Cancer Management-Current Evidence and Future Prospects. *Int. J. Mol. Sci.* **2023**, *24*, 4615. [CrossRef]
13. Bharwani, N.; Miquel, M.E.; Powles, T.; Dilks, P.; Shawyer, A.; Sahdev, A.; Wilson, P.D.; Chowdhury, S.; Berney, D.M.; Rockall, A.G. Diffusion-weighted and multiphase contrast-enhanced MRI as surrogate markers of response to neoadjuvant sunitinib in metastatic renal cell carcinoma. *Br. J. Cancer* **2014**, *110*, 616–624. [CrossRef]
14. Antunes, J.; Viswanath, S.; Rusu, M.; Valls, L.; Hoimes, C.; Avril, N.; Madabhushi, A. Radiomics Analysis on FLT-PET/MRI for Characterization of Early Treatment Response in Renal Cell Carcinoma: A Proof-of-Concept Study. *Transl. Oncol.* **2016**, *9*, 155–162. [CrossRef]
15. Duclos, V.; Iep, A.; Gomez, L.; Goldfarb, L.; Besson, F.L. PET Molecular Imaging: A Holistic Review of Current Practice and Emerging Perspectives for Diagnosis, Therapeutic Evaluation and Prognosis in Clinical Oncology. *Int. J. Mol. Sci.* **2021**, *22*, 4159. [CrossRef]
16. Lo Gullo, R.; Daimiel, I.; Morris, E.A.; Pinker, K. Combining molecular and imaging metrics in cancer: Radiogenomics. *Insights Imaging* **2020**, *11*, 1. [CrossRef] [PubMed]
17. Gopal, N.; Yazdian Anari, P.; Turkbey, E.; Jones, E.C.; Malayeri, A.A. The Next Paradigm Shift in the Management of Clear Cell Renal Cancer: Radiogenomics-Definition, Current Advances, and Future Directions. *Cancers* **2022**, *14*, 793. [CrossRef]
18. Alessandrino, F.; Shinagare, A.B.; Bossé, D.; Choueiri, T.K.; Krajewski, K.M. Radiogenomics in renal cell carcinoma. *Abdom. Radiol.* **2019**, *44*, 1990–1998. [CrossRef] [PubMed]
19. Zhong, W.; Li, Y.; Yuan, Y.; Zhong, H.; Huang, C.; Huang, J.; Lin, Y.; Huang, J. Characterization of Molecular Heterogeneity Associated With Tumor Microenvironment in Clear Cell Renal Cell Carcinoma to Aid Immunotherapy. *Front. Cell Dev. Biol.* **2021**, *9*, 736540. [CrossRef]
20. Ljungberg, B.; Albiges, L.; Abu-Ghanem, Y.; Bensalah, K.; Dabestani, S.; Fernández-Pello, S.; Giles, R.H.; Hofmann, F.; Hora, M.; Kuczyk, M.A.; et al. European Association of Urology Guidelines on Renal Cell Carcinoma: The 2019 Update. *Eur. Urol.* **2019**, *75*, 799–810. [CrossRef] [PubMed]
21. Wang, Y.; Zhang, Y.; Wang, P.; Fu, X.; Lin, W. Circular RNAs in renal cell carcinoma: Implications for tumorigenesis, diagnosis, and therapy. *Mol. Cancer* **2020**, *19*, 149. [CrossRef]
22. Klatte, T.; Rossi, S.H.; Stewart, G.D. Prognostic factors and prognostic models for renal cell carcinoma: A literature review. *World J. Urol.* **2018**, *36*, 1943–1952. [CrossRef]
23. Achrol, A.S.; Rennert, R.C.; Anders, C.; Soffietti, R.; Ahluwalia, M.S.; Nayak, L.; Peters, S.; Arvold, N.D.; Harsh, G.R.; Steeg, P.S.; et al. Brain metastases. *Nat. Rev. Dis. Primers* **2019**, *5*, 5. [CrossRef] [PubMed]
24. Linehan, W.M.; Ricketts, C.J. The Cancer Genome Atlas of renal cell carcinoma: Findings and clinical implications. *Nat. Rev. Urol.* **2019**, *16*, 539–552. [CrossRef]
25. Gui, C.P.; Wei, J.H.; Chen, Y.H.; Fu, L.M.; Tang, Y.M.; Cao, J.Z.; Chen, W.; Luo, J.H. A new thinking: Extended application of genomic selection to screen multiomics data for development of novel hypoxia-immune biomarkers and target therapy of clear cell renal cell carcinoma. *Brief Bioinform.* **2021**, *22*, bbab173. [CrossRef] [PubMed]

26. Deleuze, A.; Saout, J.; Dugay, F.; Peyronnet, B.; Mathieu, R.; Verhoest, G.; Bensalah, K.; Crouzet, L.; Laguerre, B.; Belaud-Rotureau, M.A.; et al. Immunotherapy in Renal Cell Carcinoma: The Future Is Now. *Int. J. Mol. Sci.* 2020, *21*, 2532. [CrossRef] [PubMed]
27. Chang, S.; Yim, S.; Park, H. The cancer driver genes IDH1/2, JARID1C/ KDM5C, and UTX/ KDM6A: Crosstalk between histone demethylation and hypoxic reprogramming in cancer metabolism. *Exp. Mol. Med.* 2019, *51*, 1–17. [CrossRef] [PubMed]
28. Díaz-Montero, C.M.; Rini, B.I.; Finke, J.H. The immunology of renal cell carcinoma. *Nat. Rev. Nephrol.* 2020, *16*, 721–735. [CrossRef] [PubMed]
29. Choueiri, T.K.; Kaelin, W.G., Jr. Targeting the HIF2-VEGF axis in renal cell carcinoma. *Nat. Med.* 2020, *26*, 1519–1530. [CrossRef]
30. Bradley, A.J.; MacDonald, L.; Whiteside, S.; Johnson, R.J.; Ramani, V.A. Accuracy of preoperative CT T staging of renal cell carcinoma: Which features predict advanced stage? *Clin. Radiol.* 2015, *70*, 822–829. [CrossRef]
31. Perazella, M.A.; Dreicer, R.; Rosner, M.H. Renal cell carcinoma for the nephrologist. *Kidney Int.* 2018, *94*, 471–483. [CrossRef]
32. Petejova, N.; Martinek, A. Renal cell carcinoma: Review of etiology, pathophysiology and risk factors. *Biomed. Pap. Med. Fac. Univ. Palacky Olomouc Czech Repub.* 2016, *160*, 183–194. [CrossRef]
33. Jonasch, E.; Donskov, F.; Iliopoulos, O.; Rathmell, W.K.; Narayan, V.K.; Maughan, B.L.; Oudard, S.; Else, T.; Maranchie, J.K.; Welsh, S.J.; et al. Belzutifan for Renal Cell Carcinoma in von Hippel-Lindau Disease. *N. Engl. J. Med.* 2021, *385*, 2036–2046. [CrossRef] [PubMed]
34. Leveridge, M.J.; Bostrom, P.J.; Koulouris, G.; Finelli, A.; Lawrentschuk, N. Imaging renal cell carcinoma with ultrasonography, CT and MRI. *Nat. Rev. Urol.* 2010, *7*, 311–325. [CrossRef] [PubMed]
35. Gray, R.E.; Harris, G.T. Renal Cell Carcinoma: Diagnosis and Management. *Am. Fam. Physician* 2019, *99*, 179–184. [PubMed]
36. Vander Velde, R.; Yoon, N.; Marusyk, V.; Durmaz, A.; Dhawan, A.; Miroshnychenko, D.; Lozano-Peral, D.; Desai, B.; Balynska, O.; Poleszhuk, J.; et al. Resistance to targeted therapies as a multifactorial, gradual adaptation to inhibitor specific selective pressures. *Nat. Commun.* 2020, *11*, 2393. [CrossRef] [PubMed]
37. Daugherty, M.; Daugherty, E.; Jacob, J.; Shapiro, O.; Mollapour, M.; Bratslavsky, G. Renal cell carcinoma and brain metastasis: Questioning the dogma of role for cytoreductive nephrectomy. *Urol. Oncol.* 2019, *37*, 182.e9–182.e15. [CrossRef]
38. Vuong, L.; Kotecha, R.R.; Voss, M.H.; Hakimi, A.A. Tumor Microenvironment Dynamics in Clear-Cell Renal Cell Carcinoma. *Cancer Discov.* 2019, *9*, 1349–1357. [CrossRef]
39. Makhov, P.; Joshi, S.; Ghatalia, P.; Kutikov, A.; Uzzo, R.G.; Kolenko, V.M. Resistance to Systemic Therapies in Clear Cell Renal Cell Carcinoma: Mechanisms and Management Strategies. *Mol. Cancer Ther.* 2018, *17*, 1355–1364. [CrossRef]
40. Suarez-Sarmiento, A., Jr.; Nguyen, K.A.; Syed, J.S.; Nolte, A.; Ghabili, K.; Cheng, M.; Liu, S.; Chiang, V.; Kluger, H.; Hurwitz, M.; et al. Brain Metastasis From Renal-Cell Carcinoma: An Institutional Study. *Clin. Genitourin. Cancer* 2019, *17*, e1163–e1170. [CrossRef]
41. Proescholdt, M.A.; Schödel, P.; Doenitz, C.; Pukrop, T.; Höhne, J.; Schmidt, N.O.; Schebesch, K.M. The Management of Brain Metastases-Systematic Review of Neurosurgical Aspects. *Cancers* 2021, *13*, 1616. [CrossRef]
42. Znaor, A.; Lortet-Tieulent, J.; Laversanne, M.; Jemal, A.; Bray, F. International variations and trends in renal cell carcinoma incidence and mortality. *Eur. Urol.* 2015, *67*, 519–530. [CrossRef]
43. Sankey, E.W.; Tsvankin, V.; Grabowski, M.M.; Nayar, G.; Batich, K.A.; Risman, A.; Champion, C.D.; Salama, A.K.S.; Goodwin, C.R.; Fecci, P.E. Operative and peri-operative considerations in the management of brain metastasis. *Cancer Med.* 2019, *8*, 6809–6831. [CrossRef] [PubMed]
44. Yang, D.C.; Chen, C.H. Potential New Therapeutic Approaches for Renal Cell Carcinoma. *Semin. Nephrol.* 2020, *40*, 86–97. [CrossRef] [PubMed]
45. De Meerleer, G.; Khoo, V.; Escudier, B.; Joniau, S.; Bossi, A.; Ost, P.; Briganti, A.; Fonteyne, V.; Van Vulpen, M.; Lumen, N.; et al. Radiotherapy for renal-cell carcinoma. *Lancet Oncol.* 2014, *15*, e170–e177. [CrossRef] [PubMed]
46. Dengina, N.; Tsimafeyeu, I.; Mitin, T. Current Role of Radiotherapy for Renal-Cell Carcinoma: Review. *Clin. Genitourin. Cancer* 2017, *15*, 183–187. [CrossRef]
47. D'Amico, R.S.; Aghi, M.K.; Vogelbaum, M.A.; Bruce, J.N. Convection-enhanced drug delivery for glioblastoma: A review. *J. Neurooncol.* 2021, *151*, 415–427. [CrossRef]
48. Patel, B.; Kim, A.H. Laser Interstitial Thermal Therapy. *Mo Med.* 2020, *117*, 50–55.
49. Chitti, B.; Goyal, S.; Sherman, J.H.; Caputy, A.; Sarfaraz, M.; Cifter, G.; Aghdam, H.; Rao, Y.J. The role of brachytherapy in the management of brain metastases: A systematic review. *J. Contemp. Brachytherapy* 2020, *12*, 67–83.
50. Petrelli, F.; Coinu, A.; Vavassori, I.; Cabiddu, M.; Borgonovo, K.; Ghilardi, M.; Lonati, V.; Barni, S. Cytoreductive Nephrectomy in Metastatic Renal Cell Carcinoma Treated With Targeted Therapies: A Systematic Review With a Meta-Analysis. *Clin. Genitourin. Cancer* 2016, *14*, 465–472. [CrossRef]
51. Napolitano, L.; Manfredi, C.; Cirillo, L.; Fusco, G.M.; Passaro, F.; Abate, M.; La Rocca, R.; Mastrangelo, F.; Spirito, L.; Pandolfo, S.D.; et al. Cytoreductive Nephrectomy and Metastatic Renal Cell Carcinoma: State of the Art and Future Perspectives. *Medicina* 2023, *59*, 767. [CrossRef]
52. Barbastefano, J.; Garcia, J.A.; Elson, P.; Wood, L.S.; Lane, B.R.; Dreicer, R.; Campbell, S.C.; Rini, B.I. Association of percentage of tumour burden removed with debulking nephrectomy and progression-free survival in patients with metastatic renal cell carcinoma treated with vascular endothelial growth factor-targeted therapy. *BJU Int.* 2010, *106*, 1266–1269. [CrossRef]

53. Pindoria, N.; Raison, N.; Blecher, G.; Catterwell, R.; Dasgupta, P. Cytoreductive nephrectomy in the era of targeted therapies: A review. *BJU Int.* **2017**, *120*, 320–328. [CrossRef] [PubMed]
54. Turajlic, S.; Xu, H.; Litchfield, K.; Rowan, A.; Chambers, T.; Lopez, J.I.; Nicol, D.; O'Brien, T.; Larkin, J.; Horswell, S.; et al. Tracking Cancer Evolution Reveals Constrained Routes to Metastases: TRACERx Renal. *Cell* **2018**, *173*, 581–594.e12. [CrossRef] [PubMed]
55. Méjean, A.; Ravaud, A.; Thezenas, S.; Chevreau, C.; Bensalah, K.; Geoffrois, L.; Thiery-Vuillemin, A.; Cormier, L.; Lang, H.; Guy, L.; et al. Sunitinib Alone or After Nephrectomy for Patients with Metastatic Renal Cell Carcinoma: Is There Still a Role for Cytoreductive Nephrectomy? *Eur. Urol.* **2021**, *80*, 417–424. [CrossRef]
56. Bex, A.; Mulders, P.; Jewett, M.; Wagstaff, J.; van Thienen, J.V.; Blank, C.U.; van Velthoven, R.; Del Pilar Laguna, M.; Wood, L.; van Melick, H.H.E.; et al. Comparison of Immediate vs Deferred Cytoreductive Nephrectomy in Patients With Synchronous Metastatic Renal Cell Carcinoma Receiving Sunitinib: The SURTIME Randomized Clinical Trial. *JAMA Oncol.* **2019**, *5*, 164–170. [CrossRef]
57. Kokorovic, A.; Rendon, R.A. Cytoreductive nephrectomy in metastatic kidney cancer: What do we do now? *Curr. Opin. Support Palliat. Care* **2019**, *13*, 255–261. [CrossRef] [PubMed]
58. Mazzaschi, G.; Quaini, F.; Bersanelli, M.; Buti, S. Cytoreductive nephrectomy in the era of targeted- and immuno- therapy for metastatic renal cell carcinoma: An elusive issue? A systematic review of the literature. *Crit. Rev. Oncol. Hematol.* **2021**, *160*, 103293. [CrossRef]
59. Stellato, M.; Santini, D.; Verzoni, E.; De Giorgi, U.; Pantano, F.; Casadei, C.; Fornarini, G.; Maruzzo, M.; Sbrana, A.; Di Lorenzo, G.; et al. Impact of Previous Nephrectomy on Clinical Outcome of Metastatic Renal Carcinoma Treated With Immune-Oncology: A Real-World Study on Behalf of Meet-URO Group (MeetUro-7b). *Front. Oncol.* **2021**, *11*, 682449. [CrossRef]
60. Van Praet, C.; Slots, C.; Vasdev, N.; Rottey, S.; Fonteyne, V.; Andras, I.; Albersen, M.; De Meerleer, G.; Bex, A.; Decaestecker, K. Current role of cytoreductive nephrectomy in metastatic renal cell carcinoma. *Turk. J. Urol.* **2021**, *47* (Suppl. 1), S79–S84. [CrossRef]
61. Singla, N.; Ghandour, R.A.; Margulis, V. Is cytoreductive nephrectomy relevant in the immunotherapy era? *Curr. Opin. Urol.* **2019**, *29*, 526–530. [CrossRef]
62. Motzer, R.J.; Jonasch, E.; Agarwal, N.; Bhayani, S.; Bro, W.P.; Chang, S.S.; Choueiri, T.K.; Costello, B.A.; Derweesh, I.H.; Fishman, M.; et al. Kidney Cancer, Version 2.2017, NCCN Clinical Practice Guidelines in Oncology. *J. Natl. Compr. Canc. Netw.* **2017**, *15*, 804–834. [CrossRef]
63. Kotecha, R.R.; Flippot, R.; Nortman, T.; Guida, A.; Patil, S.; Escudier, B.; Motzer, R.J.; Albiges, L.; Voss, M.H. Prognosis of Incidental Brain Metastases in Patients With Advanced Renal Cell Carcinoma. *J. Natl. Compr. Canc. Netw.* **2021**, *19*, 432–438. [CrossRef] [PubMed]
64. Du, W.; Sirbu, C.; Lucas, B.D., Jr.; Jubelirer, S.J.; Khalid, A.; Mei, L. A Retrospective Study of Brain Metastases From Solid Malignancies: The Effect of Immune Checkpoint Inhibitors. *Front. Oncol.* **2021**, *11*, 667847. [CrossRef]
65. Lin, N.U.; Lee, E.Q.; Aoyama, H.; Barani, I.J.; Barboriak, D.P.; Baumert, B.G.; Bendszus, M.; Brown, P.D.; Camidge, D.R.; Chang, S.M.; et al. Response assessment criteria for brain metastases: Proposal from the RANO group. *Lancet Oncol.* **2015**, *16*, e270–e278. [CrossRef]
66. Rathmell, W.K.; Rumble, R.B.; Van Veldhuizen, P.J.; Al-Ahmadie, H.; Emamekhoo, H.; Hauke, R.J.; Louie, A.V.; Milowsky, M.I.; Molina, A.M.; Rose, T.L.; et al. Management of Metastatic Clear Cell Renal Cell Carcinoma: ASCO Guideline. *J. Clin. Oncol.* **2022**, *40*, 2957–2995. [CrossRef] [PubMed]
67. Matsui, Y. Current Multimodality Treatments Against Brain Metastases from Renal Cell Carcinoma. *Cancers* **2020**, *12*, 2875. [CrossRef] [PubMed]
68. Hasanov, E.; Jonasch, E. Management of Brain Metastases in Metastatic Renal Cell Carcinoma. *Hematol. Oncol. Clin. N. Am.* **2023**, in press. [CrossRef] [PubMed]
69. Lang, F.F.; Wildrick, D.M.; Sawaya, R. Management of Cerebral Metastases: The Role of Surgery. *Cancer Control* **1998**, *5*, 124–129. [CrossRef]
70. Hassaneen, W.; Suki, D.; Salaskar, A.L.; Wildrick, D.M.; Lang, F.F.; Fuller, G.N.; Sawaya, R. Surgical management of lateral-ventricle metastases: Report of 29 cases in a single-institution experience. *J. Neurosurg.* **2010**, *112*, 1046–1055. [CrossRef]
71. Suki, D.; Hatiboglu, M.A.; Patel, A.J.; Weinberg, J.S.; Groves, M.D.; Mahajan, A.; Sawaya, R. Comparative risk of leptomeningeal dissemination of cancer after surgery or stereotactic radiosurgery for a single supratentorial solid tumor metastasis. *Neurosurgery* **2009**, *64*, 664–674; discussion 674–676. [CrossRef]
72. Patchell, R.A.; Tibbs, P.A.; Walsh, J.W.; Dempsey, R.J.; Maruyama, Y.; Kryscio, R.J.; Markesbery, W.R.; Macdonald, J.S.; Young, B. A randomized trial of surgery in the treatment of single metastases to the brain. *N. Engl. J. Med.* **1990**, *322*, 494–500. [CrossRef]
73. Andrews, D.W.; Scott, C.B.; Sperduto, P.W.; Flanders, A.E.; Gaspar, L.E.; Schell, M.C.; Werner-Wasik, M.; Demas, W.; Ryu, J.; Bahary, J.P.; et al. Whole brain radiation therapy with or without stereotactic radiosurgery boost for patients with one to three brain metastases: Phase III results of the RTOG 9508 randomised trial. *Lancet* **2004**, *363*, 1665–1672. [CrossRef]
74. Minniti, G.; Scaringi, C.; Paolini, S.; Lanzetta, G.; Romano, A.; Cicone, F.; Osti, M.; Enrici, R.M.; Esposito, V. Single-Fraction Versus Multifraction ($3 \times 9$ Gy) Stereotactic Radiosurgery for Large (>2 cm) Brain Metastases: A Comparative Analysis of Local Control and Risk of Radiation-Induced Brain Necrosis. *Int. J. Radiat. Oncol. Biol. Phys.* **2016**, *95*, 1142–1148. [CrossRef] [PubMed]

75. Wardak, Z.; Christie, A.; Bowman, A.; Stojadinovic, S.; Nedzi, L.; Barnett, S.; Patel, T.; Mickey, B.; Whitworth, T.; Hannan, R.; et al. Stereotactic Radiosurgery for Multiple Brain Metastases From Renal-Cell Carcinoma. *Clin. Genitourin. Cancer* **2019**, *17*, e273–e280. [CrossRef] [PubMed]
76. Bastos, D.C.A.; Fuentes, D.T.; Traylor, J.; Weinberg, J.; Kumar, V.A.; Stafford, J.; Li, J.; Rao, G.; Prabhu, S.S. The use of laser interstitial thermal therapy in the treatment of brain metastases: A literature review. *Int. J. Hyperth.* **2020**, *37*, 53–60. [CrossRef] [PubMed]
77. Hong, C.S.; Deng, D.; Vera, A.; Chiang, V.L. Laser-interstitial thermal therapy compared to craniotomy for treatment of radiation necrosis or recurrent tumor in brain metastases failing radiosurgery. *J. Neurooncol.* **2019**, *142*, 309–317. [CrossRef]
78. Pollock, B.E.; Brown, P.D.; Foote, R.L.; Stafford, S.L.; Schomberg, P.J. Properly selected patients with multiple brain metastases may benefit from aggressive treatment of their intracranial disease. *J. Neurooncol.* **2003**, *61*, 73–80. [CrossRef]
79. Kayama, T.; Sato, S.; Sakurada, K.; Mizusawa, J.; Nishikawa, R.; Narita, Y.; Sumi, M.; Miyakita, Y.; Kumabe, T.; Sonoda, Y.; et al. Effects of Surgery With Salvage Stereotactic Radiosurgery Versus Surgery With Whole-Brain Radiation Therapy in Patients with One to Four Brain Metastases (JCOG0504): A Phase III, Noninferiority, Randomized Controlled Trial. *J. Clin. Oncol.* **2018**, *36*, Jco2018786186. [CrossRef]
80. Cohen, H.T.; McGovern, F.J. Renal-cell carcinoma. *N. Engl. J. Med.* **2005**, *353*, 2477–2490. [CrossRef]
81. Jiang, H.; Muir, R.K.; Gonciarz, R.L.; Olshen, A.B.; Yeh, I.; Hann, B.C.; Zhao, N.; Wang, Y.H.; Behr, S.C.; Korkola, J.E.; et al. Ferrous iron-activatable drug conjugate achieves potent MAPK blockade in KRAS-driven tumors. *J. Exp. Med.* **2022**, *219*, e20210739. [CrossRef]
82. Khan, A.; Singh, P.; Srivastava, A. Iron: Key player in cancer and cell cycle? *J. Trace Elem. Med. Biol.* **2020**, *62*, 126582. [CrossRef]
83. Torti, S.V.; Torti, F.M. Iron and Cancer: 2020 Vision. *Cancer Res.* **2020**, *80*, 5435–5448. [CrossRef] [PubMed]
84. Crisman, C.M.; Patel, A.R.; Winston, G.; Brennan, C.W.; Tabar, V.; Moss, N.S. Clinical Outcomes in Patients with Renal Cell Carcinoma Metastases to the Choroid Plexus. *World Neurosurg.* **2020**, *140*, e7–e13. [CrossRef] [PubMed]
85. Ali, M.; Mooi, J.; Lawrentschuk, N.; McKay, R.R.; Hannan, R.; Lo, S.S.; Hall, W.A.; Siva, S. The Role of Stereotactic Ablative Body Radiotherapy in Renal Cell Carcinoma. *Eur. Urol.* **2022**, *82*, 613–622. [CrossRef]
86. All, S.; Garant, A.; Hannan, R. Stereotactic Ablative Radiation (SAbR) for Oligometastatic RCC. *Semin. Radiat. Oncol.* **2021**, *31*, 227–234. [CrossRef] [PubMed]
87. Kothari, G.; Foroudi, F.; Gill, S.; Corcoran, N.M.; Siva, S. Outcomes of stereotactic radiotherapy for cranial and extracranial metastatic renal cell carcinoma: A systematic review. *Acta Oncol.* **2015**, *54*, 148–157. [CrossRef]
88. Heng, D.Y.; Xie, W.; Regan, M.M.; Warren, M.A.; Golshayan, A.R.; Sahi, C.; Eigl, B.J.; Ruether, J.D.; Cheng, T.; North, S.; et al. Prognostic factors for overall survival in patients with metastatic renal cell carcinoma treated with vascular endothelial growth factor-targeted agents: Results from a large, multicenter study. *J. Clin. Oncol.* **2009**, *27*, 5794–5799. [CrossRef]
89. Heng, D.Y.; Xie, W.; Regan, M.M.; Harshman, L.C.; Bjarnason, G.A.; Vaishampayan, U.N.; Mackenzie, M.; Wood, L.; Donskov, F.; Tan, M.H.; et al. External validation and comparison with other models of the International Metastatic Renal-Cell Carcinoma Database Consortium prognostic model: A population-based study. *Lancet Oncol.* **2013**, *14*, 141–148. [CrossRef]
90. Hoff, C.M. Importance of hemoglobin concentration and its modification for the outcome of head and neck cancer patients treated with radiotherapy. *Acta Oncol.* **2012**, *51*, 419–432. [CrossRef] [PubMed]
91. Littlewood, T.J. The impact of hemoglobin levels on treatment outcomes in patients with cancer. *Semin. Oncol.* **2001**, *28* (Suppl. 8), 49–53. [CrossRef]
92. Edgren, G.; Bagnardi, V.; Bellocco, R.; Hjalgrim, H.; Rostgaard, K.; Melbye, M.; Reilly, M.; Adami, H.O.; Hall, P.; Nyrén, O. Pattern of declining hemoglobin concentration before cancer diagnosis. *Int. J. Cancer* **2010**, *127*, 1429–1436. [CrossRef]
93. Clarke, H.; Pallister, C.J. The impact of anaemia on outcome in cancer. *Clin. Lab. Haematol.* **2005**, *27*, 1–13. [CrossRef] [PubMed]
94. Webster, B.R.; Gopal, N.; Ball, M.W. Tumorigenesis Mechanisms Found in Hereditary Renal Cell Carcinoma: A Review. *Genes* **2022**, *13*, 2122. [CrossRef] [PubMed]
95. Yap, N.Y.; Rajandram, R.; Ng, K.L.; Pailoor, J.; Fadzli, A.; Gobe, G.C. Genetic and Chromosomal Aberrations and Their Clinical Significance in Renal Neoplasms. *Biomed. Res. Int.* **2015**, *2015*, 476508. [CrossRef] [PubMed]

**Disclaimer/Publisher's Note:** The statements, opinions and data contained in all publications are solely those of the individual author(s) and contributor(s) and not of MDPI and/or the editor(s). MDPI and/or the editor(s) disclaim responsibility for any injury to people or property resulting from any ideas, methods, instructions or products referred to in the content.

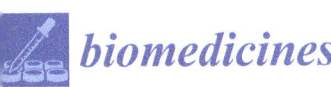 

*Article*

# Catfish Egg Lectin Enhances the Cytotoxicity of Sunitinib on Gb3-Expressing Renal Cancer Cells

Jun Ito [1,*], Shigeki Sugawara [2], Takeo Tatsuta [2], Masahiro Hosono [2] and Makoto Sato [1]

1 Department of Urology, Faculty of Medicine, Tohoku Medical and Pharmaceutical University, 1-15-1 Fukumuro, Miyagino-ku, Sendai 983-8536, Japan; ms.hifu@tohoku-mpu.ac.jp
2 Division of Cell Recognition Study, Institute of Molecular Biomembrane and Glycobiology, Tohoku Medical and Pharmaceutical University, 4-4-1 Komatsushima, Aoba-ku, Sendai 981-8558, Japan; ssuga@tohoku-mpu.ac.jp (S.S.); t-takeo@tohoku-mpu.ac.jp (T.T.); mhosono@tohoku-mpu.ac.jp (M.H.)
* Correspondence: itojun@tohoku-mpu.ac.jp; Tel.: +81-22-290-8898; Fax: +81-22-290-8860

**Abstract:** Metastatic renal cell carcinoma (RCC) is not sufficiently responsive to anticancer drugs, and thus, developing new drugs for advanced RCC remains vital. We previously reported that the treatment of globotriaosylceramide (Gb3)-expressing cells with catfish (*Silurus asotus*) egg lectin (SAL) increased the intracellular uptake of propidium iodide (PI) and sunitinib (SU). Herein, we investigated whether SAL pretreatment affects the intracellular uptake and cytotoxic effects of molecular-targeted drugs in RCC cells. We analyzed Gb3 expression in TOS1, TOS3, TOS3LN, and ACHN human RCC cells. Surface Gb3 expression was higher in TOS1 and TOS3 cells than in TOS3LN and ACHN cells. In the PI uptake assay, 41.5% of TOS1 cells and 21.1% of TOS3 cells treated with SAL were positive for PI. TOS1 cell viability decreased to 70% after treatment with 25 μM SU alone and to 48% after pretreatment with SAL (50 μg/mL). Time-series measurements of the intracellular fluorescence of SU revealed significantly enhanced SU uptake in SAL-treated TOS1 cells compared to control cells. SAL treatment did not increase PI uptake in normal renal cells. Our findings suggest that adequate cytotoxic activity may be achieved even when SU is administered at a sufficiently low dose not to cause side effects in combination with SAL.

**Keywords:** globotriaosylceramide; rhamnose-binding lectin; sunitinib; renal cell carcinoma

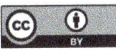

## 1. Introduction

The number of renal masses accidentally detected by ultrasound or computed tomography has increased due to the increased use of diagnostic imaging tools in patients complaining of nonspecific abdominal or back pain. Approximately 80% of renal masses are considered to be renal cell carcinoma (RCC) [1]. While early detection of renal masses has improved the overall treatment outcome of RCC, RCC is not sufficiently responsive to anticancer drugs or radiation therapy once it becomes metastatic. Therefore, new drugs for the treatment of advanced RCC are required.

Several therapeutic drugs for treating advanced RCC have been developed to meet this demand in recent years. Molecular targeting drugs exert antitumor effects by inhibiting intracellular signaling involved in the growth of tumor cells and vascular endothelial cells and therefore are a promising option. Tyrosine kinase inhibitors (TKIs) targeting the vascular endothelial growth factor (VEGF), which acts on the vascular endothelium, inhibitors of the mammalian target of rapamycin, which is involved in tumor growth, and recently, multi-tyrosine kinase inhibitors of AXL receptor tyrosine kinase (AXL) and MET receptor tyrosine kinase (MET), which are activated by the inhibition of the VEGF, have been approved and are currently being used for the treatment of unresectable/metastatic RCC [2,3]. Despite the advent of immune checkpoint agents and other drugs with novel mechanisms of action, TKIs continue to play an important role in the treatment of renal cancer [4]. However, these molecular targeting drugs can induce multiple dose-related side effects, sometimes leading to treatment discontinuation. Therefore, new therapeutic strategies are required.

Lectins, which are proteins that can bind to glycosphingolipids (GSLs), have recently received increased research interest for their role as information devices in living organisms [5]. *Silurus asotus* egg lectin (SAL) isolated from catfish eggs has been found to bind to globotriaosylceramide (Gb3) expressed on the surfaces of cells [6]. We have previously studied the effects of SAL in Gb3-expressing tumor cells [7,8]. In a study on Gb3-expressing Raji Burkitt's lymphoma cells, we found that the binding of SAL to Gb3 increased the intracellular uptake of propidium iodide (PI). Moreover, SAL induced cell permeability and enhanced the cytotoxicity of doxorubicin [7]. However, the molecular mechanism of PI and doxorubicin uptake has not been elucidated. Furthermore, our previous study showed that the binding of SAL to Gb3 expressed on the surfaces of HeLa cells promoted the cellular uptake of the tyrosine kinase inhibitor sunitinib (SU), which is used to treat RCC, and delayed its excretion, which was associated with a significant decrease in cell survival [8]. These findings suggest that SAL may enhance the uptake of therapeutic agents into Gb3-expressing tumor cells and reduce their optimal dose.

In this study, we evaluated whether the combined use of SU and SAL would reduce the viability of RCC cells. In addition, we investigated whether the increased uptake and delayed excretion of therapeutic agents in tumor cells, as observed in our previous study, would also occur in RCC cells. This study aimed to provide a new therapeutic approach to RCC treatment.

## 2. Materials and Methods

### 2.1. Lectin and Cell Lines

SAL was purified using a method described previously [6]. The TOS1, TOS3, TOS3LN, and ACHN human renal cell cancer cell lines were a gift from Dr. Makoto Sato (Department of Urology, Tohoku University, School of Medicine, Sendai, Japan). Human renal proximal tubular epithelial cells (HRPTEC) were purchased from KURABO Industries (Osaka, Japan). The renal cancer cells were cultured in Dulbecco's Modified Eagle Medium (DMEM) (Wako, Osaka, Japan) supplemented with 10% ($v/v$) fetal bovine serum (FBS) and antibiotic-antimycotic solution (penicillin (100 IU/mL), streptomycin (100 µg/mL), and amphotericin B (0.25 µg/mL); Life Technologies, Carlsbad, CA, USA) at 37 °C in a 95% air/5% $CO_2$ atmosphere. HRPTEC were cultured in a RenaLife Comp kit (KURABO Industries) supplemented with RenaLife Life Factors (KURABO Industries) at 37 °C in a 95% air/5% $CO_2$ atmosphere.

### 2.2. Flow-Cytometric Analysis of Cellular Propidium Iodide (PI) Uptake to Measure Cell Permeability

Cells ($2 \times 10^5$) were treated or not with 100 µL of SAL (50 µg/mL Dulbecco's phosphate-buffered saline (D-PBS)) at 4 °C for 30 min and washed thrice with D-PBS. PI uptake was quantified using a MEBCYTO apoptosis kit (MBL, Nagoya, Japan) and a FACSCalibur flow cytometer (BD Biosciences, Franklin Lakes, NJ, USA).

### 2.3. Cell Viability Assay

Cytotoxic activity was determined with a trypan blue (0.5% $w/v$) exclusion assay. Cell viability was determined using the cell counting kit-8 (CCK-8) assay (Dojindo Laboratories, Kumamoto, Japan). Cells were seeded into a 96-well flat-bottom plate at $5 \times 10^3$ cells/well (90 µL) and treated with SAL (final concentration, 50 µg/mL) for 24 h. Then, CCK-8 solution (10 µL) was added to each well, and the cells were incubated at 37 °C for 4 h. The absorbance at 450 nm was measured using a Tecan Infinite F200 PRO microplate reader (Tecan Austria GmbH, Männedorf, Austria).

## 2.4. Flow-Cytometric Analysis of Cell Surface Gb3 Expression

Cells ($2 \times 10^5$) were treated or not with an anti-Gb3 monoclonal antibody (mAb) (BGR23, mouse IgG2b; Tokyo Kasei, Tokyo, Japan) diluted at a 1:500 ratio in D-PBS (100 µL) at 4 °C for 30 min and washed thrice with D-PBS. Then, they were incubated with Alexa Fluor (AF) 488-conjugated goat anti-mouse IgG (H + L) (Molecular Probes, Invitrogen AG, Basel, Switzerland) diluted at a 1:2500 ratio in D-PBS (100 µL) at 4 °C for 30 min. Gb3 expression on the cell surface was quantified using a BD FACSCalibur™ Flow Cytometer (BD Biosciences).

## 2.5. Thin-Layer Chromatography (TLC) for Glycolipid Expression Analysis

Cells ($1 \times 10^6$) were suspended in a chloroform-methanol solution (2:1, $v/v$), incubated at 37 °C for 1 h, and then centrifuged at $1000 \times g$ for 10 min. The supernatant was recovered in a glass tube. The pellet was resuspended in a chloroform-methanol-water solution (1:2:0.8, $v/v/v$), incubated at 37 °C for 2 h, and centrifuged at $1000 \times g$ for 10 min. The supernatant was collected and evaporated to dryness under nitrogen gas. The residue was dissolved in 20 µL of chloroform-methanol (2:1, $v/v$), placed on a high-performance TLC plate (Merck KGaA, Darmstadt, Germany), and developed using a solvent system of chloroform-methanol-water (60:35:8, $v/v/v$). Gb3 was visualized by spraying 0.5% orcinol in 10% sulfuric acid. Neutral glycosphingolipids, including cerebrosides, lactosylceramide (LacCer), Gb3, and Gb4, were purchased from Matreya (State College, PA, USA).

## 2.6. Analysis of the Effect of a Combination of SU and SAL

To assess the effect of SU, cells ($5 \times 10^3$) were treated with SU (0, 6.25, 12.5, 25, and 50 µM) at 37 °C for 24, 48, and 72 h. To determine the effect of a combination of SU and SAL, cells were first incubated with SAL (50 µg/mL) in DMEM supplemented with FBS for 24 h and then with SU (0 and 25 µM) at 37 °C for another 24 h. Cell viability was determined using the CCK-8 assay as described above. Annexin V-positive cells were detected using the MEBCYTO apoptosis kit (MBL) as mentioned above. Bright-field images were acquired using an inverted microscope (model IX71; Olympus Corporation, Osaka, Japan) with a 10× or 100× objective lens.

## 2.7. Analysis of the Effect of a Combination of Other Molecular-Targeted Agents and SAL

To assess the effect of other molecular-targeted agents, cells ($5 \times 10^3$) were treated with pazopanib (0, 3.125, 6.25, 12.5, and 25 µM), axitinib (0, 3.125, 6.25, 12.5, and 25 µM), or everolimus (0, 5, 10, 20, 40, and 80 µM) at 37 °C for 24 or 48 h. To determine the effect of a combination of these agents and SAL, cells were first incubated with SAL (50 µg/mL) in DMEM supplemented with FBS for 24 h and then with pazopanib (0 and 25 µM), axitinib (0 and 25 µM), or everolimus (0, 35, and 40 µM) at 37 °C for another 24 or 48 h. Cell viability was determined using the CCK-8 assay as described above.

## 2.8. Efflux of SU from SAL-Treated TOS1 Cells

Cells ($5 \times 10^5$) were incubated in DMEM with (50 µg/mL) or without SAL at 37 °C in a 95% air/5% $CO_2$ atmosphere for 24 h and then treated with SU (25 µM) for another 30 min. After SU was removed from the wells, the cells were observed at 3 or 6 h intervals for 24 h. SU efflux was visualized using an Olympus FV1000 confocal scanning microscope (Olympus).

## 2.9. Time-Series Measurements of Intracellular SU Contents

Cells were seeded in a CellCarrier™ 96-well microplate (PerkinElmer Cellular Technologies Germany GmbH, Hamburg, Germany) at a density of $1 \times 10^4$ cells/well and cultured in DMEM with (50 µg/mL) or without SAL at 37 °C in a 95% air/5% $CO_2$ atmosphere. The cells were stained with Hoechst 33342 (Dojindo Laboratories), and the plate was scanned using an Operetta CLS High Content Analysis System (PerkinElmer) with a 40× objective lens in the confocal mode in a pre-warmed live cell chamber set at

37 °C in a 95% air/5% $CO_2$ atmosphere. Fluorescence images were captured using the Hoechst 33342 channel at 488 nm before and at 3 or 30 min intervals after adding SU (final concentration, 25 µM) for a total period of 1.5 h. Fluorescence signals were quantified using the Harmony 4.9 software (PerkinElmer).

*2.10. Reverse Transcription-Quantitative Real-Time Polymerase Chain Reaction (RT-qPCR)*

TOS1 and HeLa cells ($5 \times 10^5$) were cultured in Roswell Park Memorial Institute (RPMI)-1640 (Nissui Pharmaceutical Co., Tokyo, Japan) and DMEM (Wako), respectively, at 37 °C in a 95% air/5% $CO_2$ atmosphere for 24 h. Total RNA was extracted from the cells using a Direct-zol RNA MiniPrep Kit (Zymo Research, Irvine, CA, USA). cDNA was synthesized from the total RNA (1 µg) using a SuperScript VILO cDNA Synthesis Kit (Invitrogen, San Diego, CA, USA). qPCRs were run in a LightCycler 480 system using the LightCycler 480 Probes Master kit (Roche Diagnostics, Indianapolis, IN, USA). PCR primers for amplification of *VEGFR2* (forward: 5′-GAACATTTGGGAAATCTCTTGC-3′, reverse: 5′-CGGAAGAACAATGTAGTCTTTGC-3′), *PDGFRB* (forward: 5′-CATCTGCAAAACC ACCATTG-3′, reverse: 5′-GAGACGTTGATGGATGACACC-3′), *KIT* (forward: 5′-TCAGC AAATGTCACAACAACC-3′, reverse: 5′-TCTCCATCGTTTACAAATACTGTAGTG-3′), *FLT3* (forward: 5′-TGGAATTTCTGGAATTTAAGTCG-3′, reverse: 5′-TTTCCCGTGGGTGA CAAG-3′), *ABCG2* (forward: 5′-TGGCTTAGACTCAAGCACAGC-3′, reverse: 5′-TCGTCCC TGCTTAGACATCC-3′), and *GAPDH* (forward: 5′-AGCCACATCGCTCAGACAC-3′, reverse: 5′-GCCCAATACGACCAAATCC-3′) were designed using the Universal Probe Library Assay Design Center [https://www.roche-applied-science.com/sis/rtpcr/upl/acenter.jsp (accessed on 14 February 2019)]. Amplification products were separated on a 2.0% agarose gel. Bands were visualized by ethidium bromide staining.

*2.11. Statistical Analysis*

Experimental results are presented as mean ± standard error (SE). Means were compared using the two-tailed Student's *t*-test, and *p*-values < 0.05 were considered statistically significant.

## 3. Results

*3.1. Expression of Gb3 on RCC Cell Lines*

There are various types of RCC cell lines [9,10] (Table 1). Our previous studies showed that the binding of SAL to Gb3 enhances the inhibition of cell proliferation and the effects of anticancer drugs [8,9].

**Table 1.** Selected RCC cell lines currently in use.

| Cell Line | Disease | Species | Source Organ | | Sex | Established in |
|---|---|---|---|---|---|---|
| TOS1 * | Clear cell RCC | Human | Soft tissue | Metastasis | Male | 1999 |
| TOS2 * | Clear cell RCC | Human | Soft tissue | Metastasis | Male | 1999 |
| TOS3 * | Clear cell RCC | Human | Kidney | Primary | Male | 1999 |
| TOS3LN * | Clear cell RCC | Human | Lymph node | Metastasis | Male | 1999 |
| ACHN [†] | Papillary RCC | Human | Pleural effusion | Metastasis | Male | 1979 |
| caki-1 [†] | Clear cell RCC | Human | Skin | Metastasis | Male | 1971 |
| caki-2 [†] | Clear cell RCC | Human | Kidney | Primary | Male | 1971 |
| 786-O [†] | Clear cell RCC | Human | Kidney | Primary | Male | 1976 |
| 769-P [†] | Clear cell RCC | Human | Kidney | Primary | Female | 1976 |

More than 20 cell lines are widely used and stored in cell banks. Additionally, dozens of other cell lines have been established and used for research in selected laboratories. * Used in selected laboratories. [†] Available in cell banks.

Using flow cytometry and TLC, we first examined whether Gb3 is expressed on four RCC cell lines. As shown in Figure 1A,B, the surface expression of Gb3 was higher in TOS1 and TOS3 cells than in TOS3LN and ACHN cells. We previously reported that the effect of SAL depends on the expression level of Gb3 [6,8]. Therefore, we used TOS1 and TOS3 cells in subsequent experiments. Additionally, we confirmed the expression of VEGFR-2, FMS-like tyrosine kinase (FLT)-3, platelet-derived growth factor receptor (PDGFR)b, and the tyrosine-protein kinase kit (c-kit) gene on TOS1 cells (see Supplemental Figure S1).

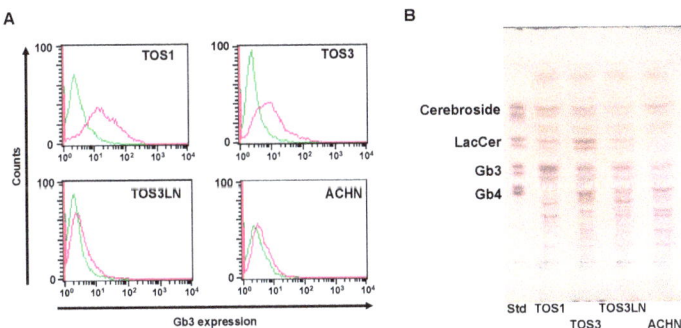

**Figure 1.** Comparison of Gb3 expression on RCC cell lines. (**A**) Flow-cytometric analysis of Gb3 expression on TOS1, TOS3, TOS3LN, and ACHN cells. Cells ($2 \times 10^5$) were treated with an anti-Gb3 mAb and an AF488-tagged goat anti-mouse mAb (red line). The level of Gb3 expression on TOS1, TOS3, TOS3LN, and ACHN cell surfaces was determined by flow cytometry. Control cells were treated with anti-Gb3 mAb alone. Fluorescence intensity of control cells: green line. (**B**) Total glycosphingolipids isolated from TOS1, TOS3, TOS3LN, and ACHN cells were separated by TLC using a solvent system as described in the Methods and were visualized by spraying orcinol-$H_2SO_4$ reagent. In the standard lane (Std), an aliquot of a standard mixture containing cerebrosides, LacCer, Gb3, and Gb4 was used.

### 3.2. PI Uptake by and Viability of SAL-Treated TOS1 and TOS3 Cells

In a previous study, SAL treatment of Raji cells (Burkitt's lymphoma cell line) expressing high levels of Gb3 at 37 °C increased the percentage of PI-positive cells with increasing treatment time, and the rate after 24 h of treatment was approximately the same as that after 30 min of treatment at 4 °C [7]. We previously reported that SAL does not reduce Raji cell viability even at concentrations of 100 µg/mL [7], and in HeLa cells, their morphology does not change until SAL concentrations of 200 µg/mL [8]. In the combined SAL and SU experiments with HeLa cells, the SAL concentration was 50 µg/mL. In this study, TOS1 and TOS3 treatments were performed using the same 50 µg/mL concentration of SAL. Additionally, RCC cell lines were treated with SAL at 4 °C for 30 min as a rapid method to determine the effect of SAL. To investigate the effect of SAL on PI uptake into RCC cells, we treated TOS1 and TOS3 cells with SAL (50 µg/mL) at 4 °C for 30 min, and then PI was added, and its uptake was observed by flow cytometry. The results showed that 41.5% of TOS1 cells and 21.1% of TOS3 cells treated with SAL were positive for PI (Figure 2A). SAL did not affect cell viability, even in the presence of PI, which normally induces apoptosis (Figure 2B). Based on these results, we decided to use TOS1, which showed a high expression of Gb3 and a high effect of SAL, in subsequent experiments.

### 3.3. Combined Effects of SAL and SU in TOS1 Cells

To confirm the cytotoxicity of SU on RCC cells, we treated TOS1 cells with SU alone and measured cell viability. The results showed that the viability of TOS1 cells decreased in a concentration- and time-dependent manner after SU treatment. At 48 h after treatment, the viability of TOS1 cells treated with 12.5 µM SU was similar to that of non-treated control cells; however, 25 µM SU moderately decreased cell viability to 70% (Figure 3A). Based on this result, we used 25 µM SU and 48 h treatment in subsequent combination treatment assays. In our previous study, SAL enhanced the cytotoxic effects of drugs [8,9]. Therefore, in this study, we observed whether the cytotoxic effect of SU on TOS1 cells was enhanced when combined with SAL pretreatment. The viability of TOS1 cells decreased to 70%

after treatment with 25 µM SU alone and further decreased to 48% upon pretreatment with SAL (50 µg/mL) (Figure 3B). In addition, the number of annexin V-positive cells was significantly increased ($p < 0.05$) in cells pretreated with SAL as compared to cells treated with SU alone (Figure 3C). Additionally, microscopic images revealed cell atrophy, suggesting decreased viability (Figure 3D).

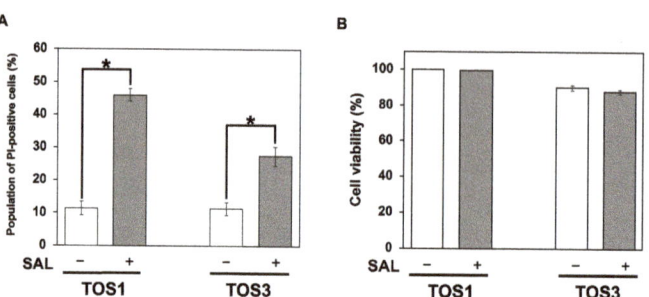

**Figure 2.** SAL enhances PI uptake but has no cytotoxic effect on TOS1 and TOS3 cells. (**A**) Cells ($1 \times 10^5$) were treated (+) or not (−) with SAL (50 µg/mL) at 37 °C for 24 h. The percentage of PI-positive cells was determined by flow cytometry. (**B**) Cells ($5 \times 10^3$) were treated (+) or not (−) with SAL (50 µg/mL) at 37 °C for 24 h. Cell viability was assessed using the trypan blue dye exclusion assay. Values represent mean values ± SEs of three independent experiments performed in triplicate. * $p < 0.05$ versus non-treated control cells.

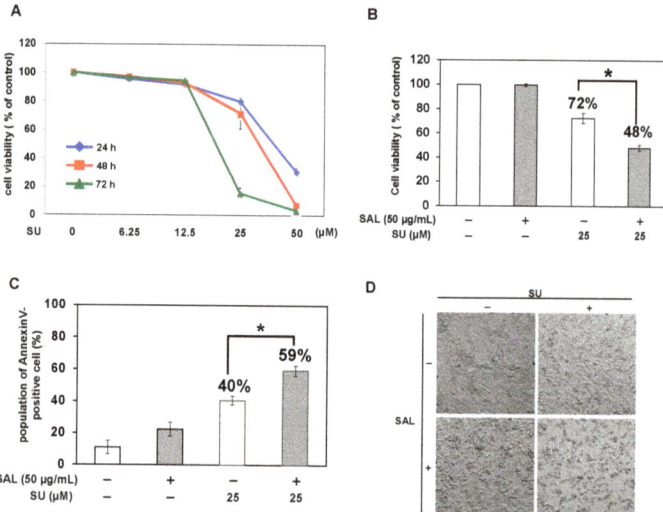

**Figure 3.** SAL enhances the antitumor effect of SU on TOS1 cells. (**A**) Cells ($5 \times 10^3$) were treated with SU (0, 6.25, 12.5, 25, and 50 µM) at 37 °C for 24, 48, and 72 h. (**B**) Cells ($5 \times 10^3$) were pretreated with SAL (0 and 50 µg/mL) at 37 °C for 24 h and then treated with SU (0 and 25 µM) at 37 °C for 48 h. Cell viability was measured using the WST-8 assay. Values represent mean values ± SEs of three independent experiments performed in triplicate. * $p < 0.05$ versus non-treated control cells. (**C**) Cells ($5 \times 10^3$) were pretreated with SAL (0 and 50 µg/mL) at 37 °C for 24 h and then treated with SU (0 and 25 µM) at 37 °C for 48 h. The percentage of annexin V-positive cells was determined by flow cytometry using a FACSCalibur™ Flow Cytometer. (**D**) Cells ($5 \times 10^3$) were pretreated (+) or not (−) with SAL (50 µg/mL) at 37 °C for 24 h and then treated with SU (0 and 25 µM) at 37 °C for 48 h. Bright-field microscopy images at a magnification of 10× are shown. Scale bar, 100 µm.

## 3.4. Effects of SAL on Intracellular Uptake and Extracellular Excretion of SU

We investigated whether the decreased viability of TOS1 cells treated with a combination of SAL and SU was due to increased SU uptake by SAL treatment. As shown in Figure 4A, based on the time-series measurements of the intracellular fluorescence of SU, the uptake of 25 µM SU was significantly enhanced in SAL-treated TOS1 cells compared to non-SAL-treated control cells. We previously reported that the extracellular excretion of SU was delayed in SAL-treated HeLa cells [9]. However, such a delay was not observed in SAL-treated TOS1 cells, and no difference with the control cells was detected (Figure 4B).

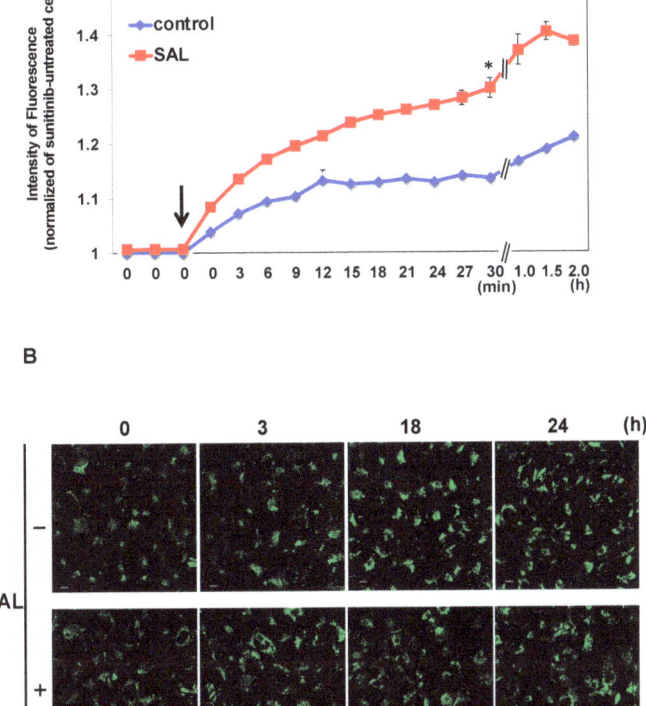

**Figure 4.** SAL promotes SU influx in TOS1 cells. (**A**) Time-course measurements of the autofluorescence of SU in cells using the Operetta CLS High Content Analysis System. TOS1 cells were treated (red squares) or not (blue rhombuses) with SAL (50 µg/mL) at 37 °C for 24 h. Subsequently, they were treated with SU (25 µM). SU influx was analyzed every 3 or 30 min after SU addition to the medium at time point 0. The arrow indicates the time immediately after SU addition. Values represent means ± SEs of three independent experiments performed in triplicate. * $p < 0.05$ versus non-treated control cells. (**B**) Cells (3 × 10$^4$) were pretreated or not with SAL (50 µg/mL) at 37 °C for 24 h. Subsequently, the cells were treated with SU (12.5 µM) at 37 °C for 30 min. After SU was removed from the medium, the residual quantity in the cells was observed using confocal laser scanning microscopy at the indicated time points. A pseudo-cyan color represents SU. Photographs were captured using a 60× objective lens. Scale bar, 10 µm.

## 3.5. Expression of ATP-Binding Cassette (ABC) Subfamily G (ABCG2) on TOS1 Cells

According to the results shown in Figure 4B, SU remained in the intracellular space of SAL-treated and non-treated TOS1 cells. SU is excreted by ABCG2 [11]. Therefore, we investigated whether ABCG2 is expressed on TOS1 cells. HeLa cells, which express ABCG2, were included as a positive control. RT-qPCR analysis confirmed the expression of *ABCG2* in HeLa cells; however, TOS1 cells did not express *ABCG2* (Figure 5).

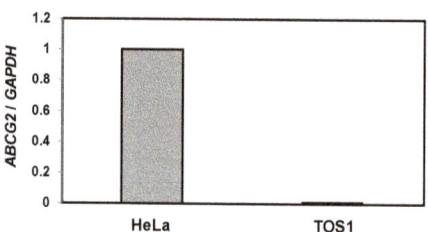

**Figure 5.** Expression of *ABCG2* in HeLa and TOS1 cells. Total RNA extracted from HeLa and TOS1 cells ($5 \times 10^4$) was analyzed by RT-qPCR using specific primers for *ABCG2* and *GAPDH* (control). Target gene expression was normalized to *GAPDH* expression, and the results are expressed as an n-fold increase over the control. Values represent means ± SEs of three independent triplicate experiments.

## 3.6. Effect of SAL on Normal Human Renal Cells

SAL enhanced the effect of SU on cancer cells; however, its effect on normal cells remained unknown. Therefore, we investigated the effect of SAL on HRPTEC. As shown in Figure 6A,B, although HRPTEC expressed Gb3, their expression level was lower than that of TOS1 cells. PI uptake assay results showed that SAL treatment did not increase PI uptake in HRPTEC (Figure 6C).

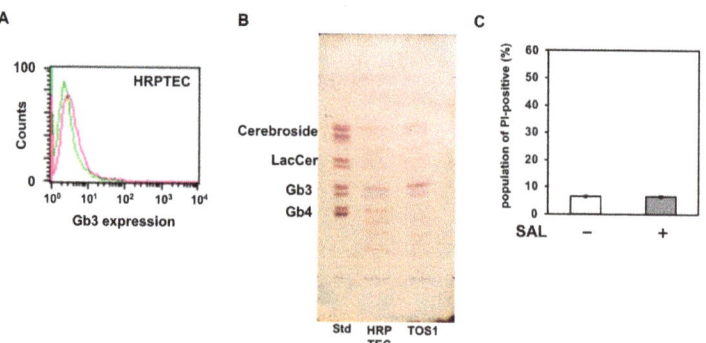

**Figure 6.** SAL does not affect normal human renal epithelial cells. (**A**) Flow-cytometric analysis of Gb3 on HRPTEC. Cells ($2 \times 10^5$) were treated with an anti-Gb3 mAb and an AF488-tagged goat anti-mouse mAb (red line). The level of Gb3 expression on surfaces of HRPTEC was determined by flow cytometry using a FACSCalibur™ Flow Cytometer. Fluorescence intensity of control cells: green line. (**B**) Total glycosphingolipids isolated from HRPTEC were separated by TLC using a solvent system as described in the Methods and visualized by spraying the orcinol-$H_2SO_4$ reagent. In the standard lane (Std), an aliquot of a standard mixture containing cerebrosides, lactosylceramide, Gb3, and Gb4 was used. (**C**) HRPTEC ($1 \times 10^5$) were treated (+) or not (−) with SAL (50 µg/mL) at 37 °C for 24 h. The population of PI-positive cells was determined by flow cytometry.

## 4. Discussion

In this study, we found that SAL recognizes and binds Gb3 on the surfaces of RCC cells, facilitating PI uptake. Although PI uptake is typically observed during the necrotic or late apoptotic phase of cell death [12], SAL enhanced PI uptake without inducing cell death. A similar observation was made in our previous studies using Raji and HeLa cells [8,9]. Moreover, the binding of SAL to Gb3 accelerated the uptake of the anti-RCC drug SU and consequently enhanced its cytotoxic activity. Based on this feature of increased cell surface permeability without the induction of apoptosis, we previously suggested that the combined use of doxorubicin and SAL in Raji cells and SU and SAL in HeLa cells increased intracellular drug concentrations and enhanced cytotoxic activity [7,8]. In the present study, we did not observe a delay in SU efflux, which can be explained by the fact that we did not observe ABCG2 expression in TOS1 cells. However, we found that SAL increased the intracellular SU concentration in TOS1 cells and decreased their viability. Importantly, SAL did not increase PI uptake in normal human renal cells. Herein, normal human renal cells were treated with SAL at a concentration of 50 µg/mL. We postulate that increasing the concentration of SAL did not enhance the effect of SAL on normal human renal cells because the amount of Gb3 in normal renal cells is lower than that in the RCC cell line. These results suggest that SAL can be used as a combination drug to enhance the efficacy of anti-RCC drugs. It is known that the therapeutic efficacy of two cancer drugs combined is higher than that of a single drug. Treatment of gastric cancer cells with the B subunit of Shiga toxin, which binds to Gb3 on the surfaces of gastric cancer cells, combined with SN38, the active metabolite of the topoisomerase inhibitor irinotecan, resulted in more than 100-fold greater cytotoxicity than treatment with irinotecan alone [13]. A combination of drugs that efficiently acts on the target cells without affecting normal cells is expected to allow drug dose reductions, thereby reducing side effects.

SU, which was used in combination with SAL in this study, has been indicated for metastatic RCC and exerts antitumor effects by inhibiting tyrosine kinases in signaling pathways, including the VEGFR-1–3, FLT-3, PDGFRb, and c-kit pathways. We confirmed that TOS1 cells express *VEGFR2, FLT3, PDGFRB,* and *KIT* (see Supplemental Figure S1). These results indicated that SU might exert cytotoxic effects by inhibiting these tyrosine kinase receptors. SU exerts cytotoxicity in various solid tumors, including gastrointestinal stromal and pancreatic neuroendocrine tumors [14–16]. However, increased plasma levels of SU increase the incidence of side effects, and many patients are forced to discontinue treatment. We found that SU alone reduced the viability of TOS1 cells in a concentration- and time-dependent manner, whereas treatment with SAL alone did not affect cell viability. This suggests that SAL is effective in enhancing the cytotoxic activity of SU without affecting cell viability and, thus, may be a suitable candidate combination drug. Although other molecular-targeted agents (e.g., pazopanib, axitinib, everolimus) reduced the survival rate of TOS1 cells when used alone, not all of them were effective when combined with SAL (see Supplemental Figures S2 and S3). Therefore, further studies are needed to determine which agents are effective in combination with SAL.

We observed that Gb3, a GSL, is expressed on the surfaces of TOS1 and TOS3 RCC cells and recognized and bound by SAL. The uptake of PI following SAL treatment was higher in TOS1 than in TOS3. This may be due to the higher Gb3 expression in TOS1 than in TOS3, which originate from human soft tissue with metastases and human kidney tissue with primary tumors, respectively. We thus speculated that the origin of the RCC cell line may be responsible for the differences in Gb3 expression levels. Although Gb3 is highly expressed in TOS1, glycosphingolipids with different mobilities, such as Gb4, are also expressed. In previous studies, we demonstrated that SAL binds strongly to Gb3 and not to other glycosphingolipids; Gb3 plays an essential role in exerting the effect of SAL [6,8]. However, functions other than those of Gb3 expressed in TOS1 remain to be elucidated. GSLs are abundant on cell surfaces and affect cell functions in various ways, including canceration, metastasis, and drug responses. Młynarczyk et al. showed that the content of Gb3 or GM3 in clear cell RCC is altered in a malignancy-grade-dependent manner [17]. Changes in the expression of GSLs on the cancer cell surface modulate genes involved in cell proliferation and apoptosis (i.e., oncogenesis), genes related to invasiveness and angiogenesis (i.e., promotion of metastasis), and drug transporter genes (i.e., drug resistance) [18]. GSLs are expressed characteristically in carcinomas, and Gb3 is particularly abundant on the surfaces of breast [19], rectal [20], testicular [21], bladder [22], lung [23], and gastric [14] cancer cells. Cancer cells expressing Gb3 show increased invasive and metastatic potential, as well as resistance to drugs, and several studies have evaluated the potential of Gb3 as a therapeutic marker or target. Tyler et al. reported that in cisplatin-resistant lung cancer, the expression of Gb3 and the drug excretion transporters MDR1 and MRP1 are upregulated, which facilitates the excretion of cisplatin from the cells, resulting in a decrease in drug concentration and the development of drug resistance [23]. Johansson et al. reported that treatment with verotoxin, which recognizes and binds Gb3, together with cisplatin, limited drug resistance to cisplatin and induced apoptosis of breast cancer cells [19]. Although the role of Gb3 in renal cancer remains to be elucidated, a combination of SAL, which recognizes and binds Gb3, and SU may be a new and useful therapeutic strategy.

Lectins, including SAL, have recently attracted molecular and cellular research attention as recipients of information from GSLs. Lectins are sugar-binding proteins widely distributed in the animal and plant kingdoms. Animal lectins have been suggested to be involved in infection, defense, cell differentiation, and cell adhesion [24]. Lectins are classified into several families based on the similarity of their carbohydrate recognition domains. Lectins widely distributed in fish eggs are characterized by their affinity for l-rhamnose and, thus, form the rhamnose-binding lectin (RBL) family. The RBL family includes not only SAL isolated from catfish (*Silurus asotus*) but also many other fish egg lectins, such as chum salmon (*Osmerus lanceoratus*, *O. keta*) lectins [25]. In addition to SAL, chum salmon egg lectin (CSL) 3 and *Crenomytilus grayanus* lectin (CGL) reportedly recognize Gb3 [26,27]. In contrast to SAL, which only reversibly increases membrane permeability when bound to Gb3, CSL3, and CGL induce cell death (i.e., apoptosis) when bound to Gb3 [26,27]. Further studies are needed to understand the changes in plasma membrane function that occur when SAL binds to Gb3 and the differential effects of lectins on Gb3-expressing cells.

## 5. Conclusions

SAL recognizes Gb3 expressed on the surfaces of RCC cells and increases the intracellular concentration of SU, a drug for RCC, enhancing its cytotoxicity to RCC cells. SAL may increase cell surface permeability and SU uptake by binding to Gb3. As SAL binds only to Gb3 and does not affect cell viability, sufficient cytotoxic activity may be achieved even when SU is administered at a sufficiently low dose not to cause side effects combined with SAL. However, there are many unknowns in the detailed molecular mechanism of SAL bound to Gb3, which requires further elucidation.

**Supplementary Materials:** The following supporting information can be downloaded at: https://www.mdpi.com/article/10.3390/biomedicines11082317/s1, Figure S1: Expression of tyrosine kinase receptor genes on HeLa and TOS1 cells; Figure S2: Cytotoxic effects of pazopanib, axitinib, and everolimus in TOS1 cells; Figure S3: Cytotoxic effects of pazopanib, axitinib, and everolimus in SAL-pretreated TOS1 cells.

**Author Contributions:** J.I. and S.S. conducted all experiments and analyzed the data. J.I. and S.S. wrote the manuscript. M.S. contributed to the manuscript revision. T.T., M.H. and M.S. supervised all experiments. All authors have read and agreed to the published version of the manuscript.

**Funding:** This work was supported by JSPS KAKENHI Grant Number 19K18619.

**Institutional Review Board Statement:** Not applicable.

**Informed Consent Statement:** Not applicable.

**Data Availability Statement:** The datasets supporting the conclusions of this article are included within the article (and its additional files). They are not deposited in publicly available repositories. The datasets used and analyzed during the current study are available from the corresponding author upon reasonable request.

**Conflicts of Interest:** The authors declare no conflict of interest.

## References

1. Almassi, N.; Gill, B.C.; Rini, B.; Fareed, K. Management of the small renal mass. *Transl. Androl. Urol.* **2017**, *6*, 923–930. [CrossRef] [PubMed]
2. Rodriguez-Vida, A.; Hutson, T.E.; Bellmunt, J.; Strijbos, M.H. New treatment options for metastatic renal cell carcinoma. *ESMO Open* **2017**, *2*, e000185. [CrossRef]
3. Singh, D. Current updates and future perspectives on the management of renal cell carcinoma. *Life Sci.* **2021**, *264*, 118632. [CrossRef] [PubMed]
4. Zhang, H.; Bai, L.; Wu, X.Q.; Tian, X.; Feng, J.; Wu, X.; Shi, G.H.; Pei, X.; Lyu, J.; Yang, G.; et al. Proteogenomics of clear cell renal cell carcinoma response to tyrosine kinase inhibitor. *Nat. Commun.* **2023**, *14*, 4274. [CrossRef]
5. Cheung, R.C.; Wong, J.H.; Pan, W.; Chan, Y.S.; Yin, C.; Dan, X.; Ng, T.B. Marine lectins and their medicinal applications. *Appl. Microbiol. Biotechnol.* **2015**, *99*, 3755–3773. [CrossRef]
6. Sugawara, S.; Im, C.; Kawano, T.; Tatsuta, T.; Koide, Y.; Yamamoto, D.; Ozeki, Y.; Nitta, K.; Hosono, M. Catfish rhamnose-binding lectin induces G(0/1) cell cycle arrest in Burkitt's lymphoma cells via membrane surface Gb3. *Glycoconj J.* **2017**, *34*, 127–138. [CrossRef]
7. Sugawara, S.; Sasaki, S.; Ogawa, Y.; Hosono, M.; Nitta, K. 2005b. Catfish (*Silurus asotus*) lectin enhances the cytotoxic effects of doxorubicin. *Yakugaku Zasshi* **2005**, *125*, 327–334. [CrossRef] [PubMed]
8. Sugawara, S.; Takayanagi, M.; Honda, S.; Tatsuta, T.; Fujii, Y.; Ozeki, Y.; Ito, J.; Sato, M.; Hosono, A.M. Catfish egg lectin affects influx and efflux rates of sunitinib in human cervical carcinoma HeLa cells. *Glycobiology* **2020**, *30*, 802–816. [CrossRef]
9. Satoh, M.; Nejad, F.M.; Nakano, O.; Ito, A.; Kawamura, S.; Ohyama, C.; Saito, S.; Orikasa, S. Four new human renal cell carcinoma cell lines expressing globo-series gangliosides. *Tohoku J. Exp. Med.* **1999**, *189*, 95–105. [CrossRef]
10. Brodaczewska, K.K.; Szczylik, C.; Fiedorowicz, M.; Porta, C.; Czarnecka, A.M. Choosing the right cell line for renal cell cancer research. *Mol. Cancer* **2016**, *15*, 83. [CrossRef]
11. Gotink, K.J.; Broxterman, H.J.; Labots, M.; de Haas, R.R.; Dekker, H.; Honeywell, R.J.; Rudek, M.A.; Beerepoot, L.V.; Musters, R.J.; Jansen, G.; et al. Lysosomal sequestration of sunitinib: A novel mechanism of drug resistance. *Clin. Cancer Res.* **2011**, *17*, 7337–7346. [CrossRef]
12. Fadok, V.A.; Voelker, D.R.; Campbell, P.A.; Cohen, J.J.; Bratton, D.L.; Henson, P.M. Exposure of phosphatidylserine on the surface of apoptotic lymphocytes triggers specific recognition and removal by macrophages. *J. Immunol.* **1992**, *148*, 2207–2216. [CrossRef] [PubMed]
13. Geyer, P.E.; Maak, M.; Nitsche, U.; Perl, M.; Novotny, A.; Slotta-Huspenina, J.; Dransart, E.; Holtorf, A.; Johannes, L.; Janssen, K.P. Gastric adenocarcinomas express the glycosphingolipid Gb3/CD77: Targeting of castric cancer cells with shiga toxin B-subunit. *Mol. Cancer Ther.* **2016**, *15*, 1008–1017. [CrossRef] [PubMed]
14. Demetri, G.D.; van Oosterom, A.T.; Garrett, C.R.; Blackstein, M.E.; Shah, M.H.; Verweij, J.; McArthur, G.; Judson, I.R.; Heinrich, M.C.; Morgan, J.A.; et al. Efficacy and safety of sunitinib in patients with advanced gastrointestinal stromal tumour after failure of imatinib: A randomised controlled trial. *Lancet* **2006**, *368*, 1329–1338. [CrossRef] [PubMed]
15. Raymond, E.; Dahan, L.; Raoul, J.L.; Bang, Y.J.; Borbath, I.; Lombard-Bohas, C.; Valle, J.; Metrakos, P.; Smith, D.; Vinik, A.; et al. Sunitinib malate for the treatment of pancreatic neuroendocrine tumors. *N. Engl. J. Med.* **2011**, *364*, 501–513. [CrossRef]
16. Boegemann, M.; Hubbe, M.; Thomaidou, D.; Blackburn, S.; Bent-Ennakhil, N.; Wood, R.; Bargo, D. Sunitinib treatment modification in first-line metastatic renal cell carcinoma: Analysis of the STAR-TOR registry. *Anticancer Res.* **2018**, *38*, 6413–6422. [CrossRef]
17. Młynarczyk, G.; Mikłosz, A.; Suchański, J.; Reza, S.; Romanowicz, L.; Sobolewski, K.; Chabowski, A.; Baranowski, M. Grade-dependent changes in sphingolipid metabolism in clear cell renal cell carcinoma. *J. Cell Biochem.* **2022**, *123*, 819–829. [CrossRef]
18. Patwardhan, G.A.; Liu, Y.Y. Sphingolipids and expression regulation of genes in cancer. *Prog. Lipid Res.* **2011**, *50*, 104–114. [CrossRef]
19. Johansson, D.; Kosovac, E.; Moharer, J.; Ljuslinder, I.; Brannstrom, T.; Johansson, A.; Behnam-Motlagh, P. Expression of verotoxin-1 receptor Gb3 in breast cancer tissue and verotoxin-1 signal transduction to apoptosis. *BMC Cancer* **2009**, *9*, 67. [CrossRef]
20. Kovbasnjuk, O.; Mourtazina, R.; Baibakov, B.; Wang, T.; Elowsky, C.; Choti, M.A.; Kane, A.; Donowitz, M. The glycosphingolipid globotriaosylceramide in the metastatic transformation of colon cancer. *Proc. Natl. Acad. Sci. USA* **2005**, *102*, 19087–19092. [CrossRef]
21. Kang, J.L.; Rajpert-De Meyts, E.; Wiels, J.; Skakkebaek, N.E. Expression of the glycolipid globotriaosylceramide (Gb3) in testicular carcinoma in situ. *Virchows Arch.* **1995**, *426*, 369–374. [CrossRef]
22. Kawamura, S.; Ohyama, C.; Watanabe, R.; Satoh, M.; Saito, S.; Hoshi, S.; Gasa, S.; Orikasa, S. Glycolipid composition in bladder tumor: A crucial role of GM3 ganglioside in tumor invasion. *Int. J. Cancer* **2001**, *94*, 343–347. [CrossRef]

23. Tyler, A.; Johansson, A.; Karlsson, T.; Gudey, S.K.; Brannstrom, T.; Grankvist, K.; Behnam-Motlagh, P. Targeting glucosylceramide synthase induction of cell surface globotriaosylceramide (Gb3) in acquired cisplatin-resistance of lung cancer and malignant pleural mesothelioma cells. *Exp. Cell Res.* **2015**, *336*, 23–32. [CrossRef]
24. Gabius, H.J. Animal lectins. *Eur. J. Biochem.* **1997**, *243*, 543–576. [CrossRef]
25. Watanabe, Y.; Tateno, H.; Nakamura-Tsuruta, S.; Kominami, J.; Hirabayashi, J.; Nakamura, O.; Watanabe, T.; Kamiya, H.; Naganuma, T.; Ogawa, T.; et al. The function of rhamnose-binding lectin in innate immunity by restricted binding to Gb3. *Dev. Comp. Immunol.* **2009**, *33*, 187–197. [CrossRef] [PubMed]
26. Shirai, T.; Watanabe, Y.; Lee, M.S.; Ogawa, T.; Muramoto, K. Structure of rhamnose-binding lectin CSL3: Unique pseudo-tetrameric architecture of a pattern recognition protein. *J. Mol. Biol.* **2009**, *391*, 390–403. [CrossRef] [PubMed]
27. Liao, J.H.; Chien, C.T.; Wu, H.Y.; Huang, K.F.; Wang, I.; Ho, M.R.; Tu, I.F.; Lee, I.M.; Li, W.; Shih, Y.L.; et al. A multivalent marine lectin from *Crenomytilus grayanus* possesses anticancer activity through recognizing globotriose Gb3. *J. Am. Chem. Soc.* **2016**, *138*, 4787–4795. [CrossRef] [PubMed]

**Disclaimer/Publisher's Note:** The statements, opinions and data contained in all publications are solely those of the individual author(s) and contributor(s) and not of MDPI and/or the editor(s). MDPI and/or the editor(s) disclaim responsibility for any injury to people or property resulting from any ideas, methods, instructions or products referred to in the content.

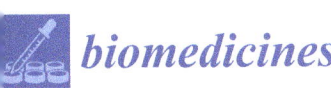 

*Article*

# Evaluation of Parameters Affecting the Occurrence of Systemic Inflammatory Response Syndrome in Patients Operated on Due to Kidney Tumors

Mateusz Marcinek [1,*], Michał Tkocz [1], Kamil Marczewski [1], Robert Partyka [2], Leszek Kukulski [3], Krystyna Młynarek-Śnieżek [4], Bogumiła Sędziak-Marcinek [5], Paweł Rajwa [6,7], Adam Berezowski [8] and Danuta Kokocińska [2]

1. Department of Urology, Faculty of Medical Sciences in Katowice, Medical University of Silesia, Plac Medyków 1, 41-200 Sosnowiec, Poland
2. Department of Emergency Medicine, Faculty of Medical Sciences in Katowice, Medical University of Silesia, Francuska 20, 40-027 Katowice, Poland
3. Department of Cardiac, Vascular and Endovascular Surgery and Transplantology, Medical University of Silesia in Katowice, Silesian Centre for Heart Diseases, Curie-Skłodowskiej 9, 41-800 Zabrze, Poland
4. Department of Urology, Voivodeship Specialised Hospital No. 3, Energetyków 46, 44-200 Rybnik, Poland
5. Department of Ophthalmology, Faculty of Medical Sciences in Zabrze, Medical University of Silesia, Panewnicka 65, 40-760 Katowice, Poland
6. Department of Urology, Faculty of Medical Sciences in Zabrze, Medical University of Silesia, 3 Maja 13/15, 41-800 Zabrze, Poland
7. Department of Urology, Medical University of Vienna, Währinger Gürtel 18-20, 1090 Vienna, Austria
8. Beskidzkie Centrum Medyczne, Młodzieżowa 21, 43-309 Bielsko-Biała, Poland
* Correspondence: mmarcinek@sum.edu.pl; Tel.: +48-32-368-25-11

**Abstract:** The application and prognostic nature of systemic inflammatory reaction syndrome (SIRS) is still being researched, as using SIRS parameters to predict patient status is cheap, efficient, fast, and easy. The study aimed to determine SIRS markers and postoperative complications occurrence in patients undergoing kidney tumor surgery, and to verify if SIRS occurrence depends on age, sex, BMI (body mass index), comorbidities, patients' general condition before the surgery, type of surgery, intraoperative blood loss, or intraoperative ischemia time. Body temperature, heart rate, respiratory rate, and leukocyte count were measured in patients ($n$ = 285) operated on due to a kidney tumor on the first (T0) and third (T3) postoperative day. Univariable and multivariable logistic regression were used to analyze the factors affecting postoperative SIRS and complications occurrence. T0: SIRS developed in patients with higher BMI, >2 ASA points, and more substantial intraoperative blood loss. T3: SIRS developed in obese or overweight patients, with >2 ASA points, significantly higher relative HR change, lower relative body temperature change, respiratory rate, and leukocyte count. BMI values, preoperative general health status, and the amount of intraoperative blood loss in patients undergoing surgery due to a kidney tumor can contribute to SIRS occurrence. Patient's sex, age, tumor size, type of surgery, operated side, and time of intraoperative ischemia do not affect SIRS occurrence.

**Keywords:** kidney tumor; systemic inflammatory response syndrome; nephrectomy

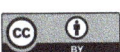

## 1. Introduction

Renal malignancies account for 2–3% of all neoplasms observed in adults, while cancers derived from renal tissue comprise 90% of all malignant tumors [1].

Environmental factors seem to significantly impact the incidence of kidney cancer; however, the etiology of renal tumor development is not yet fully defined. Among the etiological factors, the greatest impact on tumor development is smoking, being overweight or obese, long-term use of hypertension medication, painkillers, phenacetin, and thiazide drugs, and consumption of animal protein and coffee [2,3].

Numerous studies on systemic inflammatory reaction syndrome (SIRS) confirmed that its occurrence correlates with single or multiple organ failure development and an increase in deaths. Talmor et al. reported a prospective analysis of 2300 surgical ICU admissions during a 49-month period. Daily and cumulative multiple organ dysfunction scores and SIRS scores were recorded. In the presented study, defined end points were hospital mortality, days in the ICU, and organ dysfunction [4]. SIRS is related to longer hospitalization time [4,5], longer ICU hospitalization [6], and infection, sepsis, or severe sepsis development [7]. Comstedt et al. studied a 154 patients and found that SIRS status on admission was moderately associated with infection and strongly related to 28-day mortality [7]. The resolution of SIRS is also related to its increased duration and treatment results ($n = 702$) [8]. Stephenson et al. studied a total of 179 patients and showed that SIRS patients required more therapeutic interventions and surgical interventions, intensive treatments, and longer hospital stays, as well as experiencing more frequent deaths [6]. Using SIRS to predict patient status is cheap, efficient, fast, and easy. SIRS can be diagnosed when two or more of the following four criteria are met: (1) body temperature <36 °C (hypothermia) or >38 °C (fever); (2) heart rate >90/min (tachycardia); (3) respiratory rate >20/min (tachypnea) or $pCO_2 < 32$ mmHg; (4) leukocytes count <4 G/L (leukopenia) or >12 G/L (leukocytosis) or immature neutrophils count $\geq 10\%$ (bandemia) [4–8]. Evaluation of SIRS criteria allows for quickly determining the increased risk of serious complications. This enables adequate response with appropriate therapy, increased vigilance, or further extended laboratory tests [9]. The combined effect of noradrenaline and cortisol, and decreased IL-12 concentration, leads to Th1 and Th2 imbalance, namely a decrease in the activity of Th1 and an increase in the activity of Th2 [9]. That in turn causes a change in the concentrations of individual cytokines produced by them, and thus, a decrease in cellular immunity [9]. Surgeries on patients with ischemia-reperfusion syndrome have a significant impact on SIRS development increasing oxidative stress and inflammatory processes [9]. SIRS is associated with the development of single or multiple organ failure [9,10]. Since SIRS criteria monitoring is simple and enables excluding dangerous complications, SIRS could be widely used in the postoperative period, because it very well identifies a clinical condition associated with a systemic inflammatory reaction [10].

The presented study aimed to determine markers of SIRS and postoperative complications occurrence in patients undergoing kidney tumor surgery. We aimed to verify whether the SIRS occurrence depends on the following factors: age, sex, BMI (body mass index), comorbidities (such as diabetes and hypertension), patients' general condition before the surgical procedure, tumor size, operated side of the body, type of surgery (nephrectomy or organ-sparing surgery), intraoperative blood loss, or intraoperative ischemia time.

## 2. Materials and Methods

### 2.1. Study Group and Design

The study included 285 patients operated on due to kidney tumors in the Clinical Department of Urology and Urological Oncology of the 5th Specialist Hospital in Sosnowiec in 2018–2020. The study was approved by the Ethics Committee of the University of Silesia Medical Center in Katowice (No. PCN/022/KB1/73/20, date of approval: 13 October 2020) and was conducted according to the Declaration of Helsinki guidelines. Each patient was informed about the purpose, methods, risks, and benefits of the study and gave written consent to participate in the study.

The study included patients with clinically diagnosed and histopathologically confirmed kidney cancers. Patients operated on in a life-saving mode, under 18 years of age, diagnosed with other cancer(s), displaying inflammatory or autoimmune symptoms, and who did not agree to participate were excluded from the study.

Before the operation, patients were interviewed for present or past comorbidities and current medication use and examined by a urologist and anesthesiologist. Blood and urine were collected for biochemical tests. The abdominal cavity and pelvis minor were examined using ultrasonography and computed tomography or magnetic resonance imaging with contrast. Patients were evaluated by an anesthesiologist using the ASA (American Society of Anesthesiology) scale and qualified for the surgery. Depending on the examination and the imaging results, patients underwent either a nephrectomy or organ-sparing surgery [11–14].

After the operation, patients were classified according to the TNM system used for the clinical staging of tumors and assigned to relevant groups. On the first (T0) and third (T3) postoperative day, SIRS parameters, i.e., body temperature, heart rate, respiratory rate, and leukocyte count, were measured.

*2.2. Statistical Methods*

The normality of data distribution was assessed by the Shapiro–Wilk test and the quantile-quantile plot. Normally distributed interval data were presented as mean (SD). Non-normally distributed interval data were presented as median and lower and upper quartile—Me ($Q_1$; $Q_3$). Qualitative data were presented as numbers and percentages. The dichotomous variables comparison was done using $\chi^2$ test or the $\chi^2$ test with the Yates correction if the expected number was <5, or in case the data failed to meet Cochran's assumptions, with the Fisher's test. The comparison of two variables with normal or log-transformed (due to skewness) interval data was done using the Student's t-test for independent variables. The comparison of two variables with data deviating from the normal distribution was done using the Mann-Whitney U test. The analysis of variance with repeated measures and contrast analysis was used for dependent variables over time and comparisons between groups with and without SIRS.

Factors affecting the SIRS or complications occurrence after the procedure were analyzed using a univariable and multivariable logistic regression. The data for the multivariable logistic regression comprised the variables marked as significant during the univariable analysis. The results were presented as odds ratios (OR) with a 95% confidence interval (CI) and corresponding statistical significance level. Histograms and box plots were used to graphically present the results. Statistical significance was set at $p < 0.05$. All analyses were done using Statistica version 13.3 (TIBCO, Paolo Alto, USA) and R CRAN software, version 4.3.1 (R Core Team, Vienna, Austria).

## 3. Results
*3.1. Study Group Characteristics*

In total, 285 patients participated in the study, including 132 (46.3%) women and 153 (53.7%) men. The average age of the patients was 63 (11) years (range: 23–91 years), even though 49.1% of patients were above 65 years.

Histopathological assessment recognized 248 cases of ccRCC, 26 cases of pRCC, 8 cases of chRCC, and 8 cases of oncocytoma. Surgery on the right side of the body was performed in 135 (47.4%) patients, while organ-sparing surgery in 155 (54.4%) patients. The tumor diameter ranged from 0.7–15 cm with a median of 3.7 (2.5; 5.7) cm (Figure 1). In 20 cases (7%), the patients had multifocal tumors. After the procedure, the patients were discharged from the ward on the 6th day on average (range: 3–25 days).

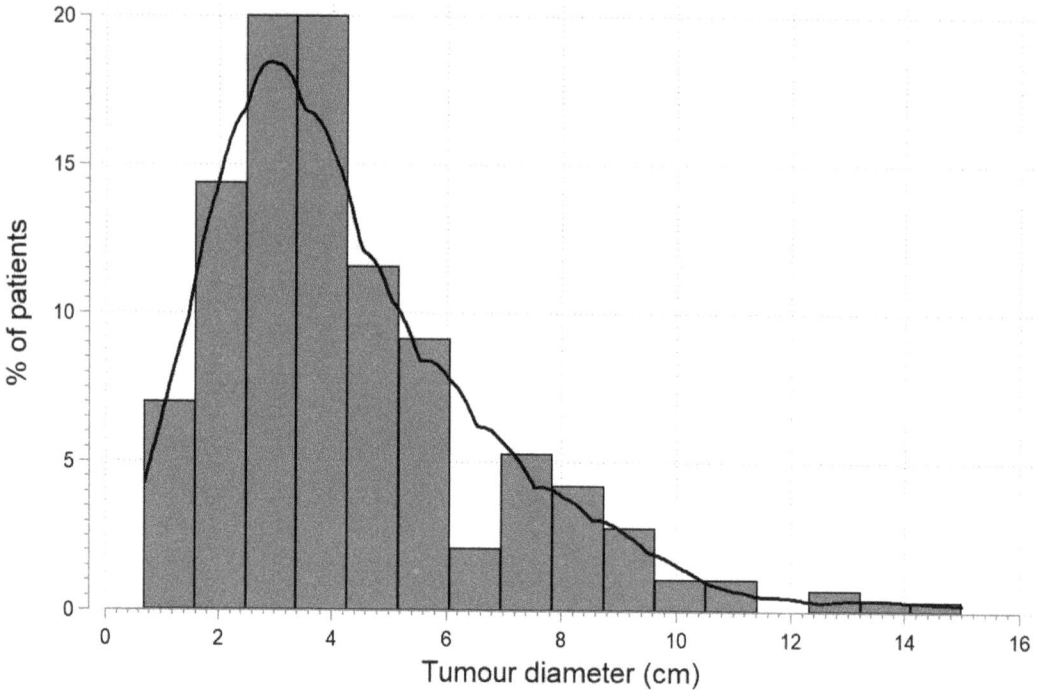

**Figure 1.** Tumor diameter distribution in patients ($n$ = 285) diagnosed with kidney tumors subjected to nephrectomy or organ-sparing surgery.

The average BMI of study participants was 25.5 (3.5) kg/m$^2$ (range: 14–32 kg/m$^2$). Overweight and obesity were diagnosed in 162 (56.8%) and 26 (9.1%) patients, respectively. Concomitant diseases were noted in 177 (62.1%) patients, including arterial hypertension in 64.6%, diabetes in 22.8%, and solitary kidney in 2.5%. Local recurrence affected 2.5% of patients.

Elevated creatinine levels were found in 26 (9.1%) patients, and 78 (27.4%) patients scored >2 on the ASA scale, indicating an increased operational risk related to serious complications or death during or after anesthesia. The average noted intraoperative blood loss was 150 (100; 210) mL, and it ranged from 50–700 mL. For patients who underwent organ-sparing surgery, the average time of intraoperative ischemia was 12 (3.9) min (range: 0–20 min). Systemic inflammatory reaction syndrome occurred in 127 (44.6%) patients on the first and in 35 (12.3%) on the third postoperative day. Postoperative complications occurred in 44 (15.4%) patients.

*3.2. SIRS Occurrence on the First Day after Surgery Due to a Kidney Tumor*

The occurrence of SIRS was not related to the sex and age of the patients, yet it depended on the operated side of the body but not on the tumor TNM classification, size, or type of the surgery, i.e., nephrectomy or organ-sparing surgery ($p$ = 0.058). The time of the intraoperative ischemia and creatinine level were also not related to SIRS occurrence (Table 1). The patients who developed SIRS had a statistically significant higher BMI, so they were more often overweight or obese, but less frequently presented comorbidities.

In addition, patients who developed SIRS after surgery more often obtained >2 points on the ASA scale, suffered from more substantial intraoperative blood loss, and had longer hospitalization time.

**Table 1.** Basic statistics describing patients with and without systemic inflammatory reaction syndrome (SIRS) on the first day after surgery due to a kidney tumor. Results are presented as mean (SD) or median (lower quartile; upper quartile).

| Study Variable | SIRS n = 127 (44.6%) | No SIRS n = 158 (55.4%) | p |
|---|---|---|---|
| Sex M/F, n (%) | 67/60 (52.8/47.2) | 86/72 (54.4/45.6) | 0.78 |
| Age, years | 62 (11) | 64 (12) | 0.25 |
| Age ≥ 65 years, n (%) | 56 (44.1) | 84 (53.2) | 0.13 |
| Comorbidities, n (%) | 68 (53.5.7) | 109 69.0) | <0.01 |
| Hypertension, n (%) | 83 (65.4) | 101 (63.9) | 0.80 |
| T2DM, n (%) | 34 (26.8) | 31 (19.6) | 0.15 |
| BMI, kg/m$^2$ | 27.3 (2.9) | 24.0 (3.2) | <0.001 |
| Overweight, n (%) | 91 (71.7) | 71 (44.9) | <0.001 |
| Obesity, n (%) | 21 (16.5) | 5 (3.3) | |
| ASA > 2, n (%) | 54 (42.5) | 24 (15.2) | <0.001 |
| Solitary kidney, n (%) | 2 (1.6) | 5 (3.2) | 0.47 |
| Cancer local recurrence, n (%) | 5 (3.9) | 2 (3.2) | 0.15 |
| Operated side: R/L, n (%) | 70/57 (55.1/44.9) | 65/93 (41.1/58.9) | <0.05 |
| Tumor diameter, cm | 4.0 (2.5; 5.0) | 3.6 (2.5; 6.0) | 0.76 |
| Multifocal tumor, n (%) | 12 (9.4) | 8 (5.1) | 0.17 |
| TNM: T1a, n (%) | 78 (61.4) | 97 (61.4) | |
| TNM: T1b, n (%) | 37 (29.1) | 46 (29.1) | |
| TNM: T2a, n (%) | 7 (5.5) | 10 (6.3) | 0.95 |
| TNM: T2b, n (%) | 3 (2.4) | 4 (2.5) | |
| TNM: T3a, n (%) | 2 (1.6) | 1 (0.7) | |
| Surgery type: NSS/nephrectomy, n (%) | 77/50 (60.6/39.4) | 78/80 (49.4/50.6) | 0.058 |
| Intraoperative blood loss, mL | 180 (120; 250) | 120 (80; 190) | <0.001 |
| Ischemia time, min | 12.1 (4.0) | 11.9 (3.8) | 0.71 |
| Creatinine, mg/dL | 1.0 (0.8; 1.1) | 1.0 (0.9; 1.1) | 0.77 |
| Creatinine > 1.1/1.4 mg/dL *, n (%) | 10 (7.9) | 16 (10.1) | 0.51 |
| HR, 1/min | 85 (11) | 80 (7) | <0.001 |
| Postoperative body temperature, °C | 36.4 (1.1) | 36.5 (0.7) | 0.47 |
| Respiratory rate, 1/min | 18 (4) | 16 (3) | <0.001 |
| Leukocytes, G/L | 14.7 (12.5; 17.0) | 11.2 (9.1; 13.6) | <0.001 |
| Leukocytes > G/L, n (%) | 109 (85.8) | 98 (62.0) | <0.001 |
| Hospitalization time, days | 6 (5; 7) | 5 (4; 7) | <0.05 |

Legend: * The value 1.1 mg/mL applies to women, and the value 1.4 mg/mL applies to men. Abbreviations: ASA—American Society of Anesthesiology system, assessing patients' general condition and the risk of severe complications or death during or after anesthesia; BMI—body mass index; HR—heart rate; F—female; M—male; NSS—nephron-sparing surgery; SIRS—systemic inflammatory response syndrome; TNM—International Union Against Cancer (UICC) renal tumor classification system; T1a—tumor limited to kidney, <4 cm; T1b—tumor limited to kidney, >4 cm and ≤7 cm; T2a—tumor limited to kidney, >7 cm and ≤10 cm; T2b—tumor limited to kidney, >10 cm; T3a—tumor infiltrating the renal vein or its branches, the pyelocaliceal system, the perirenal fat, or perirenal sinus fat, but not beyond Gerota's fascia or the adrenal gland.

### 3.3. Factors Influencing SIRS Occurrence on the First Day after Surgery Due to a Kidney Tumor

Univariable and multivariable logistic regression of the study participants' results included the patient's sex, age, and BMI, tumor size, type of surgery performed (nephron-sparing surgery (NSS) or nephrectomy), presence of comorbidities, obtaining > 2 points in the ASA classification, intraoperative blood loss, and intraoperative ischemia time. Detailed results of the univariable and multivariable analysis of the variables studied in the patients participating in the study are presented in Table 2.

**Table 2.** Results of univariable and multivariable logistic regression of factors influencing the occurrence of systemic inflammatory reaction syndrome on the first day after the procedure performed due to a kidney tumor.

| Study Variable | Univariable Analysis OR | ±95% CI | Multivariable Analysis OR | 95% CI |
|---|---|---|---|---|
| Sex F vs. M | 1.070 | 0.668–1.712 | | |
| Age | 0.988 | 0.968–1.008 | | |
| Age ≥ 65 years | 0.695 | 0.433–1.114 | | |
| Comorbidities | 0.518 ** | 0.318–0.843 | 0.359 * | 0.168–0.777 |
| BMI | 1.461 # | 1.315–1.623 | | |
| Obesity/overweight | 8.056 # | 4.310–15.057 | 4.998 # | 2.246–11.122 |
| ASA > 2 | 4.130 # | 2.355–7.243 | 7.205 # | 3.221–16.001 |
| Tumor diameter | 0.978 | 0.888–1.077 | | |
| NSS vs. nepherctomy | 1.579 | 0.982–2.541 | | |
| Intraoperative blood loss (per 100 mL) | 1.773 # | 1.351–2.326 | 2.471 # | 1.695–3.603 |
| Ischemia time | 1.016 | 0.935–1.103 | | |
| HR | 1.713 # | 1.306–2.246 | 2.143 # | 1.428–3.216 |
| Respiratory rate | 3.607 # | 2.362–5.511 | 3.211 # | 1.808–5.702 |
| Leukocytes > G/L | 3.707 # | 2.042–6.729 | 7.705 # | 3.221–18.428 |

Legend: * $p < 0.05$; ** $p < 0.01$; # $p < 0.001$; Abbreviations: ASA—American Society of Anesthesiology system assessing patients' general condition and the risk of severe complications or death during or after anesthesia; BMI—body mass index; CI—confidence interval; HR—heart rate; F—female; M—male; NSS—nephron-sparing surgery; OR—odds ratio.

The univariable analysis results showed that the odds of developing SIRS after the surgical procedure increased with the BMI (OR = 1.461), the intraoperative blood loss (OR = 1.773 for each 100 mL lost), or ASA classification > 2 (OR = 4.130) increase. Other analyzed factors, including comorbidities, did not increase the chance of SIRS occurrence after the procedure.

The multivariable analysis results confirmed the statistically significant impact on SIRS occurrence for all the factors indicated by the univariable analysis, except for BMI. The goodness of fit of the multivariable logistic regression model was moderate ($R2 = 0.422$).

### 3.4. SIRS Occurrence on the Third Day after Surgery Due to a Kidney Tumor

Patients who developed SIRS on the third day after surgery due to a kidney tumor had statistically significantly higher BMI, so they were more often obese or overweight, and more often scored >2 points on the ASA scale. We observed a more significant intraoperative blood loss and SIRS occurrence in these patients on the first day after the procedure. In addition, on average, patients who developed SIRS on the third postoperative day were discharged from the ward one day later. The analysis indicated that the size of multifocal tumors tended to be larger in male patients who developed SIRS on the third day after the surgery (tendency to statistical significance, $p = 0.062$)—see Table 3.

Patients who developed SIRS on the third day after the surgery also had significantly higher relative HR change, lower relative body temperature change, respiratory rate, and leukocyte count.

No statistically significant differences in SIRS occurrence on the third day after the surgery were found for sex, age, operated body side, tumor size, tumor TNM classification, type of surgery, concomitant diseases occurrence, intraoperative ischemia time, and baseline creatinine concentration (Table 3).

Table 3. Basic statistics describing patients with and without systemic inflammatory reaction syndrome (SIRS) on the third day after surgery due to a kidney tumor. Results are presented as mean (SD) or median (lower quartile; upper quartile).

| Study Variable | SIRS $n = 35$ (12.3%) | No SIRS $n = 250$ (87.7%) | $p$ |
|---|---|---|---|
| Sex M/F, $n$ (%) | 25/10 (71.4/28.6) | 128/122 (51.2/48.8) | 0.06 |
| Age, years | 62 (11) | 63 (12) | 0.68 |
| Age $\geq 65$ years, $n$ (%) | 14 (40.0) | 126 (50.4) | 0.25 |
| Comorbidities, $n$ (%) | 19 (54.3) | 158 (63.2) | 0.31 |
| Hypertension, $n$ (%) | 21 (60.0) | 163 (65.2) | 0.55 |
| T2DM, $n$ (%) | 12 (34.3) | 53 (21.2) | 0.084 |
| BMI, kg/m$^2$ | 27.8 (2.4) | 25.1 (3.5) | <0.001 |
| Overweight, $n$ (%) | 28 (80.0) | 134 (53.6) | <0.001 |
| Obesity, $n$ (%) | 5 (14.3) | 21 (8.4) | |
| ASA > 2, $n$ (%) | 21 (60.0) | 57 (22.8) | <0.001 |
| Solitary kidney, $n$ (%) | 1 (2.9) | 6 (2.4) | 1.00 |
| Cancer local recurrence, $n$ (%) | 2 (5.7) | 5 (2.0) | 0.21 |
| Operated side: R/L, $n$ (%) | 20/15 (57.1/42.9) | 115/135 (46.0/54.0) | 0.22 |
| Tumor diameter, cm | 4.0 (3.0; 6.0) | 3.5 (2.5; 5.5) | 0.11 |
| Multifocal tumor, $n$ (%) | 7 (20.0) | 13 (5.2) | <0.01 |
| TNM: T1a, $n$ (%) | 21 (60.0) | 154 (61.6) | |
| TNM: T1b, $n$ (%) | 7 (20.0) | 76 (30.4) | |
| TNM: T2a, $n$ (%) | 4 (11.4) | 13 (5.2) | 0.19 |
| TNM: T2b, $n$ (%) | 2 (5.7) | 5 (2.0) | |
| TNM: T3a, $n$ (%) | 1 (2.9) | 2 (0.8) | |
| Surgery type: NSS/nephrectomy, $n$ (%) | 16/19 (45.7/54.3) | 139/111 (55.6/44.4) | 0.27 |
| Intraoperative blood loss, mL | 220 (150; 250) | 140 (100; 200) | <0.001 |
| Ischemia time, min | 12.3 (4.4) | 12.0 (3.9) | 0.74 |
| Creatinine, mg/dL | 1.0 (0.8; 1.2) | 1.0 (0.8; 1.1) | 0.23 |
| Creatinine > 1.1/1.4 mg/dL *, $n$ (%) | 5 (14.3) | 21 (8.4) | 0.26 |
| Δ HR, % | 6.3 (16.0) | −5.7 (12.6) | <0.001 |
| Δ body temperature, % | −2.1 (7.4) | 0.7 (1.9) | <0.05 |
| Δ respiratory rate, % | −1.9 (23.7) | −8.7 (18.3) | 0.11 |
| Δ leukocytes, % | −12.1 (−30.0; 15.4) | −26.0 (−39.3; −11.1) | <0.01 |
| SIRS$_{T0}$, $n$ (%) | 33 (94.3) | 94 (37.6) | <0.001 |
| Leukocytes$_{T0}$ > G/L, $n$ (%) | 29 (82.9) | 178 (71.2) | 0.15 |
| Leukocytes$_{T3}$ > G/L, $n$ (%) | 31 (88.6) | 79 (31.6) | <0.001 |
| Hospitalization time, days | 7 (5; 8) | 6 (4; 6) | <0.001 |

Legend: Δ—relative parameter change; * The value 1.1 mg/mL applies to women, and the value 1.4 mg/mL applies to men. Abbreviations: ASA—American Society of Anesthesiology system assessing patients' general condition and the risk of severe complications or death during or after anesthesia; BMI—body mass index; HR—heart rate; F—female; M—male; NSS—nephron-sparing surgery; SIRS—systemic inflammatory response syndrome; TNM—International Union Against Cancer (UICC) renal tumor classification system; T0—the first day after surgery; T1a—tumor limited to kidney, <4 cm; T1b—tumor limited to kidney, >4 cm and ≤7 cm; T2a—tumor limited to kidney, >7 cm and ≤10 cm; T2b—tumor limited to kidney, >10 cm; T3—the third day after surgery; T3a—tumor infiltrating the renal vein or its branches, the pyelocaliceal system, the perirenal fat, or perirenal sinus fat, but not beyond Gerota's fascia or the adrenal gland.

We observed a significant increase in the pulse value in patients with SIRS (84 (11) vs. 88 (9) 1/min; $p < 0.01$) and a significant decrease (82 (9) vs. 76 (7) 1/min; $p < 0.001$) in the pulse value in patients without SIRS during the postoperative follow-up (Figure 2). Immediately after the procedure (T0), we found no significant difference ($p = 0.682$) between the patients with and without SIRS developed on the third day. Patients diagnosed with

SIRS on the third day after the surgery had statistically significantly higher HR ($p < 0.001$) that day than patients without SIRS.

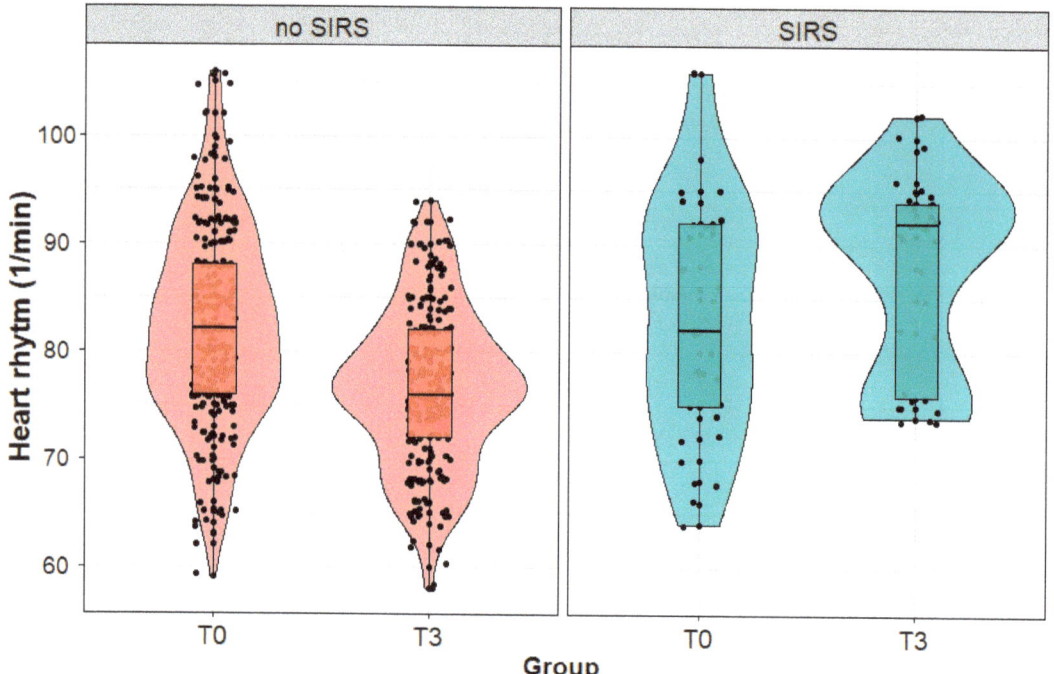

**Figure 2.** Heart rate (1/min) in patients with and without systemic inflammatory reaction syndrome (SIRS) developed on the third day after the surgery, measured immediately after (T0) and on the third day (T3) after surgery performed due to a kidney tumor. Legend: HR—heart rate.

We observed a significant decrease (36.6 (1.1) vs. 35.8 (2.6) °C; $p < 0.001$) in body temperature in patients with SIRS and no change ($p = 0.091$) in body temperature in patients without SIRS during postoperative observation (Figure 3). We observed no significant difference ($p = 0.493$) in body temperature between the patients with and without SIRS immediately after the procedure. In contrast, on the third day after the procedure, the body temperature of patients diagnosed with SIRS was statistically significantly lower ($p < 0.001$) than in patients with SIRS on the first day.

The respiratory rate of patients who developed SIRS on the third day after surgery was statistically significantly higher on the third day after surgery than in patients without SIRS (17 (4) vs. 15 (2) 1/min; $p < 0.001$), although we observed no significant difference ($p = 0.981$) between the patient groups immediately after the surgery. We observed no change ($p = 0.372$) in the respiratory rate in patients diagnosed with SIRS on the third postoperative day. On the other hand, the respiratory rate significantly decreased ($p < 0.001$) in the group of patients without SIRS (Figure 4).

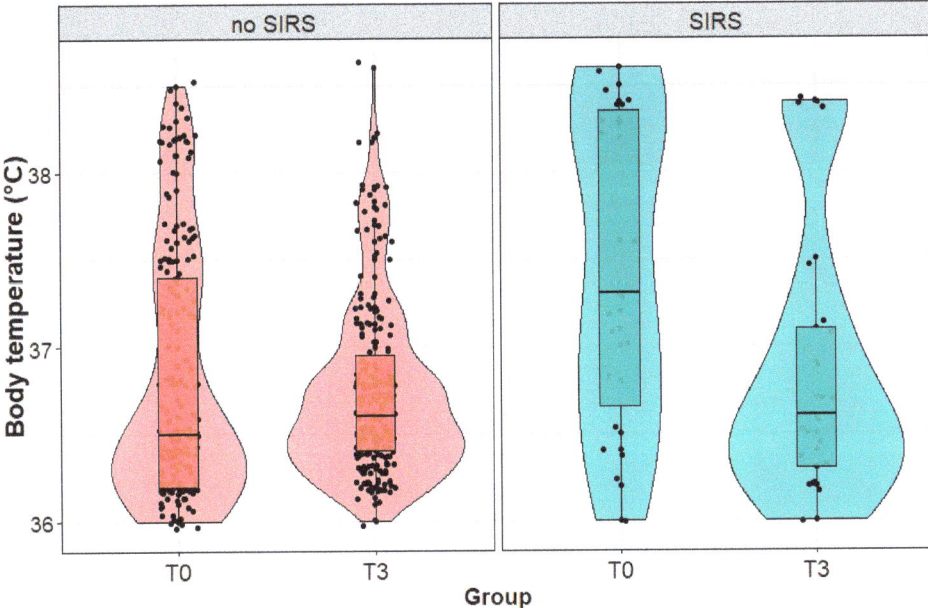

**Figure 3.** Body temperature (°C) in patients with and without systemic inflammatory reaction syndrome (SIRS) on the third day after surgery, measured immediately after (T0) and on the third day (T3) after the surgery performed due to a kidney tumor.

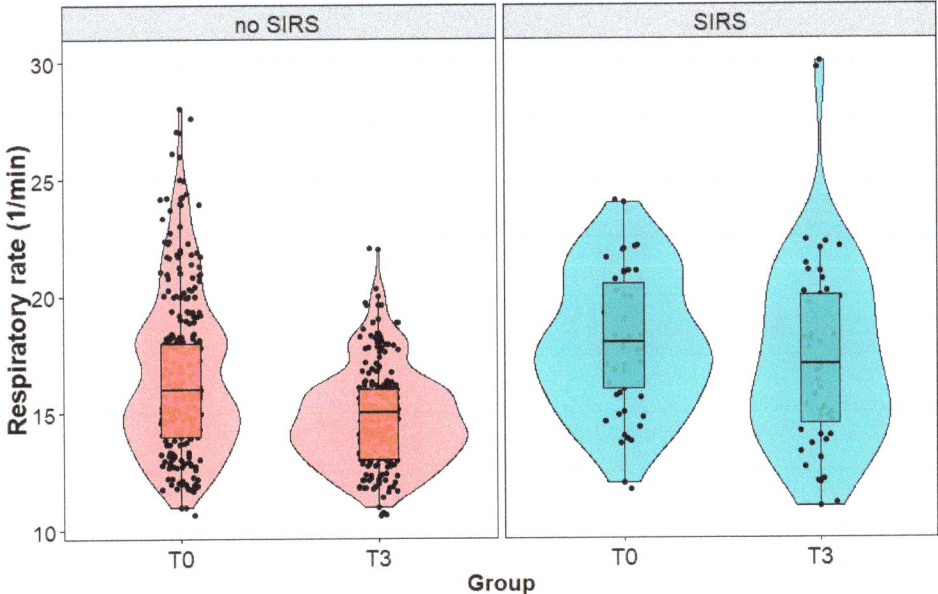

**Figure 4.** Respiratory rate (1/min) in patients with and without systemic inflammatory reaction syndrome (SIRS) on the third day after surgery, measured immediately after (T0) and on the third day (T3) after surgery performed due to a kidney tumor.

On the third day after the procedure, the leukocyte count in the serum of patients diagnosed with SIRS on the third day after the procedure was statistically significantly higher than in patients without SIRS (13.4 (12.2; 14.0) vs. 8.9 (3.6; 29.5) G/L; $p < 0.001$), although we observed no significant difference between the groups immediately after the procedure ($p = 0.581$). We noted a slight decrease in the leukocyte count in patients diagnosed with SIRS on the third day after the procedure (a statistically insignificant change), and a significant decrease in patients without SIRS (12.5 (9.8l; 15.2) vs. 8.9 (7.3; 11.2) G/L; $p < 0.001$) (Figure 5).

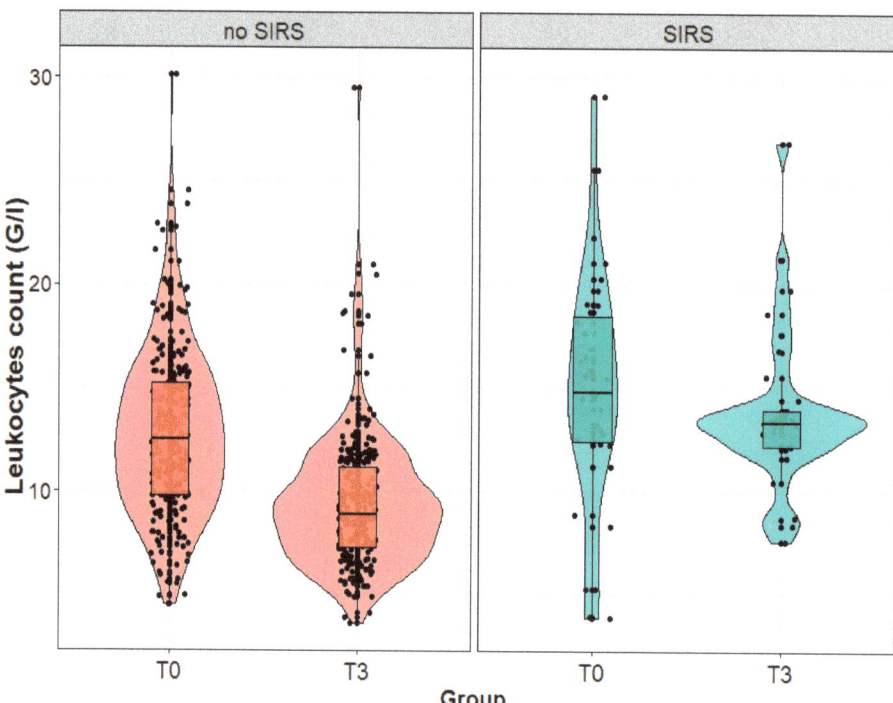

**Figure 5.** Leukocytes count (G/L) in patients with and without systemic inflammatory reaction syndrome (SIRS) on the third day after surgery, measured immediately after (T0) and on the third day (T3) after the surgical removal of the kidney tumor.

*3.5. Factors Influencing SIRS Occurrence on the Third Day after Surgery Due to a Kidney Tumor*

Univariable analysis showed that the odds ratio of developing SIRS on the third day after the surgery increased with increased BMI (OR = 1.374; 95%CI: 1.181–1.600; $p < 0.001$), increased intraoperative blood loss (OR = 1.768, per 100 mL; 95%CI: 1.332–2.348, $p < 0.001$), ASA classification >2 (OR = 5.079; 95%CI: 2.420–10.658; $p < 0.001$), and leukocytosis occurrence on the first postoperative day (OR = 27.385; 95%CI: 6.383–117.494; $p < 0.001$), while female sex decreased it (OR = 0.420; 95%CI: 0.193–0.913; $p < 0.05$). The rest of the analyzed factors did not change the patient's chances of developing systemic inflammatory reaction syndrome on the third day after the surgery.

*3.6. Complications Occurrence after Surgery Due to a Kidney Tumor*

Postoperative complications occurred in 44 (15.4%) patients enrolled in the study. Patients with complications stayed in the ward longer, were more likely to have had the right side of the body operated on, were more likely to have multifocal tumors (tendency to statistical significance, $p = 0.063$), and had higher BMI values, including overweight or obesity. Additionally, patients with complications had greater intraoperative blood loss, more frequently an ASA classification > 2, higher pulse values (on the first and third day after surgery), as well as higher respiratory rate and leukocytosis on the third day after surgery.

We also observed a statistically significantly higher incidence of SIRS occurrence immediately after and on the third day after surgery, a lower relative change in body temperature, lower leukocyte count, and a greater relative change in the respiratory rate in patients with postoperative complications.

## 4. Discussion

The presented results indicate that the occurrence of SIRS on the first and third day after surgery due to a kidney tumor mainly depends on the BMI value of patients undergoing surgery. Obesity is one of the most important risk factors for developing cancer, heart disease, and metabolic disease [15], changing current medical and surgical strategies in Western societies [16]. The relationship between obesity and chronic diseases seems clear, but the relationship between obesity and the onset of SIRS is still poorly understood. The results of this study indicate that overweight/obesity measured by BMI is the strongest factor determining SIRS occurrence in patients undergoing surgery due to a kidney tumor.

The inflammatory state itself is associated with obesity and metabolic syndrome. The clinical picture of patients with insulin resistance and abdominal obesity, regarding cytokine profile, inflammatory profile, and morbidity, is similar to that observed in Gram-negative sepsis, but the severity of symptoms is lower than in sepsis [17]. Chen et al. [18] analyzed SIRS development in patients with different visceral-to-subcutaneous adipose tissue (VAT/SAT) ratios after multiple traumas. They analyzed whether adipose tissue distribution affects SIRS development in patients with multiple traumas. They found that a lower VAT/SAT ratio was associated with increased inflammatory response and poorer clinical outcomes in patients with multiple traumas. Furthermore, the VAT/SAT ratio is an independent factor providing additional information about BMI [18]. In turn, Southern et al. [19] showed a clear relationship between elevated BMI, one of the risk factors of postoperative fever, and SIRS occurrence after ureteroscopy due to nephrolithiasis. The authors studied 2746 patients who underwent 3298 URS for stone disease at Geisinger from 2008 to 2016. In addition, this study showed that the risk of SIRS significantly depended also on the sex and age of the patients, the presence of bacteria in the patient's urine, and the duration of the surgical procedure. Older patients were more likely to have difficult hospitalization. On the other hand, female sex, longer surgery, increased BMI, and positive urine culture before surgery turned out to be significantly associated with postoperative fever/SIRS occurrence after ureteroscopy, which translated into longer hospitalization [19]. These results are consistent with the results of our study. Patients who developed SIRS on the third day after surgery due to a kidney tumor were discharged from the ward one day later on average.

Zhu et al. reported a positive correlation between the percentage of visceral fat and the stage of Fuhrman's tumor in patients with RCC classified as T1a [20]. Ladoire et al. [21] showed that visceral obesity has a significant prognostic value in patients with advanced RCC treated with targeted therapy [21], and Steffens et al. [22] confirmed that patients with metastatic RCC (mRCC) and a higher percentage of visceral fat receiving targeted therapy achieved longer tumor-specific survival and longer overall survival [22]. On the contrary, Mano et al. [23], as one of the few, showed that neither subcutaneous adipose tissue nor visceral adipose tissue correlate with RCC stage and overall survival in patients with non-metastatic clear cell carcinoma [23]. In turn, Hakimi et al. [24] showed that overweight patients diagnosed with RCC have a better prognosis than people with normal body mass or underweight [24]. Accumulation of adipose tissue, such as high levels of SFA and TFA at the time of tumor progression, may improve the survival of mRCC patients treated with tyrosine kinase inhibitors, especially those with larger tumor burdens. Moreover, the number of increased adipose tissue components is a key prognostic factor in these patients, and hence, the accumulation of adipose tissue should be considered an important parameter for assessing the survival of patients with mRCC [25]. The mechanism by which visceral fat accumulation (VFA), subcutaneous fat accumulation (SFA), or total fat accumulation (TFA) occurs, to improve the survival of patients with mRCC, is not well understood. VFA and SFA differ by the type of adipocytes (fat cells) involved, endocrine function, lipolytic activity, and response to insulin and other hormones. The impaired or changed metabolisms (mainly glucose and lipid metabolism, primarily fatty acid synthesis and β-oxidation) are observed in cancer cells and could facilitate cell growth and proliferation. Patients with visceral obesity have been reported to have an increased risk of metabolic complications, e.g., metabolic syndrome [25]. Translational studies have shown that RCC can be induced by long-term intake of a high-fat diet, which was confirmed by pathological changes observed in histological sections [26].

Interestingly, obesity is a factor that favors a good prognosis of RCC, even though it contributes to an increased risk of RCC. For patients with organ-confined but not advanced RCC, being overweight improved their tumor-specific survival [27]. Another study also found that tumor-specific survival, but not overall survival, was significantly prolonged in patients with a higher BMI (>30 kg/m$^2$) undergoing radical nephrectomy [28]. These observations partially coincide with our results presented here. Multivariable analysis showed that the comorbidities presented a protective effect (OR = 0.36) on SIRS occurrence after renal tumor surgery. In addition, it showed that people without comorbidities were almost three times more likely to develop SIRS; however, the goodness of fit of the multivariable logistic regression model was only moderate.

In the presented study, SIRS occurred in 44.6% on the first day and in 12.3% of patients on the third day after surgery. Postoperative complications were reported in 15.4%. One of the factors influencing SIRS occurrence was the higher intraoperative blood loss. Patients with heavier bleeding were by 34.8% more likely to develop SIRS. Patients who developed SIRS were also more likely to have an ASA score >2. Patients with >2 ASA score also had greater intraoperative blood loss, more frequent SIRS occurrence (94.3%) on the first postoperative day, and leukocytosis on the third postoperative day (88.6%). Every kidney-sparing surgical technique described in the literature, such as enucleation, excavation, resection of the kidney pole, extensive transverse resection, and partial ex vivo resection followed by autotransplantation, is characterized by a certain percentage of postoperative complications. Some of these techniques, such as enucleation or extracorporeal resection with autotransplantation, are performed rarely and only in special cases of large and particularly difficult-to-access tumors [29].

Intraoperative blood loss or postoperative bleeding has been associated with SIRS. Despite the relatively low incidence of bleeding after partial nephrectomy, estimated at 4.2–6% for laparoscopic partial nephrectomy [30], 6% for open procedures, and 8.1% for robotic procedures [31], postoperative bleeding remains one of the most serious complications, especially in the case of centrally located tumors [32]. Several studies have examined various factors associated with hemorrhage after partial nephrectomy, including patient demographics, surgical method, and tumor parameters [33]. Van Poppel et al. [34], in their study of open partial nephrectomy in 76 patients, suggested that larger tumor size and its central location correlate with an increased risk of postoperative hemorrhage. Similarly, Ramani et al. [33] showed that the frequency of postoperative bleeding was higher in patients with central tumors and deeper infiltration. In our study, the univariable analysis indicated that for each 100 mL lost amount of intraoperative blood the odds of developing SIRS after the procedure increased by 77.3%.

The presented results showed that patients who developed SIRS on the third day after surgery more often scored >2 on the ASA scale and were discharged from the ward one day later on average. It can be concluded that SIRS occurrence affects the length of hospitalization. Uchida et al. analyzed preoperative and intraoperative SIRS risk factors after ureteroscopy, as infectious complications are one of the most worrying problems of urolithiasis treatment [35]. Uchida et al. [35] and Martov et al. [36], in their independent studies under the CROES URS Global Study, showed that female sex, elevated ASA, high stone burden, Crohn's disease, and cardiovascular disease are significant risk factors for postoperative urinary tract infection, fever, and SIRS in patients with negative baseline urine cultures [35,36]. The analyzes of preoperative and intraoperative risk factors for SIRS development after surgical procedures used in urology and other types of surgery are abundantly available. However, no consensus among researchers on the risk factors predicting SIRS has been achieved due to the complexity of pathophysiology and surgical factors. According to Moses et al. [37], age, sex, BMI, ASA score, and duration of surgery are not risk factors for SIRS after percutaneous nephrolithotomy [37]. On the other hand, an analysis by Akdeniz et al. [38] showed that diabetes, acute phase proteins (CRP), platelet-to-lymphocyte ratio, neutrophil-to-lymphocyte count, urinary white blood cell count, stone size, mean ASA score, type of surgery, duration of surgery, mean hemoglobin drop, length of hospital stay, blood transfusion, and complication rate were associated with SIRS development after percutaneous nephrolithotomy, but age, gender, BMI, and location of stones were not [38]. Takenaka et al. [39], in turn, indicated that postoperative monitoring of acute phase parameters (IL–6 and CRP) and SIRS parameters is very important, as they correlate well with the intensity of surgical stress and the length of hospitalization. Haga et al. [40] studied the incidence of SIRS and multiple organ dysfunction in patients undergoing gastrointestinal surgery. The results showed that the length of SIRS or the number of positive SIRS criteria after surgery significantly correlated with parameters of surgical stress (blood/weight loss and duration of surgery) and CRP value. The systemic inflammatory reaction syndrome, which persisted or reappeared after the third postoperative day, was an early sign of postoperative complications. Researchers concluded that SIRS is a useful criterion for diagnosing postoperative complications. Becher et al. [41], studying the impact of the inflammatory response on the outcome of patients undergoing emergency colorectal surgery, concluded that failure to regulate the body's systemic inflammatory response was the leading cause of death in patients undergoing the unscheduled surgery and patients with SIRS or sepsis who underwent surgery shorter than 2.5 h had fewer postoperative complications. Their results further support the importance of timely surgical intervention with the best possible control of tissue manipulation, potentially reducing inflammation. Smajic et al. [42] showed that SIRS incidence in patients subjected to unscheduled surgery (86.7%) tended to decrease gradually during the postoperative period, to 60% 24 h after surgery and 40% 72 h after surgery [42]. They explained the high SIRS incidence before surgery by the already-present initial inflammatory reaction, forcing the scheduled procedure. They observed a high rate of postoperative SIRS, which gradually decreased as the root cause of the inflammatory response subsided. The following residual effects of SIRS intertwined with the effect of the surgical procedure acted as an additional stress stimulus. The SIRS criteria are a postoperative reflection of the activated inflammatory cascade that tends to decrease. Smajic et al. [42] also showed that the SIRS score correlates with the hospitalization time and slightly less with the treatment outcome, which can be explained by the resolving inflammation cascade within 72 h after surgery [42]. These results coincide with the presented observations regarding the relationship between SIRS occurrence on the third day after surgery and the hospitalization time.

In this study, SIRS occurrence was not related to the time of intraoperative ischemia. The mean intraoperative ischemia time in patients undergoing organ-sparing surgery was $12 \pm 3.9$ min (range: 0–20 min). Nephrectomy procedures should always aim at minimizing ischemic time. Research evidence and patients' observations indicate that a time interval of up to 20–25 min is the most accurate cut-off point for ischemic patients who do not develop a short-term and long-term decline in renal function after partial nephrectomy, depending on the amount of renal tissue saved. According to the latest studies, good clinical practice (i.e., achieving relatively short periods of warm ischemia) means that ischemic time is not the strongest factor influencing long-term renal function, since renal filtration depends on the quality and quantity of preserved renal parenchyma. Despite the lack of consistent data indicating a significant relationship between intraoperative ischemia and end-stage renal disease in patients with both kidneys, warm ischemic time remains a strong predictor of acute kidney injury and the need for dialysis after partial nephrectomy in solitary kidneys [43]. Thompson et al. [44] reported that warm ischemia longer than 25 min was associated with a 2.3-fold increased risk of chronic kidney disease after partial nephrectomy [44]. These data suggest that the loss of function due to limited warm ischemia is marginal; however, prolonging the duration of warm ischemia may be detrimental.

## 5. Conclusions

BMI values, preoperative general health status measured with the ASA scale, and the amount of intraoperative blood loss in patients undergoing surgery due to a kidney tumor can contribute to SIRS occurrence. On the other hand, the patient's sex, age, tumor size, type of surgery, operated side, and time of intraoperative ischemia do not affect SIRS occurrence.

**Author Contributions:** Conceptualization, M.M. and M.T.; methodology, D.K.; software, L.K.; validation, P.R.; formal analysis, K.M.-Ś.; investigation, K.M. and M.M.; resources, A.B.; data curation, M.M.; writing—original draft preparation, M.M.; writing—review and editing, M.T.; visualization, B.S.-M.; supervision, D.K.; project administration, R.P. All authors have read and agreed to the published version of the manuscript.

**Funding:** This research received no external funding.

**Institutional Review Board Statement:** The study was conducted in accordance with the Declaration of Helsinki, and approved by the Ethics Committee of the University of Silesia Medical Center in Katowice (No. PCN/022/KB1/73/20, date of approval: 13 October 2020).

**Informed Consent Statement:** Informed consent was obtained from all subjects involved in the study.

**Data Availability Statement:** The data presented in this study are available on request from the corresponding author. The data are not publicly available due to legal and ethical reasons.

**Conflicts of Interest:** The authors declare no conflict of interest.

## References

1. Bray, F.; Ferlay, J.; Soerjomataram, I.; Siegel, R.L.; Torre, L.A.; Jemal, A. Global cancer statistics 2018: GLOBOCAN estimates of incidence and mortality worldwide for 36 cancers in 185 countries. *CA Cancer J. Clin.* **2018**, *68*, 394–424. [CrossRef] [PubMed]
2. Choueiri, T.K.; Je, Y.; Cho, E. Analgesic use and the risk of kidney cancer: A meta-analysis of epidemiologic studies. *Int. J. Cancer* **2014**, *134*, 384–396. [CrossRef] [PubMed]
3. Franklin, J.R.; Figlin, R.; Belldegrun, A. Renal cell carcinoma: Basic biology and clinical behavior. *Semin. Urol. Oncol.* **1996**, *14*, 208–215.
4. Talmor, M.; Hydo, L.; Barie, P.S. Relationship of systemic inflammatory response syndrome to organ dysfunction, length of stay, and mortality in critical surgical illness: Effect of intensive care unit resuscitation. *Arch. Surg.* **1999**, *134*, 81–87. [CrossRef] [PubMed]
5. Stephenson, J.A.; Gravante, G.; Butler, N.A.; Sorge, R.; Sayers, R.D.; Bown, M.J. The systemic inflammatory response syndrome (SIRS)—Number and type of positive criteria predict interventions and outcomes in acute surgical admissions. *World J. Surg.* **2010**, *34*, 2757–2764. [CrossRef]
6. NeSmith, E.G.; Weinrich, S.P.; Andrews, J.O.; Medeiros, R.S.; Hawkins, M.L.; Weinrich, M. Systemic inflammatory response syndrome score and race as predictors of length of stay in the intensive care unit. *Am. J. Crit. Care* **2009**, *18*, 339–346. [CrossRef]
7. Comstedt, P.; Storgaard, M.; Lassen, A.T. The systemic inflammatory response syndrome (SIRS) in acutely hospitalised medical patients: A cohort study. *Scand. J. Trauma Resusc. Emerg. Med.* **2009**, *17*, 67. [CrossRef]
8. Bochicchio, G.V.; Napolitano, L.M.; Joshi, M.; Knorr, K.; Tracy, J.K.; Ilahi, O.; Scalea, T.M. Persistent systemic inflammatory response syndrome is predictive of nosocomial infection in trauma. *J. Trauma* **2002**, *53*, 245–251. [CrossRef]
9. Hadasik, G.; Hadasik, K.; Święszek, A. Usefulness of testing for the prevalence of systemic inflammatory response syndrome (SIRS) in clinical practice. *Chir. Pol.* **2014**, *16*, 12–19.
10. Karpel, E. Zespół Ogólnoustrojowej Reakcji Zapalnej w Okresie Pooperacyjnym. Habilitation Thesis, Medical University of Silesia, Katowice, Poland, 2001. (In Polish)
11. Albers, P.; Heidenreich, A.; Lech, H. *Podstawowe Operacje Urologiczne*; Czelej: Lublin, Poland, 2007. (In Polish)

12. Smith, J.A.; Howards, S.S.; Preminger, G.M.; Dmochowski, R.R. *Hinman's Atlas of Urologic Surgery*; Elsevier/Saunders: Philadelphia, PA, USA, 2012.
13. Lau, W.K.; Blute, M.L.; Weaver, A.L.; Torres, V.E.; Zincke, H. Matched comparison of radical nephrectomy vs nephron-sparing surgery in patients with unilateral renal cell carcinoma and a normal contralateral kidney. *Mayo Clin. Proc.* **2000**, *75*, 1236–1242. [CrossRef]
14. Lerner, S.E.; Hawkins, C.A.; Blute, M.L.; Grabner, A.; Wollan, P.C.; Eickholt, J.T.; Zincke, H. Disease outcome in patients with low stage renal cell carcinoma treated with nephron sparing or radical surgery. *J. Urol.* **2002**, *167*, 884–889. [CrossRef]
15. Weir, C.B.; Jan, A. *BMI Classification Percentile and Cut Off Points*; StatPearls Publishing: Treasure Island, FL, USA, 2021.
16. Quesenberry, C.P., Jr.; Caan, B.; Jacobsen, A. Obesity, health service use, and health care costs among members of a health maintenance organization. *Arch. Int. Med.* **1998**, *158*, 466–472. [CrossRef]
17. Cave, M.C.; Hurt, R.T.; Frazier, T.H.; Matheson, P.J.; Garrison, R.N.; McClain, C.J.; McClave, S.A. Obesity, inflammation, and the potential application of pharmaconutrition. *Nutr. Clin. Pract.* **2008**, *23*, 16–34. [CrossRef]
18. Chen, Z.; Wittenberg, S.; Auer, T.A.; Bashkuev, M.; Gebert, P.; Fehrenbach, U.; Geisel, D.; Graef, F.; Maerdian, S.; Tsitsilonis, S. The effect of fat distribution on the inflammatory response of multiple trauma patients—A retrospective study. *Life* **2021**, *11*, 1243. [CrossRef]
19. Southern, J.B.; Higgins, A.M.; Young, A.J.; Kost, K.A.; Schreiter, B.R.; Clifton, M.; Fulmer, B.R.; Garg, T. Risk factors for postoperative fever and systemic inflammatory response syndrome after ureteroscopy for stone disease. *J. Endourol.* **2019**, *33*, 516–522. [CrossRef]
20. Gu, W.; Zhu, Y.; Wang, H.; Zhang, H.; Shi, G.; Liu, X.; Ye, D. Prognostic value of components of body composition in patients treated with targeted therapy for advanced renal cell carcinoma: A retrospective case series. *PLoS ONE* **2015**, *10*, e0118022. [CrossRef]
21. Ladoire, S.; Bonnetain, F.; Gauthier, M.; Zanetta, S.; Petit, J.M.; Guiu, S.; Kermarrec, I.; Mourey, E.; Michel, F.; Krause, D.; et al. Visceral fat area as a new independent predictive factor of survival in patients with metastatic renal cell carcinoma treated with antiangiogenic agents. *Oncologist* **2011**, *16*, 71–81. [CrossRef]
22. Steffens, S.; Grunwald, V.; Ringe, K.I.; Seidel, C.; Eggers, H.; Schrader, M.; Wacker, F.; Kuczyk, M.A.; Schrader, A.J. Does obesity influence the prognosis of metastatic renal cell carcinoma in patients treated with vascular endothelial growth factor–targeted therapy? *Oncologist* **2011**, *16*, 1565–1571. [CrossRef]
23. Mano, R.; Hakimi, A.A.; Zabor, E.C.; Bury, M.A.; Donati, O.F.; Karlo, C.A.; Bazzi, W.M.; Furberg, H.; Russo, P. Association between visceral and subcutaneous adiposity and clinicopathological outcomes in non-metastatic clear cell renal cell carcinoma. *Can. Urol. Assoc. J.* **2014**, *8*, E675–E680. [CrossRef]
24. Hakimi, A.A.; Furberg, H.; Zabor, E.C.; Jacobsen, A.; Schultz, N.; Ciriello, G.; Mikklineni, N.; Fiegoli, B.; Kim, P.H.; Voss, M.H.; et al. An epidemiologic and genomic investigation into the obesity paradox in renal cell carcinoma. *JNCI J. Nat. Cancer Inst.* **2013**, *105*, 1862–1870. [CrossRef]
25. Dai, J.; Zhang, X.; Liu, Z.; Song, T.; Zhu, X.; Zhang, H.; Wu, M.; Li, X.; Zeng, H.; Shen, P. The prognostic value of body fat components in metastasis renal cancer patients treated with TKIs. *Cancer Manag. Res.* **2020**, *12*, 891–903. [CrossRef] [PubMed]
26. Yang, X.-F.; Ma, G.; Feng, N.-H.; Yu, D.-S.; Wu, Y.; Li, C. Twist2 and CD24 expression alters renal microenvironment in obesity associated kidney cancer. *Eur. Rev. Med. Pharmacol. Sci.* **2018**, *22*, 358–364.
27. Waalkes, S.; Merseburger, A.S.; Kramer, M.W.; Herrmann, T.R.; Wegener, G.; Rustemeier, J.; Hofmann, R.; Schrader, M.; Kuczyk, M.A.; Schrader, A.J. Obesity is associated with improved survival in patients with organ-confined clear-cell kidney cancer. *Cancer Causes Control* **2010**, *21*, 1905–1910. [CrossRef] [PubMed]
28. Rogde, A.J.; Gudbrandsdottir, G.; Hjelle, K.M.; Sand, K.E.; Bostad, L.; Beisland, C. Obesity is associated with an improved cancer-specific survival, but an increased rate of postoperative complications after surgery for renal cell carcinoma. *Scand. J. Urol. Nephrol.* **2012**, *46*, 348–357. [CrossRef] [PubMed]
29. Kupilas, A.; Fryczkowski, M. Powikłania po operacjach organooszczędzających nerki. *Przegląd. Urol.* **2007**, *5*, 31–33.
30. Montag, S.; Rais-Bahrami, S.; Seideman, C.A.; Rastinehad, A.R.; Vira, M.A.; Kavoussi, L.R.; Richstone, L. Delayed haemorrhage after laparoscopic partial nephrectomy: Frequency and angiographic findings. *BJU Int.* **2011**, *107*, 1460–1466. [CrossRef]
31. Campbell, S.C.; Novick, A.C.; Belldegrun, A.; Blute, M.L.; Chow, G.K.; Derweesh, I.H.; Faraday, M.M.; Kaouk, J.H.; Leveillee, R.J.; Matin, S.F.; et al. Guidelines for management of the clinical T1 renal mass. *J. Urol.* **2009**, *182*, 1271–1279. [CrossRef]
32. Nadu, A.; Kleinmann, N.; Laufer, M.; Dotan, Z.; Winkler, H.; Ramon, J. Laparoscopic partial nephrectomy for central tumors: Analysis of perioperative outcomes and complications. *J. Urol.* **2009**, *181*, 42–47. [CrossRef]
33. Ramani, A.P.; Desai, M.M.; Steinberg, A.P.; Ng, C.S.; Abreu, S.C.; Kaouk, J.H.; Finelli, A.; Novick, A.C.; Gill, I.S. Complications of laparoscopic partial nephrectomy in 200 cases. *J. Urol.* **2005**, *173*, 42–47. [CrossRef]
34. Van Poppel, H.; Bamelis, B.; Oyen, R.; Baert, L. Partial nephrectomy for renal cell carcinoma can achieve long-term tumor control. *J. Urol.* **1998**, *160*, 674–678. [CrossRef]
35. Uchida, Y.; Takazawa, R.; Kitayama, S.; Tsujii, T. Predictive risk factors for systemic inflammatory response syndrome following ureteroscopic laser lithotripsy. *Urolithiasis* **2018**, *46*, 375–381. [CrossRef]

36. Martov, A.; Gravas, S.; Etemadian, M.; Unsal, A.; Barusso, G.; D'Addessi, A.; Krambeck, A.; de la Rosette, J.; on behalf of the Clinical Research Office of the Endourological Society Ureteroscopy Study Group. Postoperative infection rates in patients with a negative baseline urine culture undergoing ureteroscopic stone removal: A matched case-control analysis on antibiotic prophylaxis from the CROES URS global study. *J. Endourol.* **2015**, *29*, 171–180. [CrossRef]
37. Moses, R.A.; Agarwal, D.; Raffin, E.P.; Viers, B.R.; Sharma, V.; Krambeck, A.E.; Pais, V.M. Postpercutaneous nephrolithotomy systemic inflammatory response syndrome is not associated with unplanned readmission. *Urology* **2017**, *100*, 33–37. [CrossRef]
38. Akdeniz, E.; Ozturk, K.; Ulu, M.B.; Gur, M.; Caliskan, S.T.; Sehmen, E. Risk factors for systemic inflammatory response syndrome in patients with negative preoperative urine culture after percutaneous nephrolithotomy. *J. Coll. Phys. Surg. Pak.* **2021**, *31*, 410–416.
39. Takenaka, K.; Ogawa, E.; Wada, H.; Hirata, T. Systemic inflammatory response syndrome and surgical stress in thoracic surgery. *J. Crit. Care.* **2006**, *21*, 48–53. [CrossRef] [PubMed]
40. Haga, Y.; Beppu, T.; Doi, K.; Nozawa, F.; Mugita, N.; Ikei, S.; Ogawa, M. Systemic inflammatory response syndrome and organ dysfunction following gastrointestinal surgery. *Crit. Care Med.* **1997**, *25*, 1994–2000. [CrossRef]
41. Becher, R.D.; Hoth, J.J.; Miller, P.R.; Meredith, J.W.; Chang, M.C. Systemic inflammation worsens outcomes in emergency surgical patients. *J. Trauma Acute Care Surg.* **2012**, *72*, 1140–1149. [CrossRef]
42. Smajic, J.; Tupkovic, L.R.; Husic, S.; Avdagic, S.; Hodzic, S.; Imamovic, S. Systemic inflammatory response syndrome in surgical patients. *Med. Arch.* **2018**, *72*, 116–119. [CrossRef]
43. Volpe, A.; Blute, M.L.; Ficarra, V.; Gill, I.S.; Kutikov, A.; Porpiglia, F.; Rogers, C.; Touijer, K.A.; Van Poppel, H.; Thompson, R.H. Renal ischemia and function after partial nephrectomy: A collaborative review of the literature. *Eur. Urol.* **2015**, *68*, 61–74. [CrossRef]
44. Thompson, R.H.; Lane, B.R.; Lohse, C.M.; Leibovich, B.C.; Fergany, A.; Frank, I.; Gill, I.S.; Blute, M.L.; Campbell, S.C. Renal function after partial nephrectomy: Effect of warm ischemia relative to quantity and quality of preserved kidney. *Urology* **2012**, *79*, 356–360. [CrossRef]

**Disclaimer/Publisher's Note:** The statements, opinions and data contained in all publications are solely those of the individual author(s) and contributor(s) and not of MDPI and/or the editor(s). MDPI and/or the editor(s) disclaim responsibility for any injury to people or property resulting from any ideas, methods, instructions or products referred to in the content.

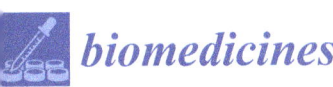 

*Article*

# Role of Nivolumab in the Modulation of PD-1 and PD-L1 Expression in Papillary and Clear Cell Renal Carcinoma (RCC)

Joanna Bialek *, Stefan Yankulov, Felix Kawan, Paolo Fornara and Gerit Theil

Medical Faculty, Clinic of Urology, Martin Luther University Halle-Wittenberg, 06120 Halle (Saale), Germany
* Correspondence: joanna.bialek@uk-halle.de

**Abstract:** The expression and cellular mechanisms of programmed cell death-1 protein (PD-1) and its ligands (PD-L1 and PD-L2) in renal cancer cells are not well known. Here, we aimed to investigate the response of renal carcinoma subtypes to the immune checkpoint inhibitor nivolumab and its impact on related signaling pathways. All cell lines analyzed (clear cell (cc)RCC (Caki-1, RCC31) and papillary (p)RCC (ACHN, RCC30)) expressed PD-1 and both ccRCC cell lines, and RCC30 expressed PD-L1. Nivolumab treatment at increasing doses led to increased PD-1 levels in analyzed cells and resulted in aggressive behavior of pRCC but diminished this behavior in ccRCC. The analysis of PD-1/PD-L1-associated signaling pathways demonstrated increased AKT activity in Caki-1 and RCC30 cells but decreased activity in ACHN and RCC31 cells, while ribosomal protein S6 remained largely unchanged. Androgen receptors are related to RCC and were predominantly increased in RCC30 cells, which were the only cells that formed nivolumab-dependent spheroids. Finally, all cell lines exhibited a complex response to nivolumab treatment. Since the pRCC cells responded with increased tumorigenicity and PD-1/PD-L1 levels while ccRCC tumorigenicity was diminished, further studies are needed to improve nivolumab-based therapy for renal carcinoma subtypes, especially the identification of response-involved molecular pathways.

**Keywords:** renal carcinoma; RCC; PD-1; PD-L1; nivolumab

## 1. Introduction

Kidney cancer is one of the most common cancers, as more than 403,000 new cases are diagnosed each year, which accounts for 2.2% of all newly diagnosed cancers worldwide [1]. The two most common variants, clear cell renal cell carcinoma (ccRCC) and papillary renal cell carcinoma (pRCC), originate from proximal tubule epithelial cells and display morphological differences [2,3]. The clinical prognosis of patients with pRCC is better than that of patients with ccRCC, who may develop metastasis to the lung, liver, bones or lymph nodes [2,3].

Tumor expansion is complex. The development of immune checkpoint inhibitors (ICIs) has transformed therapeutic options in oncology by inhibiting the survival of tumor cells through the escape from immunological destruction. Nivolumab, an agent that blocks the interaction between PD-1 and its ligands (PD-L1 and PD-L2), is approved for the treatment of many cancers, including renal carcinoma (RCC). As with other therapies, many patients experience a good quality of life during treatment; however, some patients can experience immune-related adverse events, which can induce atypical responses, such as hyperprogressive disease or pseudoprogressive disease, and increase the mortality risk [4–6]. To improve quality of life, the efficacy of combined therapy (example TKI/PD-1/PD-L1) was tested [7].

For a long time, it was believed that the PD-1 expression was limited to mature cytotoxic T lymphocytes, while its ligands were primarily expressed by tumors. Recently, Wang et al. [8] described an analysis of the intrinsic expression of PD-1 in different tumors, including renal carcinoma. Little information has been reported on the signaling pathways

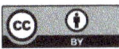

of PD-1/PD-L1 molecules. As reviewed by Han et al. [9], the silencing of cell-intrinsic PD-1 results in higher proliferation of the non-small cell lung cancer cell lines NCI-H1299 and Calu-1 as well as increased phosphorylation of protein kinase B (AKT) (p-AKT) and extracellular-signal regulated kinase (ERK1/2) (p-ERK). This suggests the involvement of pathways similar to those of T-cells [8] and indicates that intrinsic PD-1 is a potential tumor suppressor [9]. In melanoma cells, PD-L1 signaling is correlated with AKT and S6 protein phosphorylation, which suggests the activation of the mTOR pathway.

The incidence of RCC is higher in men than in women, which implies the participation of steroid hormones in tumor development. It has been suggested that supportive treatment based on steroid receptor signaling pathways should be considered for renal carcinoma [10]. Expression of androgen receptor (AR) was analyzed in many tumors [11–16] supplying information about tumor growth, survival time [12] and advancement for antiandrogen therapy [17]. The relationship between AR and RCCs was analyzed in many studies. Among others, AR has been considered as a marker of indolent RCC and is associated with tumor-suppressive activity [10]. However, its role in RCC is still controversial. In their review, Czarnecka et al. [10] discuss the utility of AR in the prognosis, diagnosis and treatment of RCC. The authors describe AR as a favorable marker in RCC that is correlated with a low stage or grade as well as with primary tumor tissues rather than metastases. However, many reports present opposed results [18–20]. In our previous studies, we found that AR was differentially expressed in different types of RCC [21].

In many gender disparity tumors, such as HCC or thyroid, AR bind the PD-L1 promotor and so downregulates PD-L1 expression [22,23]. Guan et al. [24] noted that blocking AR and PD-L1 correlated with a reduction in prostate tumor growth, which provides a connection between androgens and therapy resistance. Additionally, cathepsin B (Cath B) is correlated with therapy resistance [25], and overexpression of this protease is associated with invasive phenotypes of many cancers [26]; moreover, this protein has been demonstrated to have a tumor-protective role [27]. This is why its expression was analyzed as a marker of the effectiveness of several therapies [26].

In our study, we investigated the expression of PD-1 and PD-L1 in two ccRCC and two pRCC cell lines and the functional response of these cells to the immune checkpoint inhibitor nivolumab. Furthermore, we tested the expression of proteins such as AR as well as the typical ones of signaling pathways that were previously identified as related to PD-1/PD-L1 cascades.

## 2. Materials and Methods

### 2.1. Cell Culture

The human papillary renal carcinoma cell line ACHN and the ccRCC cell line Caki-1 obtained from American Type Culture Collection (ATCC, Manassas, VA, USA) were cultured in RPMI medium (Life Technologies Europe B.V., Bleiswijk, The Netherlands); the cell lines established from RCC tissues (the papillary RCC30 cell line and the clear cell RCC31 cell line) were obtained from the Institute of Medical Immunology MLU Halle and were cultured in glucose-high DMEM (Life Technologies). All media were enriched with 10% fetal calf serum (FCS) (Capricorn Scientific GmbH, Ebsdorfergrund, Germany), and the primary RCCs were enriched with MEM Non-Essential Amino Acid Solution (Gibco/Life Technologies Europe B.V.). All cells were cultured at an early passage. The cells were passaged every 4–5 days, and the culture medium was changed every 2–3 days. Prior to experiments, the cells were seeded in 6- or 96-well plates (Sarstedt, Nümbrecht, Germany) and allowed to adhere for 24 h. For each experiment, the cells were incubated with increasing concentrations of nivolumab (0, 12, 24, 36, 48 or 72 µg/mL), which should correspond to the monotherapy used as second-line therapy for RCC. Our experiments were performed in a monoculture (immune-independent conditions). The initial nivolumab concentration corresponds with that used in patients. Higher levels of the ICI were used to test the signals in cancer cells.

## 2.2. RNA Isolation/RT- and q-PCR

After one day of growth in 6-well plates (Sarstedt), the cells ($1 \times 10^6$) were incubated with nivolumab (OPDIVO, Bristol-Myers Squibb, Berlin, Germany) (0, 12, 24, 36, 48, 72 µg/mL) for 24 or 48 h. Subsequently, all cells were scraped off, and RNA was isolated using an RNA isolation kit (RNeasy Plus Mini Kit, Qiagen, Hilden, Germany). cDNA was synthesized using a SuperScript IV VILO Master Mix (Thermo Fisher, Dreieich, Germany) kit at 42 °C for 15 min according to the manufacturer's instructions. Quantitative PCR (qPCR) was performed using 5× Hot FirePol Eva Green qPCR Mix Plus (Solis Biodyne, Tartu, Estonia) in a QuantStudio5 Thermocycler (Thermo Fisher Scientific, Waltham, MA, USA). The expression of the target genes was analyzed using specific primers, and β-actin served as an endogenous control (Table 1). The results were calculated using the $2^{-\Delta\Delta CT}$ method.

**Table 1.** Primers used in qPCR. (*—[28], **—[29]).

| Target | Primer | Product Length (bp) |
|---|---|---|
| AR-FL * | F: CAGCCTATTGCGAGAGAGCTG<br>R: GAAAGGATCTTGGGCACTTGC | 73 |
| AR-V1 | F: AGGGAAAAAGGGCCGAGCTA<br>R: TCCTCCGAGTCTTTAGCAGC | 185 |
| AR-V3 | F: AAGAGCCGCTGAAGGGAAAC<br>R: AGGCAAGTCAGCCTTTCTTCA | 199 |
| AR-V4 | F: CTCTCAGCTGCTCATCCACA<br>R: GGTTTTCAAATGCAGCCAGGA | 74 |
| AR-V7 ** | F: AAAAGAGCCGCTGAAGGGAA<br>R: GCCAACCCGGAATTTTTCTCC | 150 |
| β-Actin | F: ATTGCCGACAGGATGCAGAA<br>R: GCTGATCCACATCTGCTGGAA | 150 |

## 2.3. Western Blot Analysis

A total of 10 µg of protein isolated with RIPA buffer (Cell Signaling, Leiden, The Netherlands) was separated in 4–12% polyacrylamide gels (Thermo Fisher), followed by a 1 h transfer at 350 mA 4 °C. The membranes were incubated in blocking solution (5% BSA/TBS-T 0.01%) for 1 h and with the primary monoclonal antibodies (PD-1, PD-L1, AKT, pAKT, S6 and pS6 rabbit antibodies all from Cell Signaling; β-actin (mouse) from Sigma, Burlington, MA, USA) overnight at 4 °C. The membranes were then incubated with the corresponding secondary antibodies (peroxidase-labeled anti-rabbit or anti-mouse antibodies) for 1 h at room temperature. The bands were visualized with Lumi-Light Western Blotting Substrate (Roche, Manheim, Germany) in a ChemiDoc™ Touch Imaging System (Bio-Rad, Feldkirchen, Germany).

## 2.4. Cell Viability Assay

One day after the cells ($1 \times 10^4$/well) were seeded in a 96-well plate (Sarstedt), the growth medium was exchanged for medium containing increasing concentrations of nivolumab (0, 12, 24, 36, 48, 72 µg/mL) after which the cells were cultured for 24 or 48 h. A WST assay (Merck/Sigma) was performed according to the manufacturer's instructions. After 4 h of incubation at 37 °C, the absorbance was measured at 450 nm using a Cytation5 instrument (Agilent Technologies, Waldbronn, Germany).

## 2.5. Scratch Assay

We seeded the cells in a 6-well plate and allowed them to grow until confluent. The monolayer was scratched with a sterile 100 µL pipette tip in the center of the well, and the growth medium was discarded. After gentle washing in PBS (Sigma), the cells were incubated with a control medium or a medium containing different concentrations of nivolumab (12, 24, 36, 48, 72 µg/mL). The 24 h assay was performed with a Cytation5 instrument (Agilent Technologies), and images were obtained every 2 min. After one day, the final images were analyzed.

### 2.6. Spheroid Formation

The 3D culture was initiated using $1 \times 10^4$ cells/well in a nonadherent round-bottom 96-well plate (Sarstedt). The control medium and medium enriched with nivolumab were changed every 4–5 days. Spheroid formation was observed for 6 weeks. Images and spheroid measurements were performed using a Cytation5 reader (Agilent Technologies). The aggregates were considered spheroids if they displayed visible 3D structures.

### 2.7. Cath B Activity

Cath B activity was measured using a fluorometric Cathepsin B Activity Assay Kit (Abcam, Berlin, Germany). All cells ($1 \times 10^5$/well) were seeded in 6-well plates (Sarstedt) and treated with increasing concentrations of nivolumab the following day. After 24 h of incubation, the cells were harvested, washed in PBS (Sigma) and resuspended in chilled Cell Lysis Buffer (4 °C), which was included in the kit, for 30 min, followed by centrifugation at 4 °C for 5 min. The activity was measured in the supernatant according to the manufacturer's instructions. The output was measured using a Cytation5 reader (Agilent Technologies) at Ex/Em = 400/505 nm.

## 3. Results

### 3.1. Intrinsic Expression of PD-1 and PD-L1

We first analyzed the expression of PD-1 and PD-L1 in all four RCC cell lines. The Western blots performed on cell lysates revealed bands with a size of approximately 55 kDa, which corresponds to PD-1, and >55 kDa, corresponding to PD-L1 (Figure 1). We observed an increase in the PD-1 expression in papillary cell lines after nivolumab treatment. The expression of PD-L1 was either weak (RCC30) or absent (ACHN). In ccRCC cells, the PD-L1 expression was increased after treatment with low concentrations of nivolumab (12–36 µg/mL) and was decreased after treatment with higher concentrations (48–72 µg/mL). PD-1 expression was increased in both ccRCC—Caki-1 (24–36 µg/mL) and RCC31 (24–48 µg/mL) cells and was decreased with the highest nivolumab concentrations, while in pRCCs was increased.

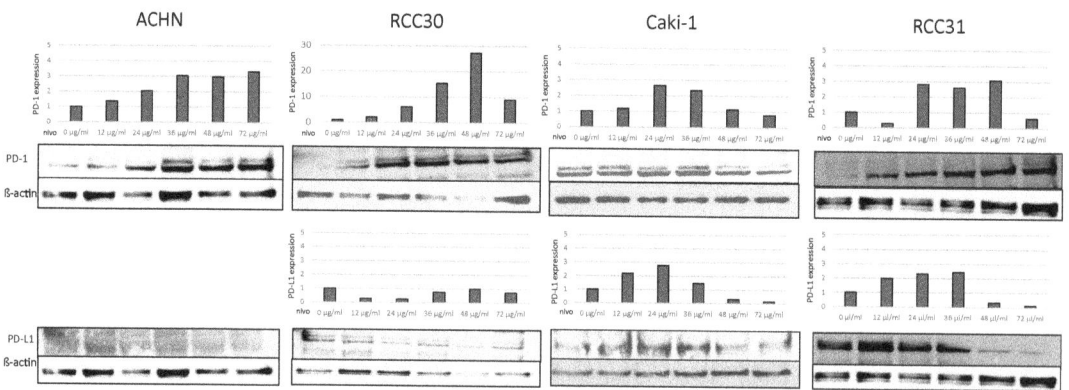

**Figure 1.** Expression of PD-1 and PD-L1 in renal carcinoma cell lines. Caki-1, RCC30, RCC31, but not ACHN cells, expressed PD-L1 when PD-1 was expressed in these cells.

## 3.2. AKT and S6 Activation

We analyzed the expression of phosphorylated (p) and total (t) AKT and S6 (Figure 2). We considered the relationship between p and t (p/t) as an indicator of protein activation. Papillary cell lines (ACHN, RCC30) reacted positively at low concentrations of nivolumab, while increasing amounts decreased AKT activity. The results obtained for ccRCC cells are inconsistent. AKT activity was increased under the influence of nivolumab in Caki-1 cells, while this activity was decreased in RCC31 cells. In addition, besides the increase induced in Caki-1 cells, no significant differences were observed in S6 protein activation.

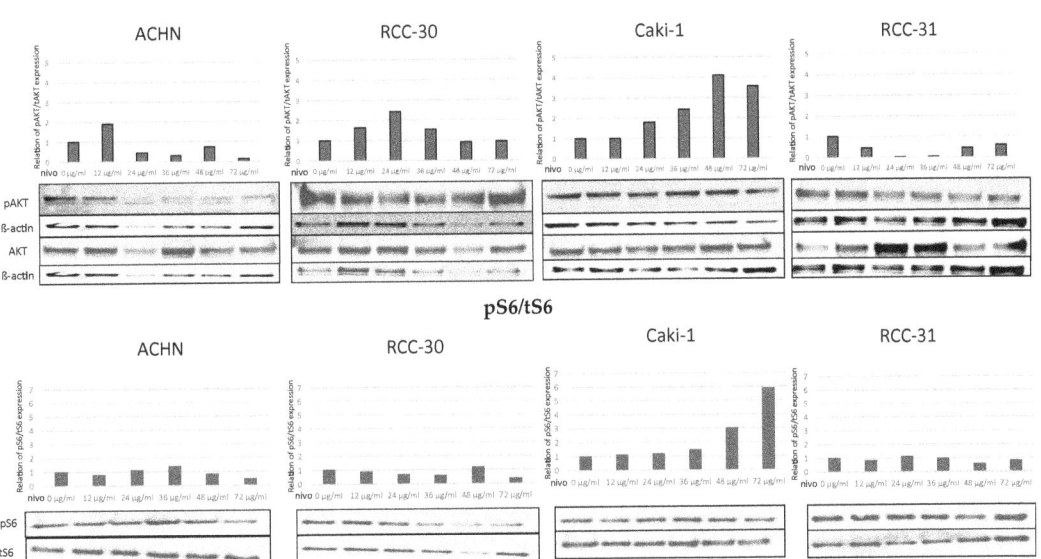

**Figure 2.** Status of AKT and S6 activation. The relationship between p/t expression of tAKT and pAKT as well as S6/pS6 in RCC cell lines was defined as the protein activation status.

## 3.3. Contribution of Nivolumab to Metabolic Activity

Using a WST assay, we analyzed the influence of nivolumab on the viability of renal carcinoma cells. The results revealed a significant response of ACHN and Caki-1 cells after 24 h (Figure 3a–d), while the tissue-derived cell lines reacted after 48 h (Figure 3e–h). Both papillary cell lines (ACHN, RCC30) responded with an increase in metabolic activity in the presence of nivolumab (Figure 3a,f). The increasing trend in ACHN cells was noted at all concentrations; however, significant differences were observed at concentrations of 36 μg/mL and 72 μg/mL (both $p > 0.05$) (Figure 3a). RCC30 cells responded with a significant increase in metabolic activity at concentrations of 24 μg/mL and 36 μg/mL ($p > 0.05$), while higher concentrations decreased the metabolic activity to the baseline level (Figure 3f). Notably, nivolumab diminished the metabolic activity of ccRCC cell lines only at higher concentrations (Figure 3c,h). Caki-1 cells exhibited significant differences at 48 μg/mL ($p > 0.05$) and 72 μg/mL ($p > 0.001$) (Figure 3c), while RCC31 cells exhibited significant differences at only 72 μg/mL ($p > 0.05$ and 0.01) (Figure 3h).

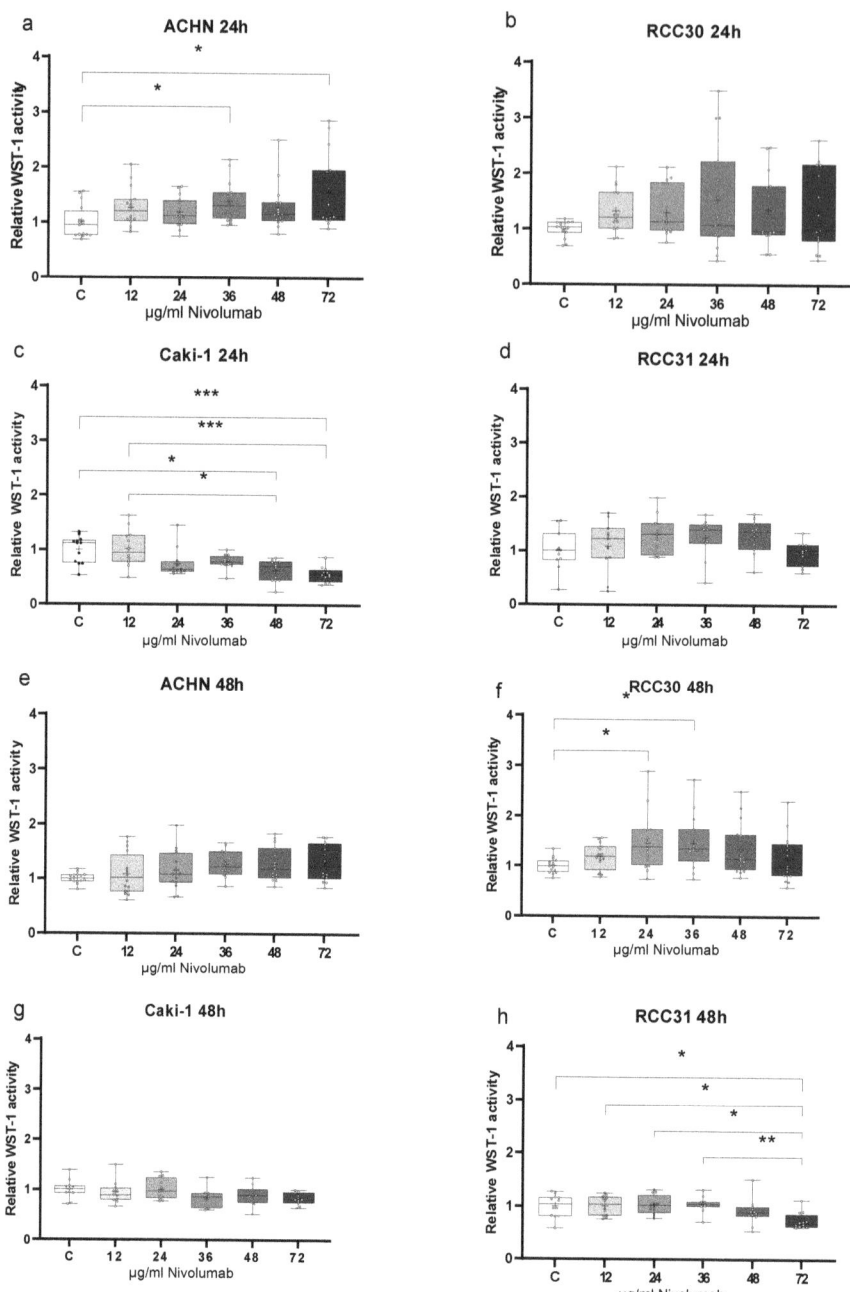

**Figure 3.** Metabolic activity of renal carcinoma cell lines. WST-1 activity was measured after 24 h (**a–d**) and 48 h (**e–h**) in papillary (**a,b,e,f**) and clear cell (**c,d,g,h**) renal carcinoma cells. * $\leq 0.05$, ** $\leq 0.01$, *** $\leq 0.001$.

## 3.4. Motility of Renal Carcinoma Cell Lines

Scratch assays were performed to examine the influence of nivolumab on cell motility. As demonstrated in Figure 4, ACHN cells reacted to the treatment by almost complete closure of the scratched area (Figure 4). The primary cell line RCC30 partially responded with increased cell motility after treatment with low concentrations of nivolumab (12–36 µg/mL). Differences in the responses of Caki-1 and RCC31 cells were not detected (not shown).

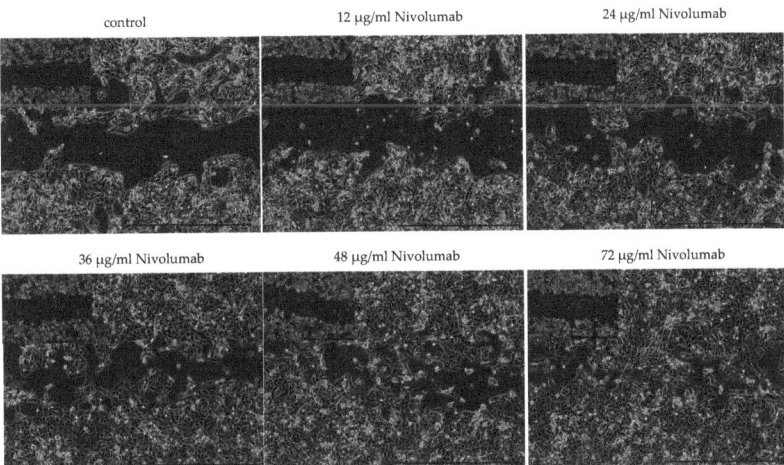

**Figure 4.** Motility of ACHN cells treated with nivolumab for 24 h; scale bars 1000 µm.

## 3.5. Spheroid Formation

The only cell line that formed spheroids upon nivolumab treatment was RCC30 (Figure 5a–c). The spheroids were detected at every concentration of nivolumab as well as in the control group. The numbers of spheroids in the control group and in the group treated with 72 µg/mL nivolumab were similar at 212 and 230, respectively, while the numbers were higher at concentrations of 12 µg/mL (390 spheroids), 24 µg/mL (381 spheroids) and 48 µg/mL (380 spheroids) (Figure 5a). The highest number (495) of spheroids was observed at 36 µg/mL nivolumab. Most spheroids in each group were relatively small, reaching up to 100 µm in diameter. The highest number of them was observed at a concentration of 36 µg/mL nivolumab (335 spheroids) compared with the control (130 spheroids). It is worth noting that spheroids greater than 400 µm were formed only at concentrations that ranged from 24–48 µg/mL (Figure 5a). During the six weeks, ACHN, Caki-1 and RCC31 cells formed aggregates of similar size but not regular spheroids, which were independent of nivolumab concentration.

## 3.6. Cath B Expression and Activity

Nivolumab did not influence the expression of Cath B in any of the cell lines (not shown). We analyzed the activity of Cath B by normalizing the results after employing the specific inhibitor (included in the kit) and defining its results as "1". Cath B activity was detected in three (RCC30, Caki-1 and RCC31) of four cell lines. The ACHN cell line showed levels equal to when the inhibitor was used. Exposure to nivolumab for 24 h had no significant influence on Cath B activity (Figure 6).

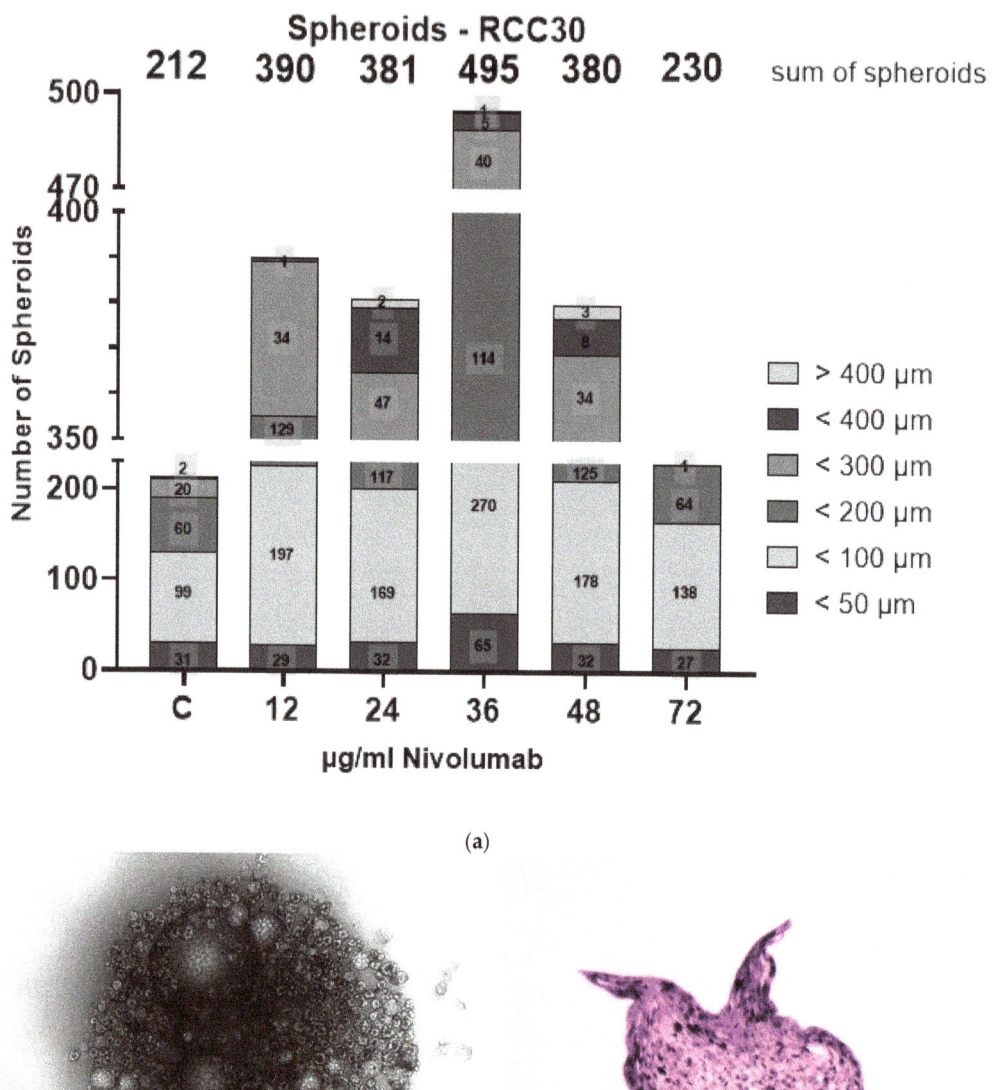

**Figure 5.** 3D culture under nivolumab treatment. Number of spheroids formed by the RCC30 cell line (a). Spheroids formed by the RCC30 cell line under bright field microscopy; the scale bar: 1000 µm (b) and after HE staining; the scale bar: 100 µm (c) at a concentration of 36 µg/mL nivolumab.

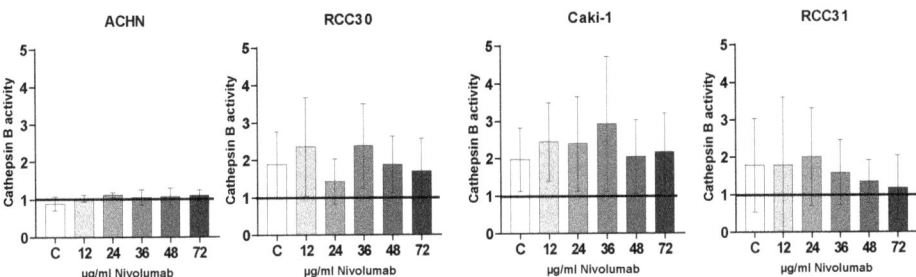

**Figure 6.** Cath B in RCC cells. Cath B activity after incubation with increasing concentrations of nivolumab. The activity in each cell line after using a specific inhibitor was defined as "1".

*3.7. AR Expression*

In our study, we noticed differences with regard to tumor type, as papillary tumor cells showed a higher expression of AR-FL (full length) and AR-SVs (splice variants) than ccRCC cells (Figure 7). Considering the results of the most well studied variants AR-FL and AR-V7 obtained in naïve cells, AR-FL was detected only in primary cells, while AR-V7 SV was present in ccRCC cells only. The three additional variants displayed similar patterns among all tested cell lines, with minimal detection of AR-V1, higher AR-V3 and the highest detection of AR-V4. Generally, except for the primary papillary RCC30 cell line, the expression of all ARs was weak in all tested cell lines (not shown). Incubation with increasing concentrations of nivolumab did not influence AR expression.

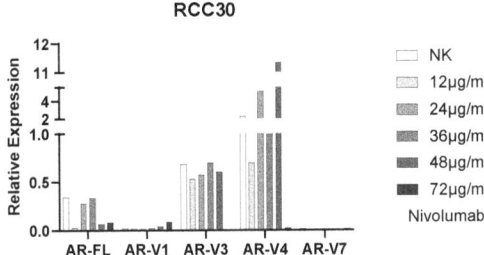

**Figure 7.** Expression of AR-FL and AR-SVs in RCC30 cells.

## 4. Discussion

This study clearly demonstrated the effects and pathways that might be involved in the response to nivolumab treatment in clear cell and papillary RCC cell lines. In an immune-independent manner, we observed that, in contrast to clear cell RCC cells, papillary RCC cells responded to nivolumab with increased aggressive behavior manifested as a dose-dependent response, higher motility and higher metabolic rates.

Treatment of RCC patients is a challenge because approximately one-third of RCC patients already present with metastasis at the initial diagnosis. After surgical resection, another one-third experience recurrence with distant metastases [3]. The management of ccRCC patients with immunotherapies shows positive effects, but knowledge of advances in nonclear cell RCC is limited.

The indication for nivolumab immune therapy is PD-L1 expression. However, the phase 3 CheckMate 025 trial demonstrated that even if the expression of PD-L1 ($\geq 1\%$) in RCC is associated with poorer survival, the benefit of therapy is independent of PD-L1 status. The PD-L1 as a marker for the treatment outcomes seems to be dependent on tumor type or histologic class [30].

PD-1 was described for the first time in murine hematopoietic progenitor and murine T-hybridoma cell lines in 1992 [31]. As reviewed by Han et al. [9], this immune response inhibitor is present in activated T-cells, natural killer cells and B lymphocytes as well as macrophages, dendritic cells and monocytes. PD-1 binds PD-L1 on cancer cells and initiates the immune escape of tumor cells. This process can be blocked with immune checkpoint inhibitors, such as nivolumab, which bind PD-1 and prevent the interaction with PD-L1.

Recently, intrinsic tumor expression of PD-1 was described in various cancer cells [32–34], including renal cancer [8]. Wang et al. [8] demonstrated PD-1 transcripts in four renal cancer cell lines (ACHN, Caki-1, 769-P, 786-O). In our study, we observed PD-1 protein in ACHN and Caki-1 cells as well as in the two in-house established cell lines RCC30 (pRCC) and RCC31 (ccRCC).

In papillary RCC, PD-1 expression is constant when PD-L1 expression is weak (RCC30) or absent (ACHN). In contrast, the clear cell carcinoma cell lines Caki-1 and RCC31 strongly express both proteins. Our study shows that exposure of tumor cells to increasing concentrations of nivolumab seems to downregulate the PD-1 expression and partially downregulate PD-L1 in ccRCC, but seems to increase PD-1 expression in pRCC. This partly coincides with our analysis of the metabolic activity in cells treated with nivolumab. At high concentrations, we observed a reduction in WST-1 generation in ccRCC cells but an increase in pRCC cells. The results obtained in our study suggest the activation of intrinsic PD-1 without the necessary involvement of PD-L1 in papillary RCCs. This lead probably to the initiation of still not known signaling cascades, which induce aggressive behavior of the cells. Lately, the results of open-label phase IIIb/IV CheckMate 374 study established monotherapy with nivolumab as the treatment option for advanced nccRCC. From the pRCC patients of the cohort and only one demonstrated partial response (PR), 9—stable disease but 11—progressive disease [35]. In other studies, in combination with ipilimumab treatment (anti-CTLA-4 antibody) also only 1/18 pRCC patients responded complete (CR) for the treatment, when 4/18 were PR [36]. Du et al. [33] observed that the NSCLC cell line M109 xenotransplanted into mice demonstrated increased viability associated with exposure to anti-PD-1 blockade. Kleffel et al. [32] and Wang et al. [8], however, noticed suppression of melanoma and lung tumor cell growth, respectively, after antibody blockade. Interestingly, the PD-1 protein differed significantly in the size and number of detected bands (~55 kDa [8] and ~32 kDa [32]) between the two studies.

The results of Denize et al. [37] raise the possibility that PD-L1 expression in ccRCC cancer cells might require intrinsic pro-oncogenic signals from tumor cells. When coexpressed in tumors, PD-L1 can activate intrinsic PD-1 in an immune-independent manner and thus modulate signaling cascades in tumor cells [38]. Considering the differential intrinsic expression and potentially differential PD-1/PD-L1 interaction intensity within the two (clear and papillary) types of renal carcinoma, one could speculate the activation of different signaling pathways (PI3K/AKT, MAPK, mTOR).

The PI3K/AKT/mTOR signaling pathway is implicated in the development of many human malignancies, including RCC [37]. The PD-1/PD-L1 cascade is thought to be involved in the initiation of mTOR signaling. Intrinsic PD-1, activated by PD-L1, activates mTOR [38], while the inhibition of mTOR increases the level of PD-L1 [39]. Kleffel et al. [32] also demonstrated a positive influence of PD-1 on the phosphorylation of ribosomal protein S6 (RPS6), a downstream signaling target of mTOR and marker of its activity, which is associated with poor prognosis in renal cancer [40] and many other cancers [41,42]. In our study, nivolumab did not change the level of pS6 in three cell lines. We detected higher S6 activity levels after nivolumab treatment only in Caki-1 cells. Moreover, contrary to PD-L1 and PD-1 expression, the increase in S6 was noticed at higher concentrations of nivolumab treatment. Additionally, we could not detect PD-L1 protein in the ACHN cell line in the presence of pS6 and increasing levels of PD-1. To implicate this signaling pathway in the treatment of RCC, additional investigations, such as determining the PD-L1 promoter activity or the perturbance of PD-L1 degradation, are planned.

The analysis of AKT activity revealed that in ACHN cells, the ratio of pAKT/AKT was decreased, while in Caki-1 cells, this ratio was elevated. The significance of AKT activity in tumor development is controversial. Since some investigators indicate a relationship between pAKT, poor differentiation and lymph node (LN) metastasis [43], others provide evidence for the association of pAKT with high differentiation and no LN metastasis [44]. In addition, the correlation of pAKT with PD-1 was also investigated. Wang et al. [8] observed an increase in pAKT after the knockdown of PDCD1 (PD-1 coding gene) and a decrease after overexpression by stable phosphorylation of the S6 protein.

In their analysis of diffuse large B-cell lymphoma (DLBCL), Dong et al. [45] described a correlation between PD-L1 and pAKT expression with clinicopathological characteristics. The detection of both proteins in tumors significantly reduced the positive prognosis of the patients compared with patients whose tumors expressed only one of the proteins. The authors suggest using a combination of PD-1/PD-L1 antibodies together with AKT/mTOR inhibitors as a novel therapeutic approach for DLBCL. In our study, three cell lines (Caki-1, RCC30 and RCC31) express both proteins when by ACHN PD-L1 is absent.

In their manuscript, Guan et al. [24] proposed that androgens may be responsible for therapy resistance in advanced prostate cancer patients. This hypothesis is based on the observation that the blockade of both AR and PD-L1 reduces tumor growth and that the inhibition of AR improves T-cell function. Our previous analysis showed differences in the frequency of AR-FL expression and that of its splice variant between ccRCC and normal tissues. We also observed an increased AR expression in pRCC compared with ccRCC [21]. Our current study confirms this observation but only for the in-house established cell lines. In our case, the cell line with the highest AR expression was pRCC30.

In further experiments, we tested the abilities of the cell lines to form aggregates. Both clear-cell carcinoma cells and ACHN cells formed masses with low cell-cell adhesion, but only RCC30 cells formed spheroids whose growth was dependent on nivolumab. In 2D culture, RCC30 displayed higher expression of AR than the other cell lines. However, still no evidence indicates a relationship between AR and spheroid formation. Nevertheless, Niture et al. [46] described an increased ability of prostate cancer cells to create spheroids after microRNA-99b-5p silencing, which was accompanied by the upregulation of the AR axis. However, the relationship between AR expression and spheroid formation remains open. Another aspect is that the growth of cells in a 3D structure may enforce morphological and transcriptional changes or hinder the diffusion of nutrients or drugs (such as nivolumab), which can influence protein expression. These questions require further investigation. Transcriptome analysis of the treated spheroids is the next step to analyze the influence of nivolumab on RCC cells.

As mentioned previously, some patients treated with an immune checkpoint inhibitor (ICI) therapy experience immune-related adverse events (irAEs), which can induce atypical responses, such as hyperprogressive disease (HPD) or pseudoprogressive disease [4–6]. A protein implicated in the prevention of the cytotoxic effects of many drugs is cathepsin B [47]. Increased expression of cathepsin B in RCC indicates its role in tumor progression [48]. Our results show that even if Cath B is expressed and active (except in ACHN cells) in RCC, nivolumab did not influence the expression or activity of this protein. This suggests its limited role in processes initiated by this immune checkpoint inhibitor blockade.

According to the S3 guideline renal cell carcinoma (S3-Leitlinie Nierenzellkarzinom) and international guidelines [49] nivolumab can be used as the first-line medicament in combination with other medicaments (ipilimumab, cabozantinib) or as the second-line therapy after the failure of the VEGF/R- or mTOR-based treatment. It is known that VEGFR TKIs affect the protein expression pattern of tumor cells [25] and metabolic cargo and activity in small extracellular vesicles of RCC [50]. Chen et al. [25] describe increased Cath B expression as a response to TKI. In our study with nivolumab, we did not notice any changes in Cath B expression. Our analysis, however, was performed as a simulation of the monotherapy without previous treatment. It is an intriguing question if previous treatment of our cells with TKI would induce similar changes and if further incubation or coincubation with nivoumab would reduce such differences. This question should be addressed in future studies.

## 5. Conclusions

This study clearly shows the intrinsic expression of PD-1 and PD-L1 in clear cell and papillary RCCs and their complex response to nivolumab treatment. Since pRCC cells reacted with elevated tumorigenicity and augmented PD-1/PD-L1 levels and ccRCC reacted with decreased tumorigenicity, further improvements in nivolumab-based therapy for renal carcinoma are needed.

## 6. Limitations

We must address some limitations to our study. Our analysis was performed in vitro, using commercial and in-house established cell lines. For a better validation of our results, the analysis of probes from patients treated with nivolumab with a combination of other medicaments or as the second-line monotherapy should be performed. To implicate signaling pathways in the treatment of RCC, additional investigations, such as determining the PD-L1 promoter activity or the perturbance of PD-L1 degradation, are planned.

**Author Contributions:** Conceptualization, J.B. and G.T.; methodology, J.B.; validation, S.Y. and F.K.; formal analysis, J.B.; investigation, J.B.; writing—original draft preparation, J.B.; writing—review and editing, J.B., G.T. and P.F. All authors have read and agreed to the published version of the manuscript.

**Funding:** This research received no external funding.

**Institutional Review Board Statement:** Not applicable.

**Informed Consent Statement:** Not applicable.

**Data Availability Statement:** Not applicable.

**Conflicts of Interest:** The authors declare no conflict of interest.

## References

1. Bray, F.; Ferlay, J.; Soerjomataram, I.; Siegel, R.L.; Torre, L.A.; Jemal, A. Global cancer statistics 2018: GLOBOCAN estimates of incidence and mortality worldwide for 36 cancers in 185 countries. *CA Cancer J. Clin.* **2018**, *68*, 394–424. [CrossRef] [PubMed]
2. Muglia, V.F.; Prando, A. Renal cell carcinoma: Histological classification and correlation with imaging findings. *Radiol. Bras.* **2015**, *48*, 166–174. [CrossRef] [PubMed]
3. Ciarimboli, G.; Theil, G.; Bialek, J.; Edemir, B. Contribution and expression of organic cation transporters and aquaporin water channels in renal cancer. *Rev. Physiol. Biochem. Pharmacol.* **2020**, *181*, 81–104. [CrossRef]
4. Johnson, D.B.; Sullivan, R.J.; Menzies, A.M. Immune checkpoint inhibitors in challenging populations. *Cancer* **2017**, *123*, 1904–1911. [CrossRef] [PubMed]
5. Ferrara, R.; Mezquita, L.; Texier, M.; Lahmar, J.; Audigier-Valette, C.; Tessonnier, L.; Mazieres, J.; Zalcman, G.; Brosseau, S.; Le Moulec, S.; et al. Hyperprogressive disease in patients with advanced non-small cell lung cancer treated with PD-1/PD-L1 inhibitors or with single-agent chemotherapy. *JAMA Oncol.* **2018**, *4*, 1543–1552. [CrossRef]
6. Kurman, J.S.; Murgu, S.D. Hyperprogressive disease in patients with non-small cell lung cancer on immunotherapy. *J. Thorac. Dis.* **2018**, *10*, 1124–1128. [CrossRef] [PubMed]
7. Dong, Q.; Diao, Y.; Sun, X.; Zhou, Y.; Ran, J.; Zhang, J. Evaluation of tyrosine kinase inhibitors combined with antiprogrammed cell death protein 1 antibody in tyrosine kinase inhibitor-responsive patients with microsatellite stable/proficient mismatch repair metastatic colorectal adenocarcinoma: Protocol for open-label, single-arm trial. *BMJ Open* **2022**, *12*, e049992. [CrossRef] [PubMed]
8. Wang, X.; Yang, X.; Zhang, C.; Wang, Y.; Cheng, T.; Duan, L.; Tong, Z.; Tan, S.; Zhang, H.; Saw, P.E.; et al. Tumor cell-intrinsic PD-1 receptor is a tumor suppressor and mediates resistance to PD-1 blockade therapy. *Proc. Natl. Acad. Sci. USA* **2020**, *117*, 6640–6650. [CrossRef]
9. Han, Y.; Liu, D.; Li, L. PD-1/PD-L1 pathway: Current researches in cancer. *Am. J. Cancer Res.* **2020**, *10*, 727–742.
10. Czarnecka, A.M.; Niedzwiedzka, M.; Porta, C.; Szczylik, C. Hormone signaling pathways as treatment targets in renal cell cancer (Review). *Int. J. Oncol.* **2016**, *48*, 2221–2235. [CrossRef]
11. Pisano, C.; Tucci, M.; Di Stefano, R.F.; Turco, F.; Scagliotti, G.V.; Di Maio, M.; Buttigliero, C. Interactions between androgen receptor signaling and other molecular pathways in prostate cancer progression: Current and future clinical implications. *Crit. Rev. Oncol. Hematol.* **2021**, *157*, 103185. [CrossRef]
12. Boorjian, S.; Ugras, S.; Mongan, N.P.; Gudas, L.J.; You, X.; Tickoo, S.K.; Scherr, D.S. Androgen receptor expression is inversely correlated with pathologic tumor stage in bladder cancer. *Urology* **2004**, *64*, 383–388. [CrossRef]
13. Gonzalez, L.O.; Corte, M.D.; Vazquez, J.; Junquera, S.; Sanchez, R.; Alvarez, A.C.; Rodriguez, J.C.; Lamelas, M.L.; Vizoso, F.J. Androgen receptor expresion in breast cancer: Relationship with clinicopathological characteristics of the tumors, prognosis, and expression of metalloproteases and their inhibitors. *BMC Cancer* **2008**, *8*, 149. [CrossRef]

14. Corbishley, T.P.; Iqbal, M.J.; Wilkinson, M.L.; Williams, R. Androgen receptor in human normal and malignant pancreatic tissue and cell lines. *Cancer* **1986**, *57*, 1992–1995. [CrossRef]
15. Zhang, H.; Li, X.X.; Yang, Y.; Zhang, Y.; Wang, H.Y.; Zheng, X.F.S. Significance and mechanism of androgen receptor overexpression and androgen receptor/mechanistic target of rapamycin cross-talk in hepatocellular carcinoma. *Hepatology* **2018**, *67*, 2271–2286. [CrossRef]
16. Zhu, H.; Zhu, X.; Zheng, L.; Hu, X.; Sun, L.; Zhu, X. The role of the androgen receptor in ovarian cancer carcinogenesis and its clinical implications. *Oncotarget* **2017**, *8*, 29395–29405. [CrossRef]
17. Yuan, Y.; Lee, J.S.; Yost, S.E.; Frankel, P.H.; Ruel, C.; Egelston, C.A.; Guo, W.; Gillece, J.D.; Folkerts, M.; Reining, L.; et al. A Phase II Clinical Trial of Pembrolizumab and Enobosarm in Patients with Androgen Receptor-Positive Metastatic Triple-Negative Breast Cancer. *Oncologist* **2021**, *26*, 99-e217. [CrossRef]
18. Bennett, N.C.; Rajandram, R.; Ng, K.L.; Gobe, G.C. Evaluation of steroid hormones and their receptors in development and progression of renal cell carcinoma. *J. Kidney Cancer VHL* **2014**, *1*, 17–25. [CrossRef]
19. Zhu, G.; Liang, L.; Li, L.; Dang, Q.; Song, W.; Yeh, S.; He, D.; Chang, C. The expression and evaluation of androgen receptor in human renal cell carcinoma. *Urology* **2014**, *83*, 510.e19–510.e24. [CrossRef]
20. Langner, C.; Ratschek, M.; Rehak, P.; Schips, L.; Zigeuner, R. Steroid hormone receptor expression in renal cell carcinoma: An immunohistochemical analysis of 182 tumors. *J. Urol.* **2004**, *171*, 611–614. [CrossRef]
21. Bialek, J.; Piwonka, M.; Kawan, F.; Fornara, P.; Theil, G. Differential expression of the androgen receptor, splice variants and relaxin 2 in renal cancer. *Life* **2021**, *11*, 731. [CrossRef] [PubMed]
22. Jiang, G.; Shi, L.; Zheng, X.; Zhang, X.; Wu, K.; Liu, B.; Yan, P.; Liang, X.; Yu, T.; Wang, Y.; et al. Androgen receptor affects the response to immune checkpoint therapy by suppressing PD-L1 in hepatocellular carcinoma. *Aging* **2020**, *12*, 11466–11484. [CrossRef] [PubMed]
23. O'Connell, T.J.; Dadafarin, S.; Jones, M.; Rodríguez, T.; Gupta, A.; Shin, E.; Moscatello, A.; Iacob, C.; Islam, H.; Tiwari, R.K.; et al. Androgen Activity Is Associated With PD-L1 Downregulation in Thyroid Cancer. *Front. Cell Dev. Biol.* **2021**, *9*, 663130. [CrossRef] [PubMed]
24. Guan, X.; Polesso, F.; Wang, C.; Sehrawat, A.; Hawkins, R.M.; Murray, S.E.; Thomas, G.V.; Caruso, B.; Thompson, R.F.; Wood, M.A.; et al. Androgen receptor activity in T cells limits checkpoint blockade efficacy. *Nature* **2022**, *606*, 791–796. [CrossRef] [PubMed]
25. Chen, C.H.; Bhasin, S.; Khanna, P.; Joshi, M.; Joslin, P.M.; Saxena, R.; Amin, S.; Liu, S.; Sindhu, S.; Walker, S.R.; et al. Study of cathepsin B inhibition in VEGFR TKI treated human renal cell carcinoma xenografts. *Oncogenesis* **2019**, *8*, 15. [CrossRef]
26. Gondi, C.S.; Rao, J.S. Cathepsin B as a cancer target. *Expert Opin. Ther. Targets* **2013**, *17*, 281–291. [CrossRef]
27. Shree, T.; Olson, O.C.; Elie, B.T.; Kester, J.C.; Garfall, A.L.; Simpson, K.; Bell-McGuinn, K.M.; Zabor, E.C.; Brogi, E.; Joyce, J.A. Macrophages and cathepsin proteases blunt chemotherapeutic response in breast cancer. *Genes Dev.* **2011**, *25*, 2465–2479. [CrossRef]
28. Antonarakis, S.E.; Lu, C.; Wang, H.; Luber, B.; Nakazawa, M.; Roeser, J.C.; Chen, Y.; Mohammad, T.A.; Chen, Y.; Fedor, H.L.; et al. AR-V7 and resistance to enzalutamide and abiraterone in prostate cancer. *N. Engl. J. Med.* **2014**, *371*, 1028–1038. [CrossRef]
29. Xia, H.; Hu, C.; Bai, S.; Lyu, J.; Zhang, B.Y.; Yu, X.; Zhan, Y.; Zhao, L.; Dong, Y. Raddeanin A down-regulates androgen receptor and its splice variants in prostate cancer. *J. Cell. Mol. Med.* **2019**, *23*, 3656–3664. [CrossRef]
30. Motzer, R.J.; Escudier, B.; McDermott, D.F.; George, S.; Hammers, H.J.; Srinivas, S.; Tykodi, S.S.; Sosman, J.A.; Procopio, G.; Plimack, E.R.; et al. Nivolumab versus everolimus in advanced renal-cell carcinoma. *N. Engl. J. Med.* **2015**, *373*, 1803–1813. [CrossRef]
31. Ishida, Y.; Agata, Y.; Shibahara, K.; Honjo, T. Induced expression of PD-1, a novel member of the immunoglobulin gene superfamily, upon programmed cell death. *EMBO J.* **1992**, *11*, 3887–3895. [CrossRef]
32. Kleffel, S.; Posch, C.; Barthel, S.R.; Mueller, H.; Schlapbach, C.; Guenova, E.; Elco, C.P.; Lee, N.; Juneja, V.R.; Zhan, Q.; et al. Melanoma cell-intrinsic PD-1 receptor functions promote tumor growth. *Cell* **2015**, *162*, 1242–1256. [CrossRef]
33. Du, S.; McCall, N.; Park, K.; Guan, Q.; Fontina, P.; Ertel, A.; Zhan, T.; Dicker, A.P.; Lu, B. Blockade of Tumor-Expressed PD-1 promotes lung cancer growth. *Oncoimmunology* **2018**, *7*, e1408747. [CrossRef]
34. Li, H.; Li, X.; Liu, S.; Guo, L.; Zhang, B.; Zhang, J.; Ye, Q. Programmed cell death-1 (PD-1) checkpoint blockade in combination with a mammalian target of rapamycin inhibitor restrains hepatocellular carcinoma growth induced by hepatoma cell-intrinsic PD-1. *Hepatology* **2017**, *66*, 1920–1933. [CrossRef]
35. Vogelzang, N.J.; Olsen, M.R.; McFarlane, J.J.; Arrowsmith, E.; Bauer, T.M.; Jain, R.K.; Somer, B.; Lam, E.T.; Kochenderfer, M.D.; Molina, A.; et al. Safety and Efficacy of Nivolumab in Patients With Advanced Non-Clear Cell Renal Cell Carcinoma: Results From the Phase IIIb/IV CheckMate 374 Study. *Clin. Genitourin. Cancer* **2020**, *18*, 461–468.e3. [CrossRef]
36. Tykodi, S.S.; Gordan, L.N.; Alter, R.S.; Arrowsmith, E.; Harrison, M.R.; Percent, I.; Singal, R.; Van Veldhuizen, P.; George, D.J.; Hutson, T.; et al. Safety and efficacy of nivolumab plus ipilimumab in patients with advanced non-clear cell renal cell carcinoma: Results from the phase 3b/4 CheckMate 920 trial. *J. Immunother. Cancer* **2022**, *10*, e003844. [CrossRef]
37. Denize, T.; Hou, Y.; Pignon, J.C.; Walton, E.; West, D.J.; Freeman, G.J.; Braun, D.A.; Wu, C.J.; Gupta, S.; Motzer, R.J.; et al. Transcriptomic correlates of tumor cell PD-L1 expression and response to nivolumab monotherapy in metastatic clear cell renal cell carcinoma. *Clin. Cancer Res.* **2022**, *28*, 4045–4055. [CrossRef]

38. Yao, H.; Wang, H.; Li, C.; Fang, J.Y.; Xu, J. Cancer cell-intrinsic PD-1 and implications in combinatorial immunotherapy. *Front. Immunol.* **2018**, *9*, 1774. [CrossRef]
39. Sun, S.Y. Searching for the real function of mTOR signaling in the regulation of PD-L1 expression. *Transl. Oncol.* **2020**, *13*, 100847. [CrossRef]
40. Hager, M.; Haufe, H.; Alinger, B.; Kolbitsch, C. pS6 expression in normal renal parenchyma, primary renal cell carcinomas and their metastases. *Pathol. Oncol. Res.* **2012**, *18*, 277–283. [CrossRef]
41. Jung, E.J.; Suh, J.H.; Kim, W.H.; Kim, H.S. Clinical significance of PI3K/Akt/mTOR signaling in gastric carcinoma. *Int. J. Clin. Exp. Pathol.* **2020**, *13*, 995–1007. [PubMed]
42. Muñoz-Cordero, M.G.; López, F.; García-Inclán, C.; López-Hernández, A.; Potes-Ares, S.; Fernández-Vañes, L.; Llorente, J.L.; Hermsen, M. Predictive value of EGFR-PI3K-pAKT-mTOR-pS6 pathway in sinonasal squamous cell carcinomas. *Acta Otorrinolaringol. Esp. (Engl. Ed.)* **2019**, *70*, 16–24. [CrossRef] [PubMed]
43. Yun, F.; Jia, Y.; Li, X.; Yuan, L.; Sun, Q.; Yu, H.; Shi, L.; Yuan, H. Clinicopathological significance of PTEN and PI3K/AKT signal transduction pathway in non-small cell lung cancer. *Int. J. Clin. Exp. Pathol.* **2013**, *6*, 2112–2120. [PubMed]
44. Mukohara, T.; Kudoh, S.; Matsuura, K.; Yamauchi, S.; Kimura, T.; Yoshimura, N.; Kanazawa, H.; Hirata, K.; Inoue, K.; Wanibuchi, H.; et al. Activated Akt expression has significant correlation with EGFR and TGF-alpha expressions in stage I NSCLC. *Anticancer Res.* **2004**, *24*, 11–17. [PubMed]
45. Dong, L.; Lv, H.; Li, W.; Song, Z.; Li, L.; Zhou, S.; Qiu, L.; Qian, Z.; Liu, X.; Feng, L.; et al. Co-expression of PD-L1 and p-AKT is associated with poor prognosis in diffuse large B-cell lymphoma via PD-1/PD-L1 axis activating intracellular AKT/mTOR pathway in tumor cells. *Oncotarget* **2016**, *7*, 33350–33362. [CrossRef] [PubMed]
46. Niture, S.; Tricoli, L.; Qi, Q.; Gadi, S.; Hayes, K.; Kumar, D. MicroRNA-99b-5p targets mTOR/AR axis, induces autophagy and inhibits prostate cancer cell proliferation. *Tumour Biol.* **2022**, *44*, 107–127. [CrossRef]
47. Mijanović, O.; Branković, A.; Panin, A.N.; Savchuk, S.; Timashev, P.; Ulasov, I.; Lesniak, M.S. Cathepsin B: A sellsword of cancer progression. *Cancer Lett.* **2019**, *449*, 207–214. [CrossRef]
48. Rudzinska-Radecka, M.; Frolova, A.S.; Balakireva, A.V.; Gorokhovets, N.V.; Pokrovsky, V.S.; Sokolova, D.V.; Korolev, D.O.; Potoldykova, N.V.; Vinarov, A.Z.; Parodi, A.; et al. In silico, in vitro, and clinical investigations of cathepsin B and stefin A mRNA expression and a correlation analysis in kidney cancer. *Cells* **2022**, *11*, 1455. [CrossRef]
49. Fontes-Sousa, M.; Magalhães, H.; Oliveira, A.; Carneiro, F.; Dos Reis, F.P.; Madeira, P.S.; Meireles, S. Reviewing Treatment Options for Advanced Renal Cell Carcinoma: Is There Still a Place for Tyrosine Kinase Inhibitor (TKI) Monotherapy? *Adv. Ther.* **2022**, *39*, 1107–1125. [CrossRef]
50. Lim, A.R.; Vincent, B.G.; Weaver, A.M.; Rathmell, W.K. Sunitinib and Axitinib increase secretion and glycolytic activity of small extracellular vesicles in renal cell carcinoma. *Cancer Gene Ther.* **2022**, *29*, 683–696. [CrossRef]

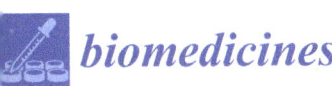 

*Article*

# High Pretreatment Serum PD-L1 Levels Are Associated with Muscle Invasion and Shorter Survival in Upper Tract Urothelial Carcinoma

Ádám Széles [1,2], Petra Terézia Kovács [1], Anita Csizmarik [1], Melinda Váradi [1], Péter Riesz [1], Tamás Fazekas [1,2], Szilárd Váncsa [2,3,4], Péter Hegyi [2,3,4], Csilla Oláh [5], Stephan Tschirdewahn [5], Christopher Darr [5], Ulrich Krafft [5], Viktor Grünwald [5], Boris Hadaschik [5], Orsolya Horváth [6], Péter Nyirády [1] and Tibor Szarvas [1,5,*]

[1] Department of Urology, Semmelweis University, Ulloi ut 78/b, 1082 Budapest, Hungary
[2] Centre for Translational Medicine, Ulloi ut 26, 1085 Budapest, Hungary
[3] Institute for Translational Medicine, Medical School, University of Pécs, Szigeti út 12., 7624 Pécs, Hungary
[4] Division of Pancreatic Diseases, Heart and Vascular Center, Semmelweis University, 1085 Budapest, Hungary
[5] Department of Urology, University of Duisburg-Essen, German Cancer Consortium (DTKK)-University Hospital Essen, Hufelandstraße 55, D-45147 Essen, Germany
[6] Department of Genitourinary Medical Oncology and Clinical Pharmacology, National Institute of Oncology, Ráth György utca 7-9., 1122 Budapest, Hungary
\* Correspondence: szarvas.tibor@med.semmelweis-univ.hu

**Citation:** Széles, Á.; Kovács, P.T.; Csizmarik, A.; Váradi, M.; Riesz, P.; Fazekas, T.; Váncsa, S.; Hegyi, P.; Oláh, C.; Tschirdewahn, S.; et al. High Pretreatment Serum PD-L1 Levels Are Associated with Muscle Invasion and Shorter Survival in Upper Tract Urothelial Carcinoma. *Biomedicines* **2022**, *10*, 2560. https://doi.org/10.3390/biomedicines10102560

Academic Editors: Łukasz Zapała and Paweł Rajwa

Received: 8 September 2022
Accepted: 6 October 2022
Published: 13 October 2022

**Publisher's Note:** MDPI stays neutral with regard to jurisdictional claims in published maps and institutional affiliations.

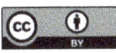

**Copyright:** © 2022 by the authors. Licensee MDPI, Basel, Switzerland. This article is an open access article distributed under the terms and conditions of the Creative Commons Attribution (CC BY) license (https://creativecommons.org/licenses/by/4.0/).

**Simple Summary:** This study aimed to assess the prognostic relevance of soluble serum PD-L1 in upper tract urothelial carcinoma (UTUC) patients who underwent surgical or systemic (chemo- or immune checkpoint inhibitor) therapy. We found that high preoperative sPD-L1 levels were correlated with higher pathological tumor stage, grade and the presence of metastasis. In addition, higher pretreatment serum PD-L1 concentrations were associated with shorter survival in both surgically and chemotherapy-treated UTUC patients. We detected a characteristic increase in serum PD-L1 levels in UTUC patients after 3 months of anti-PD-L1 therapy. Based on these results sPD-L1 is a promising prognostic biomarker in UTUC.

**Abstract:** Programmed death ligand-1 (PD-L1) is an immune checkpoint molecule and a widely used therapeutic target in urothelial cancer. Its circulating, soluble levels (sPD-L1) were recently suggested to be associated with the presence and prognosis of various malignancies but have not yet been investigated in upper tract urothelial carcinoma (UTUC). In this study, we assessed sPD-L1 levels in 97 prospectively collected serum samples from 61 UTUC patients who underwent radical nephroureterectomy (RNU), chemotherapy (CTX), or immune checkpoint inhibitor (ICI) therapy. In addition to pretreatment samples, postoperative and on-treatment sPD-L1 levels were determined in some patients by using ELISA. In the RNU group, elevated preoperative sPD-L1 was associated with a higher tumor grade ($p = 0.019$), stage ($p < 0.001$) and the presence of metastasis ($p = 0.002$). High sPD-L1 levels were significantly associated with worse survival in both the RNU and CTX cohorts. sPD-L1 levels were significantly elevated in postoperative samples ($p = 0.011$), while they remained unchanged during CTX. Interestingly, ICI treatment caused a strong, 25-fold increase in sPD-L1 ($p < 0.001$). Our results suggest that elevated preoperative sPD-L1 level is a predictor of higher pathological tumor stage and worse survival in UTUC, which therefore may help to optimize therapeutic decision-making. The observed characteristic sPD-L1 flare during immune checkpoint inhibitor therapy may have clinical significance.

**Keywords:** upper tract urothelial carcinoma; UTUC; sPD-L1; soluble programmed death ligand-1; biomarker; prognosis; immune checkpoint inhibitor therapy; chemotherapy; radical nephroureterectomy

## 1. Introduction

Urothelial carcinoma is most commonly localized in the urinary bladder; however, it can occur in every part of the urinary tract. Approximately 5–10% of all urothelial carcinomas are located in the upper urinary tract, including the ureters and pelvicalyceal system [1]. Pelvicalyceal localization of upper tract urothelial carcinoma (UTUC) is twice as frequent as the ureteral form [2]. The incidence of UTUC is approximately 1–2 cases per 100,000 each year and the 5-year disease-free survival rate ranges between 40–90% [3]. Considering their similar etiologies and therapeutic sensitivities, UTUC and urothelial bladder cancer (UBC) were considered the same disease in different anatomic locations. However, in recent years, a growing body of evidence has revealed disparities between UTUC and UBC [4]. Therefore, UTUC and UBC are now considered different tumor entities with substantial similarities. The gold standard treatment for clinically localized UTUC is surgery. In some rather rare and low-risk cases, when the biopsy confirms a small low-grade and localized tumor, endoluminal surgery or segmental resection of the ureter can be performed [5]. In the majority of cases, however, radical nephroureterectomy (RNU) with or without lymph node dissection remains the standard of care [6]. Due to the difficult anatomical features and location of UTUC, biopsy only provides a limited value for the evaluation of tumor stage [7]. As a consequence, some RNUs are performed unnecessarily, which represents an overtreatment. Therefore, preoperatively available prognostic markers are needed to reduce overtreatment of UTUC and to stratify patients for neoadjuvant systemic therapy.

In advanced cases of UTUC, systemic treatment with platinum-based chemotherapy (CTX) is the first choice in either adjuvant or neoadjuvant settings [5]. Platinum-based CTX increases both disease-free and metastasis-free survival by ~50% compared to surveillance [8]. However, after surgical removal of the kidney, the rate of cisplatin-eligible patients after RNU is only 20% [9]. For those patients who are ineligible for cisplatin, immune checkpoint inhibitors (ICI) can be administered [10]. The IMvigor 210 trial assessed the benefit of ICI therapy in cisplatin-ineligible urothelial cancer patients and revealed a never-before-seen improvement of 39% in the overall response rate [11]. However, UTUC patients show large individual differences in their responses to both CTX and ICI therapies. Therefore, pretreatment prognostication is a great unmet clinical need in UTUC.

Programmed-death ligand-1 (PD-L1) is a co-inhibitory membrane-bound protein expressed mainly by hematopoietic cells such as T-cells, B-cells, dendritic cells, and macrophages, but it is also produced by non-hematopoietic normal cells. Its receptor, programmed death protein-1 (PD-1), is primarily expressed by activated T-cells. PD-L1 is overexpressed in several cancer types. The binding of PD-1 and PD-L1 causes immune suppression, allowing tumor cells to escape from the cytotoxic effect of CD8 positive T-cells [12]. In UTUC, higher PD-L1 tissue expression levels were shown to be associated with a higher pathological tumor stage, poor survival and better response to ICI therapy [13–15]. Matrix metalloproteases are able to cleave the extracellular domain of PD-L1, leading to the appearance of soluble PD-L1 (sPD-L1) in the serum [16]. While sPD-L1 has recently been found to be prognostic in various malignancies, its potential clinical value in UTUC has not yet been assessed [17]. In this study, we aimed to assess the prognostic value of sPD-L1 and its changes in different treatment settings of UTUC. Therefore, in a post hoc pilot study, we determined sPD-L1 levels in prospectively collected pretreatment and on-treatment serum samples of UTUC patients who underwent either surgical or systemic (CTX or ICI) treatment.

## 2. Materials and Methods

### 2.1. Patient Cohort

Pretreatment serum samples were collected from an overall number of 61 UTUC patients (44 males, 17 females) who underwent surgical (RNU cohort; $n = 37$), postoperative platinum (CTX cohort; $n = 25$), or second-line immunotherapy (ICI cohort; $n = 6$) at the Department of Urology at Semmelweis University between August 2014 and July 2020. Six patients were included in more than one cohort (three patients were in both the RNU and CTX cohorts, two patients in the CTX and ICI cohorts, while one patient was in all three treatment groups). In addition to pretreatment samples, we collected samples following the start of therapy at predefined time points. For 14 patients of the RNU cohort, serum samples from the first postoperative day were available. Eighteen samples from the CTX cohort from the first day of the second CTX cycle, and four samples from the ICI cohort after three months of therapy were available for analysis.

Blood samples were collected in 9 mL tubes (Vacuette®, Greiner, Bio-One, Mosonmagyaróvár, Hungary) and left at room temperature for 30–90 min, then centrifuged with an Eppendorf 5702R centrifuge at $1500 \times g$ for 10 min, and finally aliquoted and kept at $-80\ °C$ until further analysis. The primary endpoint of this study was overall survival (OS), which was calculated as the period between initiation of therapy (RNU, CTX, or ICI) and the last follow-up (January 2022) or death. The secondary endpoint was progression-free survival (PFS). The study was conducted in accordance with the Declaration of Helsinki and was approved by the institutional ethics committee (TUKEB 256/2014). All patients provided a written informed consent to participate in this study.

### 2.2. Serum PD-L1 and MMP-7 Analyses

Quantitative sPD-L1 analyses were performed by using the sandwich ELISA method (PD-L1/B7-H1 Quantikine ELISA kit, DB7H10, R&D Systems, Wiesbaden, Germany), according to the manufacturer's instructions. To exclude possible interference between the therapeutic anti-PD-L1 antibody and the used ELISA assay, we also analyzed atezolizumab (anti-PD-L1) and pembrolizumab (anti-PD-1) on our ELISA plates by adding these substances as samples to the plate. Furthermore, we added different concentrations of atezolizumab and pembrolizumab to serum samples with low and high levels of sPD-L1 to check whether the addition of therapeutic antibodies would increase sPD-L1 signals.

Serum MMP-7 levels were formerly measured by using the Human Total MMP-7 Quantikine ELISA kit (R&D Systems, Wiesbaden, Germany, Catalog Number: DMP700), according to the product instructions. In this study, MMP-7 concentrations were used for testing for a possible correlation between sPD-L1 and MMP-7. Detailed results of the MMP-7 analysis were provided in an earlier published study [18].

### 2.3. Statistical Analysis

The non-parametric two-sided Wilcoxon rank-sum test (Mann–Whitney test) was used for group comparisons. Univariate OS and PFS analyses were performed using the Kaplan–Meier log-rank test and univariate Cox analysis. Low event numbers in each cohort did not allow the performance of multivariate analyses. Receiver operating characteristics (ROC) curves were applied for the RNU and CTX treatment groups to determine sPD-L1 cut-off values with the highest sensitivity and specificity for the dichotomized endpoint of death during the follow-up period. Spearman's rank correlation analysis was used to test for the correlation between formerly determined serum MMP-7 and sPD-L1 levels [18]. A $p$-value of $< 0.05$ was considered significant. All statistical analyses were performed with the IBM SPSS Statistics software (v. 27.0; IBM Corp., Armonk, NY, USA).

## 3. Results

### 3.1. Clinical Background

The median age in the RNU, CTX and ICI cohorts was 69, 72 and 65 years and the median follow-up times were 24, 18 and 20 months, respectively. In three patients, histological evaluation after RNU revealed a pT0 stage. Further patients' characteristics and baseline sPD-L1 levels are given in Table 1.

**Table 1.** Patients' characteristics for RNU, CTX and ICI treatment groups. * Non-malignant—in three cases of RNU histological examination resulted in a pT0 finding, RNU—radical nephroureterectomy, CTX—chemotherapy, ICI—immun checkpoint inhibitor therapy, ECOG PS—Eastern Cooperative Oncology Group performance status, R+—positive surgical margin, N+—lymph node metastasis, M+—distant metastasis, n. a.—not available, bold font significant value.

| General data | | | RNU | | | CTX | | | ICI | |
|---|---|---|---|---|---|---|---|---|---|---|
| | | n | median (range) | p | n | median (range) | p | n | median (range) | |
| Age at baseline, median (range) | | 34 | 68.9 (46.0–90.0) | - | 25 | 72.0 (46.0–84.0) | - | 6 | 64.5 (50.0–76.0) | |
| Follow-up in months, median (range) | | 34 | 24.2 (1.1–81.9) | - | 25 | 17.6 (1.1–67.7) | - | 6 | 20.4 (2.6–28.3) | |
| Number of patients died | | 11 | - | - | 13 | - | - | 2 | - | |
| **Parameters/sPD-L1 concentrations** | | n | sPD-L1 cc. | p | n | sPD-L1 cc. | p | n | sPD-L1 cc. | |
| Total No. of patients, median (range) | | 34 | 84.0 (49.9–172.3) | 0.347 | 25 | 96.1 (53.1–152.9) | - | 6 | 78.3 (42.17–192.1) | |
| Non-malignant * | | 3 | 68.4 (65.6–83.2) | | | | | | | |
| Age ≤ 65 | | 10 | 77.3 (49.9–162.4) | 0.183 | 5 | 78.6 (53.1–139.5) | 0.408 | 3 | 94.8 (61.9–122.9) | |
| Age > 65 | | 24 | 91.4 (59.3–172.3) | | 20 | 99.4 (65.0–152.9) | | 3 | 57.2 (42.2–192.1) | |
| Sex | male | 21 | 93.7 (49.9–172.3) | 0.600 | 21 | 102.7 (53.1–152.9) | 0.452 | 5 | 94.8 (57.2–192.1) | |
| | female | 13 | 80.7 (57.9–166.1) | | 4 | 93.9 (65.0–106.8) | | 1 | 42.2 | |
| ECOG PS | 0 | 19 | 80.6 (50.1–166.1) | - | 11 | 89.0 (53.1–128.8) | - | 5 | 61.9 (42.2–192.1) | |
| | 1 | 10 | 89.8 (49.9–162.4) | - | 10 | 103.9 (65.0–139.5) | - | 0 | - | |
| | 2 | 4 | 98.4 (73.1–172.3) | - | 4 | 107.7 (105.6–152.9) | - | 0 | - | |
| | 3 | 1 | 119.6 | - | 0 | - | - | 1 | 122.9 | |
| ECOG PS | 0–1 | 29 | 80.7 (49.9–166.1) | 0.149 | 21 | 91.8 (53.1–139.5) | 0.132 | 5 | 61.9 (42.2–192.1) | |
| ECOG PS | 2–3 | 5 | 106.7 (73.1–172.3) | | 4 | 107.7 (105.6–152.9) | | 1 | 122.9 | |
| Localization | Ureter | 17 | 70.2 (50.1–166.1) | 0.088 | 13 | 90.82 (53.1–152.9) | 0.298 | 2 | 68.5 (42.2–94.8) | |
| | Pyelon | 10 | 90.9 (61.7–172.3) | | 12 | 106.2 (65.0–139.5) | | 3 | 122.9 (61.9–192.1) | |
| | Both | 7 | 97.4 (49.9–155.3) | | 0 | | | 1 | 57.2 | |
| **RNU data** | | | | | | | | | | |
| pT0 | | 3 | 68.4 (65.6–83.2) | - | - | - | - | - | - | |
| pTa | | 7 | 70.2 (50.1–111.7) | - | 0 | - | - | - | - | |
| CIS | | 1 | 57.9 | - | 0 | - | - | 1 | 57.2 | |
| pT1 | | 9 | 68.9 (49.9–113.3) | - | 1 | 135.3 | - | 1 | 122.9 | |
| pT2 | | 2 | 110.0 (64.1–155.3) | - | 6 | 80.0 (68.3–128.8) | - | 1 | 94.78 | |
| pT3 | | 14 | 102.0 (72.7–172.3) | - | 14 | 99.4 (53.1–152.9) | - | 3 | 61.9 (42.2–192.1) | |
| pT4 | | 1 | 126.8 | - | 2 | 92.5 (89.02–96.1) | - | 0 | - | |
| n.a. | | 0 | | | 2 | | | 0 | | |
| pTa-pT1-CIS (non-invasive) | | 17 | 69.4 (49.9–113.3) | <0.001 | 1 | 135.3 | | 2 | 90 (57.2–122.9) | |
| pT2-pT4 (invasive) | | 17 | 106.7 (64.6–172.3) | | 22 | 93.9 (53.1–152.9) | | 4 | 78.3 (42.2–192.1) | |
| G1 | | 7 | 62.5 (49.9–85.9) | - | 0 | - | - | 0 | - | |
| G2 | | 12 | 87.3 (59.3–117.3) | - | 5 | 96.1 (68.3–135.3) | 0.951 | 3 | 94.8 (61.9–122.9) | |
| G3 | | 15 | 97.4 (57.9–172.3) | - | 16 | 99.4 (53.1–152.9) | - | 2 | 124.6 (57.2–192.1) | |
| n.a. | | 0 | | | 4 | | | 1 | | |
| G1–G2 | | 19 | 80.6 (49.9–117.3) | 0.019 | | - | - | 3 | 94.8 (61.9–122.9) | |
| G3 | | 15 | 97.4 (57.9–172.3) | | | - | | 2 | 124.6 (57.2–192.1) | |
| R0 | | 26 | 81.3 (49.9–166.1) | 0.368 | 14 | 104.2 (65.0–139.5) | 0.305 | 4 | 76.0 (42.2–192.1) | |
| R+ | | 8 | 91.9 (64.6–172.3) | | 9 | 89.0 (53.1–152.9) | | 1 | 61.9 | |
| n.a. | | 0 | | | 2 | | | 1 | 122.9 | |
| **Metastatic status at RNU** | | | | | | | | | | |
| N0/M0 | | 25 | 76.8 (49.9–155.3) | 0.002 | 14 | 86.0 (53.1–134.5) | 0.096 | 2 | 76.0 (57.2–94.8) | |
| N+ or M+ | | 9 | 119.6 (73.1–172.3) | | 9 | 102.7 (78.6–152.9) | | 3 | 61.9 (42.2–192.1) | |
| n.a. | | 0 | | | 2 | | | 1 | | |
| **Metastatic status at CTX baseline** | | | | | | | | | | |
| M0 | | - | - | - | 10 | 76.2 (53.1–134.5) | <0.001 | - | - | |
| M+ | | - | - | - | 14 | 110.2 (78.6–152.9) | | - | - | |
| n.a. | | - | - | - | 1 | - | | - | - | |
| **CTX regimen** | | | | | | | | | | |
| Gem/Cis | | - | - | - | 14 | 89.9 (53.1–125.9) | 0.013 | - | - | |
| Gem/Carbo | | - | - | - | 11 | 111.8 (78.6–152.9) | | - | - | |

## 3.2. Correlations of PD-L1 Concentrations with Clinicopathological Parameters

We observed no differences in the pretreatment levels of sPD-L1 between the RNU vs. CTV, RNU vs. ICI and CTX vs. ICI cohorts ($p = 0.203$, $p = 0.391$, $p = 0.698$, respectively). For the RNU cohort, age, sex, ECOG performance status and tumor localization showed no significant association with preoperative sPD-L1 levels. Higher sPD-L1 levels were found in muscle-invasive, high grade (G3) cases as well as in lymph node and/or distant metastatic cases ($p < 0.001$, $p = 0.019$ and $p = 0.002$ respectively) (Table 1, Figure 1).

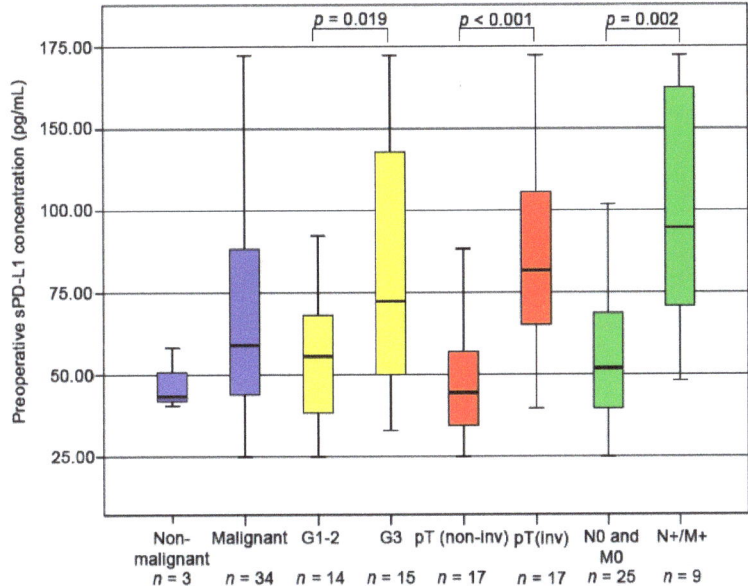

**Figure 1.** Association of preoperative sPD-L1 concentrations and clinicopathological parameters in the RNU cohort. pT(non-inv): pTa-pT1, pT(inv): pT2–pT4.

For the CTX cohort, similar to the findings in the RNU cohort, baseline sPD-L1 levels were higher in metastatic cases ($p < 0.001$) (Table 1). Furthermore, patients who received gemcitabine/carboplatin instead of gemcitabine/cisplatin had significantly elevated sPD-L1 levels ($p = 0.013$). As low case numbers of the ICI cohort did not allow the performance of a valid statistical evaluation, we provided patients' characteristics on an individual patient level in Table 2.

## 3.3. Correlation of Pretreatment sPD-L1 Levels with Patients' Prognosis

For the RNU cohort, three patients with pT0 histopathological findings were excluded from survival analyses. Muscle-invasive disease ($\geq$pT2) and the presence of lymphatic or distant metastases at RNU were associated with shorter OS (HR: 7.115; 95% CI 1.504–33.659; $p = 0.013$ and HR: 4.891; 95% CI 1.379–17.345; $p = 0.014$, respectively). Similarly, shorter PFS was significantly associated with the same factors: $\geq$pT2 stage (HR: 10.836; 95% CI 2.865–40.978; $p < 0.001$), lymph node or distant metastasis (HR: 6.185; 95% CI 2.199–17.397; $p = 0.001$) (Supplementary Materials, Table S1).

In addition, high sPD-L1 levels were associated with shorter OS, both when using the median (84.0 pg/mL; $p = 0.041$) or the ROC-based cut-off value (118.5 pg/mL; $p < 0.001$) (Figure 2A,B) (Supplementary Materials, Figure S5).

**Table 2.** Characteristics of ICI-treated patients. ICI—immune checkpoint inhibitor therapy, N—lymph node metastasis, M—distant metastasis, Gem/Carb—gemcitabine + carboplatin, Gem/Cis—gemcitabine + cisplatin, n. a.—not available, OS—overall survival, Atezo—atezolizumab, Pembro—pembrolizumab.

|  | Pat. 1 | Pat. 2 | Pat. 3 | Pat. 4 | Pat. 5 | Pat. 6 |
|---|---|---|---|---|---|---|
| Age | 76 | 64 | 64 | 75 | 65 | 50 |
| Sex | Female | Male | Male | Male | Male | Male |
| **Clinicopath. parameters at RNU** | | | | | | |
| Stage (pT) | 3 | 2 | 3 | CIS | 3 | 1 |
| Grade (G) | - | 2 | 2 | 3 | 3 | 2 |
| N+ | yes | no | yes | no | Yes | no |
| M+ | no | no | no | no | No | unknown |
| Pre-ICI CTX treatment | Gem/Car | Gem/Cis | Gem/Car | n.a. | Gem/Car | Gem/Cis |
| **Clinicopath. parameters at ICI baseline** | | | | | | |
| ICI-treatment | Atezo | Atezo | Atezo | Atezo | Atezo | Pembro |
| N+ | yes | yes | yes | no | Yes | unknown |
| M+ | yes | yes | no | no | Yes | yes |
| sPD-L1 at baseline (pg/mL) | 42.2 | 94.8 | 61.9 | 57.2 | 192.1 | 122.9 |
| sPD-L1 at 3 months (pg/mL) | 1903 | 1939 | 1993 | Unknown | 1972 | n.a. |
| OS (months) | 14.4 | 30.2 | 28.4 | 28.0 | 9.9 | 2.6 |
| status | alive | alive | alive | alive | dead | dead |
| Objective response | PD | PD | PD | PD | PD | unknown |

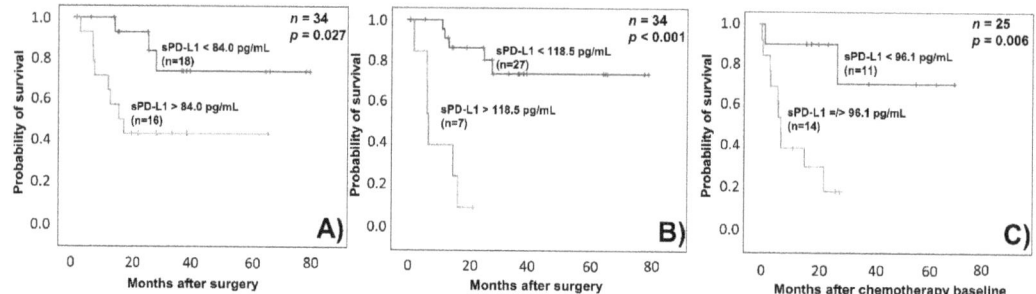

**Figure 2.** Kaplan–Meier OS analyses with log-rank tests (**A**) for the RNU cohort using the median (84.0 pg/mL) as the cut-off, (**B**) for the RNU cohort applying the ROC-based (118.5 pg/mL) cut-off, (**C**) for the CTX cohort with the median (96.1 pg/mL) cut-off (in this cohort, median- and ROC-based cut-off values resulted the same groups) (blue line—low sPD-L1 cc., green line—high sPD-L1 cc., cut-off values are shown on each line).

For the CTX cohort, the presence of lymph node or distant metastasis at CTX baseline was found to be a significant predictor of shorter OS (HR: 14.737; 95% CI 1.810–119.987; $p = 0.012$) (Supplementary Materials, Table S1). The median sPD-L1 cut-off value for the CTX cohort was 96.1 pg/mL, which is close to the ROC cut-off of 93.9 pg/mL and therefore both cut-offs divided the CTX cohort into the very same groups (Supplementary Materials, Figure S5). High sPD-L1 levels were significantly associated with shorter OS (HR: 6.956; 95% CI 1.461–33.110; $p= 0.015$) (Table 3, Figure 2). In this cohort, shorter PFS was only associated with the presence of lymph node or distant metastasis at CTX baseline (HR: 7.638; CI 95% 2.218–26.301; $p = 0.001$) (Supplementary Materials, Table S1). Survival analysis for the ICI cohort could not be performed because of low patient numbers.

**Table 3.** Correlation of pretreatment sPD-L1 concentrations with patients' prognosis *—median cut-off value for RNU is 84.0 pg/mL, median cut-off value for CTX is 96.1 pg/mL; **—ROC cut-off value for RNU is 118.5 pg/mL, ROC cut-off value for CTX is 93.9 pg/mL; RNU—radical nephroureterectomy, CTX—chemotherapy; OS—overall survival; PFS—progression-free survival, bold font significant value.

| | | RNU | | | | | | | CTX | | | | | |
| --- | --- | --- | --- | --- | --- | --- | --- | --- | --- | --- | --- | --- | --- | --- |
| | | OS | | | PFS | | | | OS | | | PFS | | |
| | n | HR | 95% CI | p | HR | 95% CI | p | n | HR | 95% CI | p | HR | 95% CI | p |
| Pretreatment sPD-L1 | | | | | | | | | | | | | | |
| median cut-off * | 17 | ref. | | | ref. | | | 11 | ref. | | | ref. | | |
| median cut-off * | 17 | 4.023 | 1.060–15.269 | 0.041 | 2.793 | 1.011–7.716 | 0.048 | 14 | 6.956 | 1.461–33.110 | 0.015 | 1.584 | 0.560–4.478 | 0.386 |
| ROC cut-off ** | 27 | ref. | | | ref. | | | 11 | ref. | | | ref. | | |
| ROC cut-off ** | 7 | 12.114 | 2.990–49.082 | <0.001 | 6.667 | 2.140–20.764 | 0.001 | 14 | 6.956 | 1.461–33.110 | 0.015 | 1.584 | 0.560–4.478 | 0.386 |

*3.4. Changes in sPD-L1 Levels during and after Therapy*

In the RNU cohort, the median preoperative sPD-L1 concentration was 84.0 pg/mL. In 14 cases, postoperative (first day after RNU) sPD-L1 levels were available, with a median of 114.5 pg/mL, which was significantly higher than the pretreatment serum concentrations ($p = 0.011$) (Figure 3A,D).

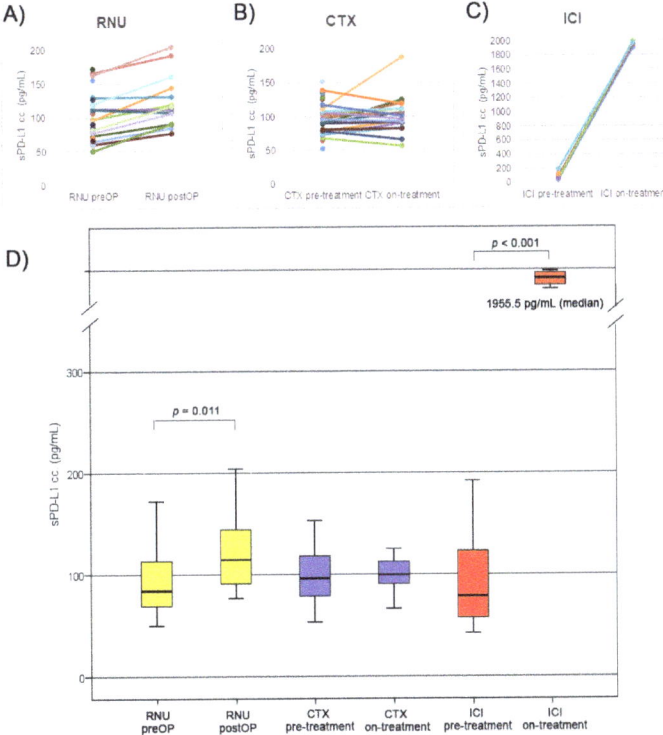

**Figure 3.** Box-plot presentation of sPD-L1 concentration changes in the RNU, CTX and ICI cohorts. (**A**) RNU cohort (preop. and postop. values), (**B**) CTX cohort (at chemotherapy baseline and on the first day of cycle 2), (**C**) ICI cohort (pretreatment and on-treatment values at 3 months), (**D**). We observed no differences in the pretreatment levels of sPD-L1 between the RNU vs. CTV, RNU vs. ICI and CTX vs. ICI cohorts ($p = 0.203$, $p = 0.391$, $p = 0.698$, respectively). RNU—radical nephroureterectomy; CTX—chemotherapy; ICI—immune checkpoint inhibitor therapy.

In the CTX cohort, the baseline median of sPD-L1 level was 96.1 pg/mL which remained unchanged (99.4 pg/mL, $n = 18$) after the first treatment cycle (Figure 3B,D).

Interestingly, we observed a remarkable, 25-fold increase in sPD-L1 levels after 3 months of ICI treatment from 78.3 pg/mL to 1955.5 pg/mL ($p < 0.001$) (Figure 3C,D). In addition, we measured atezolizumab and pembrolizumab directly on our assay plates and found no detectable signals. Furthermore, addition of various concentrations of atezolizumab and pembrolizumab to serum samples with low and high sPD-L1 levels did not significantly influence the detected signals. These, results show that the therapeutic antibodies do not directly interfere with the ELISA assay.

### 3.5. Correlation between sPD-L1 and sMMP-7 Levels

MMP-7 has been formerly shown to proteolytically cleave membrane-bound PD-L1 releasing sPD-L1 into the circulation and we formerly determined serum MMP-7 concentrations in a largely overlapping UTUC patient cohorts [18]. Therefore, we performed an exploratory Spearmen's rank correlation analysis between sPD-L1 and MMP-7 in the RNU, CTX and ICI cohorts, which revealed a significant positive correlation between the concentrations of these two serum proteins in the RNU cohort ($n = 34$, rs = 0.445, $p = 0.008$) but not in the ICI cohort ($n = 5$, rs = 0.900, $p = 0.307$) and CTX cohorts ($n = 25$, rs = 0.217, $p = 0.297$) (Supplementary Materials, Figures S1–S3).

## 4. Discussion

In this pilot study, we assessed the prognostic value and changes in sPD-L1 in various treatment settings of UTUC. In the surgical treatment cohort, elevated preoperative sPD-L1 was associated with the muscle-invasive stage (pT2–pT4), higher tumor grade, the presence of metastasis and poor survival. Similarly, in the CTX cohort, higher pretreatment sPD-L1 levels were associated with shorter survival. In addition, we observed a moderate but significant sPD-L1 increase in postoperative samples of the RNU cohort and a strong 25-fold increase at 3 months of ICI treatment, while sPD-L1 levels remained unchanged during CTX treatment.

Because of inaccurate preoperative biopsy and large individual differences in therapy sensitivities, clinical decision-making in UTUC is challenging. Various studies have compared the preoperative (biopsy-based) and postoperative (definitive) stage findings in UTUC, showing both high upstaging and downstaging rates of up to 60% [19,20]. Therefore, preoperative staging often cannot provide a reliable prognostic stratification. In contrast to staging, preoperative grading was found to be more consistent with postoperative histological findings, showing 97% and 62% agreement for high and low tumor grades, respectively [21]. Accordingly, biopsy grading is considered a more reliable source for prognostication. Other known preoperative prognostic factors in UTUC are advanced age, multifocality, hydronephrosis, ECOG PS $\geq 1$, tobacco consumption, and delayed surgical treatment [5]. These factors, however, have only a limited value for the prediction of the clinical behavior of UTUC. Therefore, additional molecular markers that better reflect the tumor's biological features are needed. In recent years, many potential prognostic tissue biomarkers have been investigated in UTUC including those involved in cell differentiation (Ki67, CDCA5, PAK1, INHBA, PTP4A3), cell cycle regulation (PAK1, Bcl-xL) and antitumoral immunity such as CD204+ macrophages [22]. On the one hand, these tissue markers reflect the biological behavior of cancer and could provide insight into the pathogenesis of the disease, while on the other hand, the evaluability of these biomarkers is strongly dependent on the quality of the biopsy and has not yet been prospectively validated. Much fewer studies are available on circulating biomarkers in UTUC. Promising results have been published on the prognostic relevance of preoperative serum MMP-7, neutrophil-to-lymphocyte ratio and CRP levels; however, larger validation studies are missing and therefore these markers are to be considered as experimental [18,23,24]. Preoperative sPD-L1 levels have recently been shown to be independently associated with shorter survival in colorectal and gastric cancers [25,26]. Accordingly, in the present study, we observed poor survival rates in UTUC patients with high preoperative sPD-L1 levels. Furthermore, in our RNU cohort, high sPD-L1 levels were associated with muscle-invasive tumor stage ($p < 0.001$), high (G3) tumor grade ($p = 0.019$) and the presence of metastasis ($p = 0.002$). These findings suggest sPD-L1 as a potential biomarker for the preoperative prediction of muscle-invasive disease, which may help to decide on the extent of surgical management. In addition, patients with high pretreatment sPD-L1 levels who are at higher risk of disease progression may benefit from a more aggressive therapeutic strategy (e.g., perioperative adjuvant or neoadjuvant systemic therapy). However, our results need to be confirmed in larger patient cohorts before being applied in practice.

In high-risk locally advanced UTUC cases, neoadjuvant CTX provided 47–52% pathological objective response rates and 8–10% pathological complete response rates [27], while in the metastatic setting first-line CTX provided 35–46% overall response rates [28]. These numbers reflect a considerable heterogeneity of therapy response to CTX in UTUC patients. In cisplatin-ineligible and tissue PD-L1 positive cases, first-line ICI provided improved survival with great individual differences [29]. Our present analysis revealed a significant unfavorable prognostic effect for higher baseline sPD-L1 levels in CTX-treated patients, while the limited size of the ICI cohort did not allow the performance of statistically valid survival analyses. Therefore, we could not compare the prognostic value of sPD-L1 between CTX and ICI-treated patients, which precludes a valid conclusion regarding the therapy predictive value of sPD-L1. Recently, conflicting results have been published regarding the prognostic value of baseline sPD-L1 in ICI-treated patients with various tumors [30–35]. Increased sPD-L1 levels were associated with better outcomes in esophageal and renal cell cancer patients, while in contrast in NSCLC and melanoma, high sPD-L1 levels were associated with poor survival [30,31,34,35]. Based on these results, the ICI predictive value of sPD-L1 seems to be tumor type-dependent. In addition, the associations we found between sPD-L1 with shorter survival in both the RNU and CTX cohorts suggest that sPD-L1 is prognostic rather than therapy predictive.

The origin of circulating sPD-L1 is not fully understood. Interestingly, recent studies found no correlation between soluble and tissue PD-L1 levels, suggesting that increased tissue expression is not the primary source of sPD-L1 [30,32,33]. Some members of the matrix metalloproteinase family, such as MMP-7, -9, -10, and -13 were shown to proteolytically cleave membrane-bound PD-L1, releasing the extracellular domain of the molecule into the blood circulation [36,37]. We recently assessed MMP-7 levels in serum samples of a largely overlapping UTUC cohort and found higher MMP-7 levels to be associated with higher tumor stages and the presence of metastasis [18]. Correlation analysis between serum MMP-7 and PD-L1 levels in the same samples revealed a significant direct correlation in the treatment-naive preoperative RNU samples. This finding is in line with our former observation in UBC and confirms the involvement of MMP-7 in the proteolytic degradation of sPD-L1 at a systemic level [32]. Considering the lack of association between the tissue and serum sPD-L1 levels on the one hand and the significant correlation between serum MMP-7 and sPD-L1 on the other hand, we hypothesize that the increased sPD-L1 levels are the consequence of an enhanced proteolytic tumor milieu rather than an increased PD-L1 expression of the tumor tissue.

Comparing the pre- and postoperative sPD-L1 levels, we detected a mild but significant increase after RNU, which suggests that tumor cells are not the predominant sources of sPD-L1. After surgery, patients have an elevated level of circulating damage-associated molecular patterns, which triggers a local and systemic inflammation [38]. As sPD-L1 levels were shown to be associated with the presence of severe inflammation, we hypothesize that the postoperative sPD-L1 elevation we observed may be a consequence of an inflammatory response to the surgical procedure itself [39].

In the CTX cohort, no differences were detected between the baseline and on-treatment sPD-L1 levels. In contrast, we found strong, 25-fold elevated sPD-L1 concentrations after three months of ICI treatment. These striking results are in line with our former observation made in UBC, showing a similar increase in sPD-L1 levels in PD-L1 inhibitor-treated (atezolizumab) patients after three months of therapy [32]. Interestingly, in PD-1 inhibitor-treated (pembrolizumab) UBC patients no sPD-L1 increase could be detected, suggesting that the detected sPD-L1 flare may be therapy-specific. Similar observations were described for PD-1 and PD-L1 inhibitor-treated NSCLC patients with strong sPD-L1 elevation in some cases, while in tyrosine kinase inhibitor-treated NSCLC cases, no such increase could be observed [40]. In addition, Chiarucci et al., using the same ELISA assay, found a similar increase in sPD-L1 levels (from a median of 70 pg/mL to 1850 pg/mL) in anti-PD-L1 treated mesothelioma patients, while in the anti-CTLA-4 and anti-PD-1 treated patients no such increase could be observed [41]. Based on these findings, it appears that only PD-L1 but not PD-1 inhibitors provoke an sPD-L1 increase; however, the exact mechanism of this sPD-L1 flare-up remains to be elucidated. A possible explanation for this phenomenon might be the presence of various sPD-L1 antibody complexes. Atezolizumab as an antigenic molecule may induce a significant anti-drug antibody response and the presence of this antibody might have a neutralizing effect on atezolizumab [42]. Our study has some limitations inherent to its retrospective nature and limited cohort sizes, which did not allow us to perform multivariate analyses. This limitation, however, should be judged in relation to the low incidence of UTUC. A further limitation of our study is that tumor samples were not available for correlation analysis between tissue and serum PD-L1 levels. However, data based on a large number of cases in various cancers uniformly showed no correlation between serum and tissue PD-L1 levels [30,33].

## 5. Conclusions

Assessing sPD-L1 for the first time in UTUC, we found significantly increased levels in advanced tumor stages and high pretreatment concentrations were associated with shorter survival in both RNU and CTX-treated patients. These findings, when confirmed in larger studies, may help to improve risk-stratification and to optimize therapeutic decision-making in UTUC. The characteristic sPD-L1 flare-up observed in UTUC seems to be therapy-specific and its biological and clinical relevance needs to be further evaluated.

**Supplementary Materials:** The following supporting information can be downloaded at: https://www.mdpi.com/article/10.3390/biomedicines10102560/s1, Figure S1: Correlation analysis between sPD-L1 and MMP-7 levels in the RNU cohort. Figure S2: Correlation analysis between sPD-L1 and MMP-7 levels in the CTX cohort. Figure S3: Correlation analysis between sPD-L1 and MMP7 levels in the ICI cohort. Figure S4: Scatter plot of the association of preoperative sPD-L1 concentration and clinicopathological parameters in the RNU cohort. Figure S5: Receiver operating characteristic (ROC) analysis of the cut-off levels in the RNU and CTX cohorts. Table S1: Correlation of clinicopathological parameters and pretreatment sPD-L1 concentrations with patients' prognosis.

**Author Contributions:** Conceptualization, Á.S., T.F., S.V., C.O., S.T. and T.S.; Data curation, P.T.K., A.C., M.V. and U.K.; Formal analysis, P.T.K., T.F., C.O., C.D., V.G. and O.H.; Funding acquisition, P.N.; Investigation, Á.S., C.D. and O.H.; Methodology, T.F., S.V., S.T., U.K. and V.G.; Resources, P.H. and T.S.; Software, A.C. and C.O.; Supervision, P.R., P.H., B.H., P.N. and T.S.; Validation, P.R.; Visualization, M.V.; Writing—original draft, Á.S.; Writing—review and editing, P.H., B.H., P.N. and T.S. All authors have read and agreed to the published version of the manuscript.

**Funding:** This work has been supported by the Ministry for Innovation and Technology from the source of the National Research Development and Innovation Fund (K139059) and by Wilhelm-Sander Stiftung (D/106-22012) and IFORES (D/107-137709). T.S. was supported by a János Bolyai Research Scholarship from the Hungarian Academy of Sciences (BO/00451/20/5) and by the New National Excellence Program (ÚNKP-21-5-SE-3).

**Institutional Review Board Statement:** The study was conducted in accordance with the Helsinki Declaration and approved by the institutional ethics committee (TUKEB 55/2014 and 256/2014).

**Informed Consent Statement:** Informed consent prior to each treatment was obtained from every patient.

**Data Availability Statement:** The data that support the findings of this study are available from the corresponding author upon reasonable request.

**Conflicts of Interest:** Boris Hadaschik reports advisory roles for ABX, Bayer, Lightpoint Medical, Inc., Janssen R&D, Bristol-Myers-Squibb, Pfizer and Astellas; research funding from the German Research Foundation, AAA/Novartis, Janssen R&D, Bristol-Myers-Squibb, Pfizer and Astellas; and travel assistance from AstraZeneca, Janssen R&D, and Astellas.

## References

1. Visser, O.; Adolfsson, J.; Rossi, S.; Verne, J.; Gatta, G.; Maffezzini, M.; Franks, K.N.; The RARECARE Working Group. Incidence and survival of rare urogenital cancers in Europe. *Eur. J. Cancer* **2012**, *48*, 456–464. [CrossRef]
2. Petros, F.G. Epidemiology, clinical presentation, and evaluation of upper-tract urothelial carcinoma. *Transl. Androl. Urol.* **2020**, *9*, 1794–1798. [CrossRef]
3. Craig Hall, M.W.S.; Sagalowsky, I.A.; Carmody, T.; Erickstad, M.D.; Roehrborn, C.G. Prognostic factors, recurrence, and survival in transitional cell carcinoma of the upper urinary tract: A 30-year experience in 252 patients PATIENTS. *Urology* **1998**, *52*, 594–601. [CrossRef]
4. Szarvas, T.; Modos, O.; Horvath, A.; Nyirady, P. Why are upper tract urothelial carcinoma two different diseases? *Transl. Androl. Urol.* **2016**, *5*, 636–647. [CrossRef]
5. Roupret, M.; Babjuk, M.; Comperat, E.; Zigeuner, R.; Sylvester, R.J.; Burger, M.; Cowan, N.C.; Gontero, P.; Van Rhijn, B.W.G.; Mostafid, A.H.; et al. European Association of Urology Guidelines on Upper Urinary Tract Urothelial Carcinoma: 2017 Update. *Eur. Urol.* **2018**, *73*, 111–122. [CrossRef] [PubMed]
6. Margulis, V.; Shariat, S.F.; Matin, S.F.; Kamat, A.M.; Zigeuner, R.; Kikuchi, E.; Lotan, Y.; Weizer, A.; Raman, J.D.; Wood, C.G.; et al. Outcomes of radical nephroureterectomy: A series from the Upper Tract Urothelial Carcinoma Collaboration. *Cancer* **2009**, *115*, 1224–1233. [CrossRef] [PubMed]
7. Clements, T.; Messer, J.C.; Terrell, J.D.; Herman, M.P.; Ng, C.K.; Scherr, D.S.; Scoll, B.; Boorjian, S.A.; Uzzo, R.G.; Wille, M.; et al. High-grade ureteroscopic biopsy is associated with advanced pathology of upper-tract urothelial carcinoma tumors at definitive surgical resection. *J. Endourol.* **2012**, *26*, 398–402. [CrossRef]
8. Birtle, A.; Johnson, M.; Chester, J.; Jones, R.; Dolling, D.; Bryan, R.T.; Harris, C.; Winterbottom, A.; Blacker, A.; Catto, J.W.F.; et al. Adjuvant chemotherapy in upper tract urothelial carcinoma (the POUT trial): A phase 3, open-label, randomised controlled trial. *Lancet* **2020**, *395*, 1268–1277. [CrossRef]
9. Zhang, J.; Ye, Z.W.; Tew, K.D.; Townsend, D.M. Cisplatin chemotherapy and renal function. *Adv. Cancer Res.* **2021**, *152*, 305–327. [CrossRef]
10. Califano, G.; Ouzaid, I.; Verze, P.; Hermieu, J.F.; Mirone, V.; Xylinas, E. Immune checkpoint inhibition in upper tract urothelial carcinoma. *World J. Urol.* **2021**, *39*, 1357–1367. [CrossRef] [PubMed]
11. Balar, A.V.; Galsky, M.D.; Rosenberg, J.E.; Powles, T.; Petrylak, D.P.; Bellmunt, J.; Loriot, Y.; Necchi, A.; Hoffman-Censits, J.; Perez-Gracia, J.L.; et al. Atezolizumab as first-line treatment in cisplatin-ineligible patients with locally advanced and metastatic urothelial carcinoma: A single-arm, multicentre, phase 2 trial. *Lancet* **2017**, *389*, 67–76. [CrossRef]
12. Sun, C.; Mezzadra, R.; Schumacher, T.N. Regulation and Function of the PD-L1 Checkpoint. *Immunity* **2018**, *48*, 434–452. [CrossRef] [PubMed]
13. Ward, M.; Albertson, D.; Furtado, L.V.; Deftereos, G. PD-L1 Tumor Cell Expression in Upper Tract Urothelial Carcinomas is Associated with Higher Pathological Stage. *Appl. Immunohistochem. Mol. Morphol.* **2022**, *30*, 56–61. [CrossRef] [PubMed]
14. Lu, Y.; Kang, J.; Luo, Z.; Song, Y.; Tian, J.; Li, Z.; Wang, X.; Liu, L.; Yang, Y.; Liu, X. The Prevalence and Prognostic Role of PD-L1 in Upper Tract Urothelial Carcinoma Patients Underwent Radical Nephroureterectomy: A Systematic Review and Meta-Analysis. *Front. Oncol.* **2020**, *10*, 1400. [CrossRef]
15. Rouanne, M.; Radulescu, C.; Adam, J.; Allory, Y. PD-L1 testing in urothelial bladder cancer: Essentials of clinical practice. *World J. Urol.* **2021**, *39*, 1345–1355. [CrossRef]
16. Dezutter-Dambuyant, C.; Durand, I.; Alberti, L.; Bendriss-Vermare, N.; Valladeau-Guilemond, J.; Duc, A.; Magron, A.; Morel, A.P.; Sisirak, V.; Rodriguez, C.; et al. A novel regulation of PD-1 ligands on mesenchymal stromal cells through MMP-mediated proteolytic cleavage. *Oncoimmunology* **2016**, *5*, e1091146. [CrossRef]
17. Huang, P.; Hu, W.; Zhu, Y.; Wu, F.; Lin, H. The Prognostic Value of Circulating Soluble Programmed Death Ligand-1 in Cancers: A Meta-Analysis. *Front. Oncol.* **2020**, *10*, 626932. [CrossRef] [PubMed]
18. Kovacs, P.T.; Mayer, T.; Csizmarik, A.; Varadi, M.; Olah, C.; Szeles, A.; Tschirdewahn, S.; Krafft, U.; Hadaschik, B.; Nyirady, P.; et al. Elevated Pre-Treatment Serum MMP-7 Levels Are Associated with the Presence of Metastasis and Poor Survival in Upper Tract Urothelial Carcinoma. *Biomedicines* **2022**, *10*, 698. [CrossRef] [PubMed]
19. Dev, H.S.; Poo, S.; Armitage, J.; Wiseman, O.; Shah, N.; Al-Hayek, S. Investigating upper urinary tract urothelial carcinomas: A single-centre 10-year experience. *World J. Urol.* **2017**, *35*, 131–138. [CrossRef]
20. Mori, K.; Katayama, S.; Laukhtina, E.; Schuettfort, V.M.; Pradere, B.; Quhal, F.; Sari Motlagh, R.; Mostafaei, H.; Grossmann, N.C.; Rajwa, P.; et al. Discordance Between Clinical and Pathological Staging and Grading in Upper Tract Urothelial Carcinoma. *Clin. Genitourin. Cancer* **2022**, *20*, 95.e1–95.e6. [CrossRef] [PubMed]
21. Simon, C.T.; Skala, S.L.; Weizer, A.Z.; Ambani, S.N.; Chinnaiyan, A.M.; Palapattu, G.; Hafez, K.; Magers, M.J.; Kaffenberger, S.D.; Spratt, D.E.; et al. Clinical utility and concordance of upper urinary tract cytology and biopsy in predicting clinicopathological features of upper urinary tract urothelial carcinoma. *Hum. Pathol.* **2019**, *86*, 76–84. [CrossRef] [PubMed]

22. Mbeutcha, A.; Roupret, M.; Kamat, A.M.; Karakiewicz, P.I.; Lawrentschuk, N.; Novara, G.; Raman, J.D.; Seitz, C.; Xylinas, E.; Shariat, S.F. Prognostic factors and predictive tools for upper tract urothelial carcinoma: A systematic review. *World J. Urol.* **2017**, *35*, 337–353. [CrossRef]
23. Dalpiaz, O.; Pichler, M.; Mannweiler, S.; Martin Hernandez, J.M.; Stojakovic, T.; Pummer, K.; Zigeuner, R.; Hutterer, G.C. Validation of the pretreatment derived neutrophil-lymphocyte ratio as a prognostic factor in a European cohort of patients with upper tract urothelial carcinoma. *Br. J. Cancer* **2014**, *110*, 2531–2536. [CrossRef]
24. Obata, J.; Kikuchi, E.; Tanaka, N.; Matsumoto, K.; Hayakawa, N.; Ide, H.; Miyajima, A.; Nakagawa, K.; Oya, M. C-reactive protein: A biomarker of survival in patients with localized upper tract urothelial carcinoma treated with radical nephroureterectomy. *Urol. Oncol.* **2013**, *31*, 1725–1730. [CrossRef] [PubMed]
25. Omura, Y.; Toiyama, Y.; Okugawa, Y.; Yin, C.; Shigemori, T.; Kusunoki, K.; Kusunoki, Y.; Ide, S.; Shimura, T.; Fujikawa, H.; et al. Prognostic impacts of tumoral expression and serum levels of PD-L1 and CTLA-4 in colorectal cancer patients. *Cancer Immunol. Immunother.* **2020**, *69*, 2533–2546. [CrossRef] [PubMed]
26. Shigemori, T.; Toiyama, Y.; Okugawa, Y.; Yamamoto, A.; Yin, C.; Narumi, A.; Ichikawa, T.; Ide, S.; Shimura, T.; Fujikawa, H.; et al. Soluble PD-L1 Expression in Circulation as a Predictive Marker for Recurrence and Prognosis in Gastric Cancer: Direct Comparison of the Clinical Burden between Tissue and Serum PD-L1 Expression. *Ann. Surg. Oncol.* **2019**, *26*, 876–883. [CrossRef] [PubMed]
27. Grossmann, N.C.; Pradere, B.; D'Andrea, D.; Schuettfort, V.M.; Mori, K.; Rajwa, P.; Quhal, F.; Laukhtina, E.; Katayama, S.; Fankhauser, C.D.; et al. Neoadjuvant Chemotherapy in Elderly Patients With Upper Tract Urothelial Cancer: Oncologic Outcomes From a Multicenter Study. *Clin. Genitourin. Cancer* **2022**, *20*, 227–236. [CrossRef]
28. Kikuchi, E.; Miyazaki, J.; Yuge, K.; Hagiwara, M.; Ichioka, D.; Inoue, T.; Kageyama, S.; Sugimoto, M.; Mitsuzuka, K.; Matsui, Y.; et al. Do metastatic upper tract urothelial carcinoma and bladder carcinoma have similar clinical responses to systemic chemotherapy? A Japanese multi-institutional experience. *Jpn. J. Clin. Oncol.* **2016**, *46*, 163–169. [CrossRef] [PubMed]
29. Park, J.C.; Hahn, N.M. Emerging role of immunotherapy in urothelial carcinoma-Future directions and novel therapies. *Urol. Oncol.* **2016**, *34*, 566–576. [CrossRef]
30. Costantini, A.; Julie, C.; Dumenil, C.; Helias-Rodzewicz, Z.; Tisserand, J.; Dumoulin, J.; Giraud, V.; Labrune, S.; Chinet, T.; Emile, J.F.; et al. Predictive role of plasmatic biomarkers in advanced non-small cell lung cancer treated by nivolumab. *Oncoimmunology* **2018**, *7*, e1452581. [CrossRef]
31. Ugurel, S.; Schadendorf, D.; Horny, K.; Sucker, A.; Schramm, S.; Utikal, J.; Pfohler, C.; Herbst, R.; Schilling, B.; Blank, C.; et al. Elevated baseline serum PD-1 or PD-L1 predicts poor outcome of PD-1 inhibition therapy in metastatic melanoma. *Ann. Oncol.* **2020**, *31*, 144–152. [CrossRef] [PubMed]
32. Krafft, U.; Olah, C.; Reis, H.; Kesch, C.; Darr, C.; Grunwald, V.; Tschirdewahn, S.; Hadaschik, B.; Horvath, O.; Kenessey, I.; et al. High Serum PD-L1 Levels Are Associated with Poor Survival in Urothelial Cancer Patients Treated with Chemotherapy and Immune Checkpoint Inhibitor Therapy. *Cancers* **2021**, *13*, 2548. [CrossRef]
33. Castello, A.; Rossi, S.; Toschi, L.; Mansi, L.; Lopci, E. Soluble PD-L1 in NSCLC Patients Treated with Checkpoint Inhibitors and Its Correlation with Metabolic Parameters. *Cancers* **2020**, *12*, 1373. [CrossRef]
34. Ji, S.; Chen, H.; Yang, K.; Zhang, G.; Mao, B.; Hu, Y.; Zhang, H.; Xu, J. Peripheral cytokine levels as predictive biomarkers of benefit from immune checkpoint inhibitors in cancer therapy. *Biomed. Pharmacother.* **2020**, *129*, 110457. [CrossRef]
35. Incorvaia, L.; Fanale, D.; Badalamenti, G.; Porta, C.; Olive, D.; De Luca, I.; Brando, C.; Rizzo, M.; Messina, C.; Rediti, M.; et al. Baseline plasma levels of soluble PD-1, PD-L1, and BTN3A1 predict response to nivolumab treatment in patients with metastatic renal cell carcinoma: A step toward a biomarker for therapeutic decisions. *Oncoimmunology* **2020**, *9*, 1832348. [CrossRef] [PubMed]
36. Aguirre, J.E.; Beswick, E.J.; Grim, C.; Uribe, G.; Tafoya, M.; Chacon Palma, G.; Samedi, V.; McKee, R.; Villeger, R.; Fofanov, Y.; et al. Matrix metalloproteinases cleave membrane-bound PD-L1 on CD90+ (myo-)fibroblasts in Crohn's disease and regulate Th1/Th17 cell responses. *Int. Immunol.* **2020**, *32*, 57–68. [CrossRef] [PubMed]
37. Hira-Miyazawa, M.; Nakamura, H.; Hirai, M.; Kobayashi, Y.; Kitahara, H.; Bou-Gharios, G.; Kawashiri, S. Regulation of programmed-death ligand in the human head and neck squamous cell carcinoma microenvironment is mediated through matrix metalloproteinase-mediated proteolytic cleavage. *Int. J. Oncol.* **2018**, *52*, 379–388. [CrossRef] [PubMed]
38. Tang, F.; Tie, Y.; Tu, C.; Wei, X. Surgical trauma-induced immunosuppression in cancer: Recent advances and the potential therapies. *Clin. Transl. Med.* **2020**, *10*, 199–223. [CrossRef]
39. Sun, S.; Chen, Y.; Liu, Z.; Tian, R.; Liu, J.; Chen, E.; Mao, E.; Pan, T.; Qu, H. Serum-soluble PD-L1 may be a potential diagnostic biomarker in sepsis. *Scand. J. Immunol.* **2021**, *94*, e13049. [CrossRef]
40. Oh, S.Y.; Kim, S.; Keam, B.; Kim, T.M.; Kim, D.W.; Heo, D.S. Soluble PD-L1 is a predictive and prognostic biomarker in advanced cancer patients who receive immune checkpoint blockade treatment. *Sci. Rep.* **2021**, *11*, 19712. [CrossRef]
41. Chiarucci, C.; Cannito, S.; Daffina, M.G.; Amato, G.; Giacobini, G.; Cutaia, O.; Lofiego, M.F.; Fazio, C.; Giannarelli, D.; Danielli, R.; et al. Circulating Levels of PD-L1 in Mesothelioma Patients from the NIBIT-MESO-1 Study: Correlation with Survival. *Cancers* **2020**, *12*, 361. [CrossRef] [PubMed]
42. Wu, B.; Sternheim, N.; Agarwal, P.; Suchomel, J.; Vadhavkar, S.; Bruno, R.; Ballinger, M.; Bernaards, C.A.; Chan, P.; Ruppel, J.; et al. Evaluation of atezolizumab immunogenicity: Clinical pharmacology (part 1). *Clin. Transl. Sci.* **2022**, *15*, 130–140. [CrossRef] [PubMed]

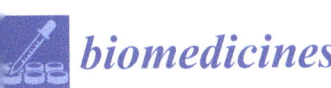 

*Article*

# The Four-Feature Prognostic Models for Cancer-Specific and Overall Survival after Surgery for Localized Clear Cell Renal Cancer: Is There a Place for Inflammatory Markers?

Łukasz Zapała *, Aleksander Ślusarczyk *, Rafał Wolański, Paweł Kurzyna, Karolina Garbas, Piotr Zapała and Piotr Radziszewski

Clinic of General, Oncological and Functional Urology, Medical University of Warsaw, Lindleya 4, 02-005 Warsaw, Poland; rafalwolanski7@gmail.com (R.W.); paw.kurzyna@gmail.com (P.K.); trelkowa98@gmail.com (K.G.); zapala.piotrek@gmail.com (P.Z.); pradziszewski@wum.edu.pl (P.R.)
* Correspondence: lzapala@wum.edu.pl (Ł.Z.); slusarczyk.aleksander@gmail.com (A.Ś.)

**Abstract:** We aimed at a determination of the relevance of comorbidities and selected inflammatory markers to the survival of patients with primary non-metastatic localized clear cell renal cancer (RCC). We retrospectively analyzed data from a single tertiary center on 294 patients who underwent a partial or radical nephrectomy in the years 2012–2018. The following parameters were incorporated in the risk score: tumor stage, grade, size, selected hematological markers (SIRI—systemic inflammatory response index; SII—systemic immune-inflammation index) and a comorbidities assessment tool (CCI—Charlson Comorbidity Index). For further analysis we compared our model with existing prognostic tools. In a multivariate analysis, tumor stage ($p = 0.01$), tumor grade ($p = 0.03$), tumor size ($p = 0.006$) and SII ($p = 0.02$) were significant predictors of CSS, while tumor grade ($p = 0.02$), CCI ($p = 0.02$), tumor size ($p = 0.01$) and SIRI ($p = 0.03$) were significant predictors of OS. We demonstrated that our model was characterized by higher accuracy in terms of OS prediction compared to the Leibovich and GRANT models and outperformed the GRANT model in terms of CSS prediction, while non-inferiority to the VENUSS model was revealed. Four different features were included in the predictive models for CSS (grade, size, stage and SII) and OS (grade, size, CCI and SIRI) and were characterized by adequate or even superior accuracy when compared with existing prognostic tools.

**Keywords:** renal cell carcinoma; risk models; survival analysis; charlson comorbidity index; systemic inflammatory markers

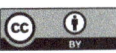

## 1. Introduction

The routine management of localized renal cell cancer (RCC) is radical or partial nephrectomy [1]. However, it should be emphasized that approximately 20–40% of cases become metastatic during the course of the disease, even given successful initial treatment [2]. Therefore, determining the key factors that affect postsurgical prognosis would allow early risk-stratification.

Oncological outcomes are routinely estimated based on the TNM classification and pathological features of a tumor [3]. According to the American Urological Association, the establishment of a prognosis should rely on TNM staging, while localized disease is connected with nearly 90% of cancer-specific survival [4]. On the other hand, there is a strong recommendation from the European Urological Association (EAU) to focus on more sophisticated tools along with a statement that new models should be compared to already existing tools prior to their introduction into the clinic [5,6]. Although it is obviously included in all the models, TNM staging proved to have restricted accuracy if selected as a single prognostic factor [2]. Additional information has been routinely gathered from pathological examination, i.e., grading or presence of tumor necrosis or sarcomatoid features [2].

Among other clinical parameters, a prognosis is often assessed using gender [7] or age [8]. It is thought that male patients may present with worse prognoses, similar to elderly people [7,8]. Interestingly, the observation that comorbidities may have even greater significance is often connected with the fact that urological cancers are diagnosed frequently in the geriatric population [3]. Consequently, despite curative surgery, other causes of mortality in RCC cases may be of crucial importance.

Among several others, three models have been validated in the literature on localized RCC, i.e., VENUSS (VEnous extension, NUclear grade, Size, Stage) [9], GRANT (GRade, Age, Nodes and Tumor) [10] and Leibovich (tumor stage, regional lymph node status, tumor size, nuclear grade and histologic tumor necrosis) [11]. Although their prognostic accuracies have already been documented, they are not commonly implemented in everyday practice. Furthermore, the EAU does not place one particular tool above the others and leaves the choice up to the clinician.

One can observe a recent growing interest in the novel inflammatory markers that can be easily obtained from preoperative complete blood counts and incorporated into clinical models for prognostic purposes [12]. Recently, we compared the accuracy of different inflammatory markers in the prognostic assessment of RCC and proved that these clinical parameters may enrich existing models [13]. However, the common clinicopathological features remained the pillars of risk stratification, as described by other authors [14].

The aim of the present study was to determine the relevance of comorbidities and selected inflammatory markers to the survival of patients with localized RCC treated by partial and radical nephrectomy in the search for a prognostic model. Here, we focused on a cohort of clear cell RCC patients as a predominant subtype, taking into consideration that the majority of clinical trials enroll these particular patients. The identification of the most efficient model seems to be of greatest importance in terms of both recruiting for future clinical trials and identifying the optimal candidates for adjuvant therapy.

## 2. Materials and Methods

### 2.1. Study Population

We collected and retrospectively analyzed the data from a single tertiary center on patients who underwent partial or radical nephrectomy in the years 2012–2018. We identified 645 patients treated with surgery due to renal cell carcinoma (RCC). We excluded patients who underwent nephrectomy for papillary RCC ($n = 97$) or chromophobe RCC ($n = 31$) or metastatic RCC ($n = 46$) and individuals with missing baseline clinical data ($n = 138$) or who were lost to follow-up shortly after surgery ($n = 39$). Finally, 294 patients with primary non-metastatic localized and locally advanced clear cell carcinoma treated with nephrectomy in our center were enrolled for further analyses.

Information about demographic, clinical and pathological features were collected. No previous cancer management was initiated prior to the radical surgery in all cases. The following clinical parameters were obtained: (a) demographic: age, sex; (b) body mass index (BMI), clinical staging based on available imaging, i.e., computed tomography or magnetic resonance of chest, abdomen and pelvis according to the 2017 TNM classification [15], comorbidities (including diabetes, hypertension, heart disease, autoimmune diseases) and Charlson Comorbidity Index (CCI) calculated according to Charlson ME et al. [16], chronic drug uptake (statins and beta-adrenolytics), preoperative laboratory findings of full blood count, surgery type (partial or radical nephrectomy); and (c) pathological: tumor stage and histological diagnosis, including grading and presence of potential necrosis or sarcomatoid components (according to Fuhrman and/or WHO/ISUP, when adequate) of clear cell carcinoma.

In the further analyses, we included two most promising inflammatory markers based on neutrophil, lymphocyte, platelet or monocyte counts, i.e., systemic inflammatory response index—SIRI—and systemic immune-inflammation index—SII. Based on the c-indexes obtained in the preliminary calculations and our previous paper on inflammatory biomarkers [13], we included SIRI and SII in the respective survival models. SIRI was calculated as follows: SIRI = neutrophil × monocyte/lymphocyte; SII was calculated as: SII = neutrophil × platelet/lymphocyte. Prior to the construction of a local risk model for patient survival after radical surgery, we performed analyses aimed at the validation of the available tools designed to be used in localized settings, i.e., VENUSS [9], GRANT [10] and Leibovich [11].

Information on cancer-specific survival (CSS), overall survival (OS) and recurrence-free survival (RFS) was included in the follow-up analysis. The study was conducted under the Ethics Committee vote AKBE/72/2021 of the Medical University of Warsaw. All patients signed informed consent.

## 2.2. Statistical Analysis

Statistical analysis was performed in SAS software (version 9.4., SAS Institute Inc., Cary, NC, USA). Baseline patient characteristics were presented as medians with interquartile ranges for continuous variables and numbers with percentages for categorized variables. Differences in continuous variables were compared using the Mann–Whitney U test, while categorized variables were evaluated with Fisher's exact test. Categorization of continuous variables (e.g., Charlson Comorbidity Index, SIRI, SII) was performed using the optimal cut-off values based on receiver operating curve (ROC) statistics. Logistic regression was utilized for uni- and multivariate analyses. Univariate analyses provided factors for stepwise selection in the development of the multivariate model. Odds ratios with 95% confidence intervals were derived via logistic regression. Two-sided $p$-values $< 0.05$ denoted statistical significance.

The VENUSS, GRANT and Leibovich models were externally validated with our patient sample using logistic regression and respective area under the curves with c-index for each risk model. The accuracy of the above risk scores was compared with our newly derived model. The differences in survival according to the risk classification based on the VENUSS, GRANT and Leibovich tools and our risk score were analyzed using the Kaplan–Meier method and evaluated with log-rank tests.

## 3. Results

### 3.1. Basic Characteristics of the Cohort

The majority of the cohort were males (n = 185) (please refer to Table 1). The patients were diagnosed mainly with T1 tumors (83.7%) of Fuhrman 1–2 (86%) grade. As for CCI, we stratified patients into ≤4 (57%) and >4 points. The greater percentage of patients underwent partial nephrectomy (65%). The details of patients' comorbidities are presented in Table 1 in detail. Additionally, a division into different risk groups according to the Leibovich, GRANT and VENUSS models is also presented in Table 1. For the median follow-up period of 53 months (IQR 42.5–61), patient survival values were determined: CSS, 94.6%; OS, 89%; and RFS, 86%.

**Table 1.** General characteristics of the studied cohort of patients with clear cell renal cell carcinoma (ccRCC).

| Characteristics | | No./Median | %/IQR |
|---|---|---|---|
| Gender | Female | 109 | 37.07 |
| | Male | 185 | 62.93 |
| Age | | 63 | 55–70 |
| BMI | kg/m$^2$ | 27.7 | 24.4–30.7 |
| Stage | T1 | 246 | 83.67 |
| | T2 | 20 | 6.80 |
| | T3 | 26 | 8.84 |
| | T4 | 2 | 0.68 |
| Grade | 1–2 | 254 | 86.39 |
| | 3–4 | 40 | 13.61 |
| Charlson Comorbidity Index | | 4 | 3–5 |
| CCI | ≤4 | 169 | 57.48 |
| | >4 | 125 | 42.52 |

Table 1. Cont.

| Characteristics | | No./Median | %/IQR |
|---|---|---|---|
| Tumor diamater | <7 cm | 247 | 84.01 |
| | ≥7 cm | 47 | 15.99 |
| SIRI | >2.15 | 170 | 57.82 |
| | ≤2.15 | 124 | 42.18 |
| SII | >660 | 189 | 64.29 |
| | ≤660 | 105 | 35.71 |
| Surgical treatment | RN | 101 | 34.35 |
| | NSS | 193 | 65.65 |
| Surgical modality | Lumbotomy | 155 | 53 |
| | Laparotomy | 62 | 21 |
| | Laparoscopy | 77 | 26 |
| Diabetes | Yes | 39 | 13.36 |
| | No | 253 | 86.64 |
| Hypertension | Yes | 180 | 61.43 |
| | No | 113 | 38.57 |
| Heart disease | Yes | 38 | 13.01 |
| | No | 254 | 86.99 |
| Autoimmune diseases | Yes | 14 | 4.79 |
| | No | 278 | 95.21 |
| Past MI | Yes | 17 | 5.82 |
| | No | 275 | 94.18 |
| Statins | Yes | 56 | 19 |
| | No | 176 | 59.86 |
| | Unknown | 62 | 21.14 |
| Beta-blockers | Yes | 80 | 27.2 |
| | No | 152 | 51.7 |
| | Unknown | 62 | 21.1 |
| GRANT risk group | Favourable | 271 | 92.18 |
| | Unfavourable | 23 | 7.82 |
| Leibovich risk group | Low | 253 | 86.05 |
| | Intermediate | 31 | 10.54 |
| | High | 10 | 3.40 |
| VENUSS risk group | Low | 244 | 82.99 |
| | Intermediate | 24 | 8.16 |
| | High | 26 | 8.84 |
| Outcomes | | | |
| Recurrence | No | 253 | 86.05 |
| | Yes | 41 | 13.95 |
| Death | No | 262 | 89.12 |
| | Yes | 32 | 10.88 |
| Cancer Death | No | 278 | 94.56 |
| | Yes | 16 | 5.44 |

### 3.2. Univariate and Multivariate Analyses of Factors Predictive for Cancer-Specific Survival in Patients with Clear Cell Renal Cell Carcinoma (ccRCC)

Associations between CSS and clinicopathological variables or laboratory parameters are shown in Tables 2 and 3. Univariate analysis revealed associations between CSS and high SII ($p = 0.0025$), high SIRI ($p = 0.0115$), tumor grade ($p < 0.001$), tumor stage ($p < 0.001$), tumor size $\geq 7$ cm ($p < 0.001$) and surgery type ($p = 0.0006$) (Table 2). In multivariate analysis, tumor stage ($p = 0.0128$), tumor grade ($p = 0.0354$), tumor size ($p = 0.0063$) and SII ($p = 0.0262$) were significant predictors of CSS (Table 3).

**Table 2.** Univariate analyses of factors predictive for cancer-specific survival in patients with clear cell renal cell carcinoma (ccRCC).

| Factors Predicting Cancer-Specific Survival—Univariate Analyses | | | | | |
|---|---|---|---|---|---|
| Variables | Reference | OR | LL 95% CI | UL 95% CI | p-Value |
| Age | >60 vs. ≤60 | 3.057 | 0.852 | 10.969 | 0.0866 |
| Gender | Male vs. female | 0.437 | 0.158 | 1.209 | 0.1108 |
| Charlson Comorbidity | >4 vs. ≤4 | 2.362 | 0.835 | 6.683 | 0.1052 |
| SII | High vs. low | 5.968 | 1.873 | 19.012 | 0.0025 |
| SIRI | High vs. low | 4.446 | 1.399 | 14.137 | 0.0115 |
| Tumor grade | High- vs. low-grade | 10.244 | 3.564 | 29.450 | <0.0001 |
| Stage T3–T4 | T1–T2 | 17.526 | 5.880 | 52.236 | <0.0001 |
| Tumor size | ≥7 cm vs. <7 cm | 20.829 | 6.363 | 68.176 | <0.0001 |
| Surgery type | NSS vs. NR | 0.107 | 0.030 | 0.385 | 0.0006 |
| Hypertension | Yes vs. no | 1.406 | 0.475 | 4.157 | 0.5382 |
| Diabetes | Yes vs. no | 0.418 | 0.054 | 3.253 | 0.4045 |
| Statins | Yes vs. no | 0.273 | 0.034 | 2.161 | 0.2186 |
| Beta-adrenolytics | Yes vs. no | 0.619 | 0.163 | 2.354 | 0.4816 |

**Table 3.** Multivariate analyses of factors predictive for cancer-specific survival in patients with clear cell renal cell carcinoma (ccRCC).

| Factors Predicting Cancer-Specific Survival—Multivariate Analysis | | | | | |
|---|---|---|---|---|---|
| Variables | Reference | OR | LL 95% CI | UL 95% CI | p-Value |
| Stage T3–T4 | T1–T2 | 5.101 | 1.414 | 18.396 | 0.0128 |
| Tumor grade | High- vs. low-grade | 3.948 | 1.099 | 14.188 | 0.0354 |
| Tumor size | ≥7 cm vs. <7 cm | 6.420 | 1.693 | 24.351 | 0.0063 |
| SII | High * vs. low | 4.547 | 1.196 | 17.280 | 0.0262 |

* High defined as SII > 660.

### 3.3. Univariate and Multivariate Analyses of Factors Predictive for Overall Survival in Patients with Clear Cell Renal Cell Carcinoma (ccRCC)

In the univariate analysis, the following associations between OS and clinicopathologic or laboratory factors were revealed: age ($p = 0.03$), CCI > 4 ($p = 0.045$), high SII ($p = 0.033$), high SIRI ($p = 0.006$), tumor grade ($p = 0.0006$), tumor stage ($p = 0.0005$), tumor size ≥ 7 cm ($p = 0.0002$) and type of surgery ($p = 0.02$). We failed to confirm the associations between survival and statins and beta-adrenolytics uptake (Table 4). In the multivariate analysis we found that tumor grade ($p = 0.0265$), CCI ($p = 0.0293$), tumor size ($p = 0.0156$) and SIRI ($p = 0.0334$) were significant predictors of OS (Table 5).

**Table 4.** Univariate analyses of factors predictive for overall survival in patients with clear cell renal cell carcinoma (ccRCC).

| Factors Predicting Overall Survival—Univariate Analyses | | | | | |
|---|---|---|---|---|---|
| Variables | Reference | OR | LL 95% CI | UL 95% CI | p-Value |
| Age | >60 vs. ≤60 | 2.625 | 1.096 | 6.286 | 0.03 |
| Gender | Male vs. female | 1.141 | 0.528 | 2.467 | 0.73 |
| Charlson Comorbidity | >4 vs. ≤4 | 2.151 | 1.019 | 4.542 | 0.045 |
| SII | High vs. low | 2.241 | 1.069 | 4.697 | 0.033 |
| SIRI | High vs. low | 2.947 | 1.364 | 6.368 | 0.006 |
| Tumor grade | High- vs. low-grade | 4.209 | 1.844 | 9.606 | 0.0006 |
| Stage T3–T4 | T1–T2 | 5.005 | 2.033 | 12.324 | 0.0005 |
| Tumor size | ≥7 cm vs. <7 cm | 4.588 | 2.078 | 10.132 | 0.0002 |
| Surgery type | NSS vs. NR | 0.416 | 0.198 | 0.874 | 0.02 |
| Hypertension | Yes vs. no | 0.908 | 0.430 | 1.919 | 0.80 |

Table 4. Cont.

| Variables | Factors Predicting Overall Survival—Univariate Analyses | | | | |
|---|---|---|---|---|---|
| | Reference | OR | LL 95% CI | UL 95% CI | p-Value |
| Diabetes | Yes vs. no | 0.402 | 0.092 | 1.753 | 0.23 |
| Statins | Yes vs. no | 0.687 | 0.247 | 1.906 | 0.47 |
| Beta-adrenolytics | Yes vs. no | 0.778 | 0.324 | 1.865 | 0.57 |

**Table 5.** Multivariate analyses of factors predictive for overall survival in patients with clear cell renal cell carcinoma (ccRCC).

| Variables | Factors Predicting Overall Survival—Multivariate Analysis | | | | |
|---|---|---|---|---|---|
| | Reference | OR | LL 95% CI | UL 95% CI | p-Value |
| Tumor grade | High- vs. low-grade | 2.964 | 1.135 | 7.740 | 0.0265 |
| Charlson Comorbidity | >4 vs. ≤4 | 2.473 | 1.095 | 5.583 | 0.0293 |
| Tumor size | ≥7 cm vs. <7 cm | 3.179 | 1.245 | 8.116 | 0.0156 |
| SIRI | High * vs. low | 2.453 | 1.073 | 5.609 | 0.0334 |

* High defined as SIRI > 2.15.

### 3.4. Multivariate Analyses of Factors Predictive for Recurrence-Free-Specific Survival in Patients with Clear Cell Renal Cell Carcinoma (ccRCC)

In the multivariate analysis, tumor grade ($p = 0.004$) and tumor size ($p = 0.0015$) were the only variables associated significantly with RFS (Table 6). No statistical significance was noted for CCI or any hematological marker.

**Table 6.** Multivariate analyses of factors predictive for recurrence-free survival in patients with clear cell renal cell carcinoma (ccRCC).

| Variables | Factors Predicting Recurrence-Specific Survival—Multivariate Analysis | | | | |
|---|---|---|---|---|---|
| | Reference | OR | LL 95% CI | UL 95% CI | p-Value |
| Tumor grade | High- vs. low-grade | 3.373 | 1.473 | 7.719 | 0.0040 |
| Tumor size | ≥7 cm vs. <7 cm | 3.605 | 1.634 | 7.954 | 0.0015 |

### 3.5. Proposal of Novel Scoring System for the Risk of Cancer-Specific Death (CSD) and Overall Mortality (OM) after Surgical Treatment of Clear Cell Renal Cell Carcinoma

The following parameters were incorporated in the risk score assessment (Table 7):

- Tumor stage T1–T2 vs. T3–T4;
- Low grade (G1–2) vs. high grade (G3–4);
- Tumor size (<7 cm vs. ≥7 cm);
- SIRI > 2.15 vs. ≤ 2.15 or SII > 660 vs. ≤ 660;
- CCI > 4 vs. ≤4.

Patients received one point for each unfavorable feature (T3–T4, high-grade, tumor size ≥ 7 cm and SII > 660), as for cancer-specific death analysis, for high-grade tumor, tumor size ≥ 7 cm, SIRI > 2.15 and CCI for overall mortality. Then, patients were stratified into low- (0 points), intermediate- (1–2 points) or high- (3–4 points) risk groups. Using respective stratification, we found that the cohort was comprised of mainly low- and intermediate-risk individuals (CSD—92%, OM—93.5%) (Table 8).

**Table 7.** Scoring system for the risk of cancer-specific death (CSD) and overall mortality (OM) after surgical treatment of clear cell renal cell carcinoma. n/a—not applicable.

| | Scoring System | |
|---|---|---|
| **Variable** | **CSD** | **OM** |
| | Score | Score |
| Stage | | |
| T1–T2 | 0 | n/a |
| T3–T4 | 1 | n/a |
| Grade | | |
| Low-grade | 0 | 0 |
| High-grade | 1 | 1 |
| Tumor size | | |
| <7 cm | 0 | 0 |
| ≥7 cm | 1 | 1 |
| SIRI | | |
| ≤2.15 | n/a | 0 |
| >2.15 | n/a | 1 |
| SII | | |
| ≤660 | 0 | n/a |
| >660 | 1 | n/a |
| Charlson Comorbidity Index | | |
| ≤4 | n/a | 0 |
| >4 | n/a | 1 |
| Risk group | | |
| Low | 0 | 0 |
| Intermediate | 1–2 | 1–2 |
| High | 3–4 | 3–4 |

**Table 8.** Risk groups for cancer-specific death and all-cause mortality after surgical treatment of clear cell renal cell carcinoma.

| | CSD Scoring | | OM Scoring | |
|---|---|---|---|---|
| **Risk Group** | No. Pts. | % | No. Pts. | % |
| Low | 151 | 51.36 | 82 | 27.89 |
| Intermediate | 122 | 41.50 | 193 | 65.65 |
| High | 21 | 7.14 | 19 | 6.46 |

*3.6. Cancer-Specific Survival According to Risk Stratification in Local and External Models*

Cancer-specific survival was significantly different among individuals stratified according to the respective model risk groups, as presented in Figure 1.

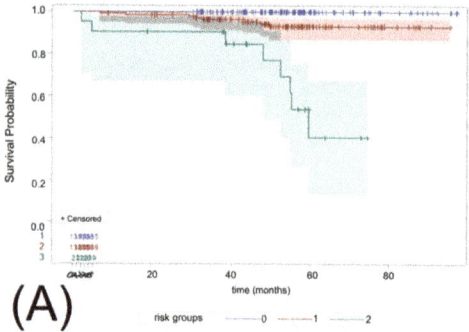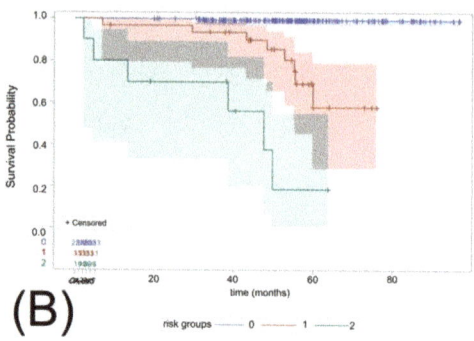

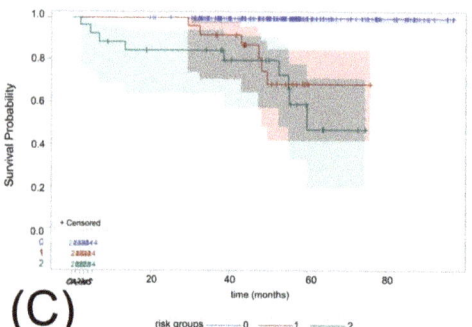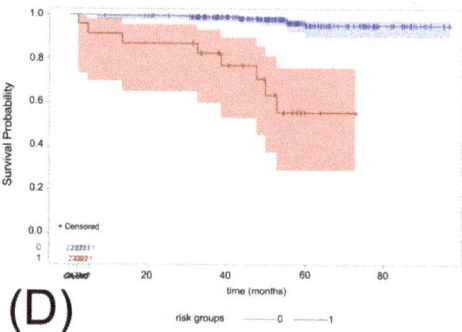

**Figure 1.** Kaplan–Meier curves representing cancer-specific survival according to the risk stratification as determined by our classification (**A**), and Leibovich (**B**), VENUSS (**C**) and GRANT (**D**) models. $p$-Values < 0.0001 were reached in all the respective models between the risk groups. Respective risk groups (0–2) were presented in different colors (**A–D**).

*3.7. Overall Survival According to Risk Stratification in Local and External Models*

The respective subgroups of all models, including our classification, were proved to be significantly associated with OS (Figure 2).

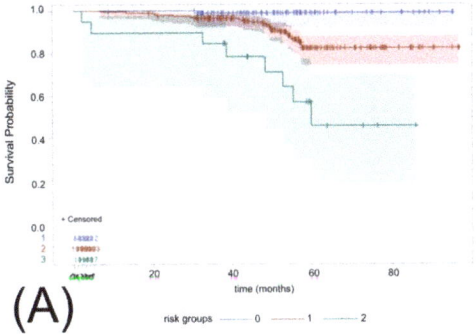
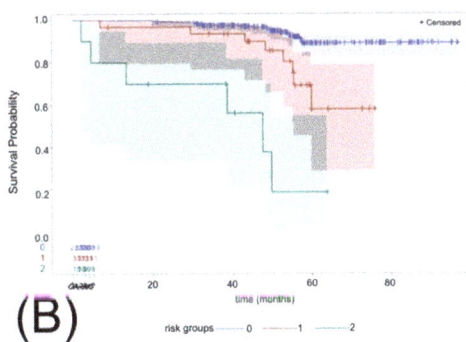
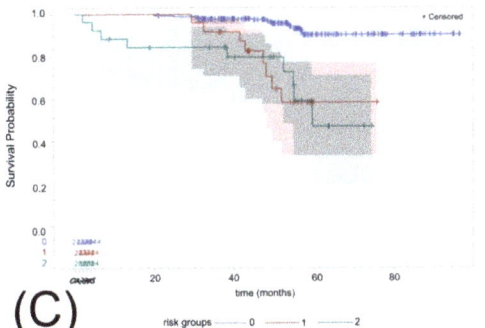
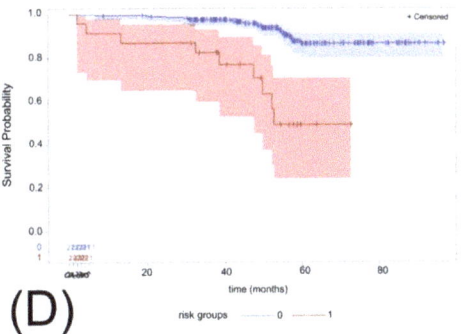

**Figure 2.** Kaplan–Meier curves representing overall survival according to the risk stratification as determined by our classification (**A**), and Leibovich (**B**), VENUSS (**C**) and GRANT (**D**) models. $p$-Values < 0.0001 were reached in all the respective models between the risk groups. Respective risk groups (0–2) were presented in different colors (**A**–**D**).

### 3.8. External Validation of the Established Risk Models (Leibovich, VENUSS and GRANT) and Comparison with Our Model

Using receiver operating curves (ROCs), we performed an analysis of the performance of the already used clinical models for non-metastatic disease (Figure 3A,B). Our model demonstrated higher accuracy in terms of OS prediction compared to Leibovich and GRANT and outperformed GRANT in CSS prediction, while non-inferiority to VENUSS with respect to both endpoints was revealed. External validation of the above-mentioned models indicated their high accuracy in terms of CSS prediction and moderate accuracy in terms of OS prediction.

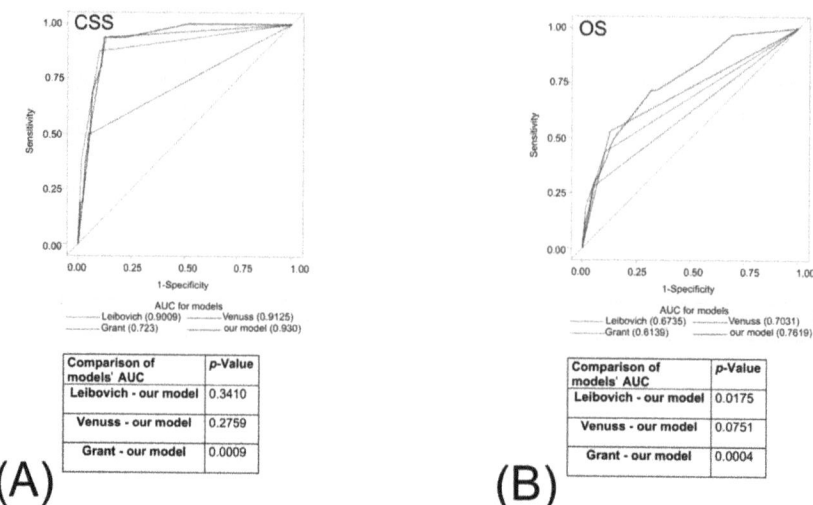

**Figure 3.** External validation of the previously established risk models: Leibovich, VENUSS and GRANT and comparison with our model. ROC curves for all the models were shown in different colors, representing prognostic values of the respective models for overall survival (**A**), and cancer-specific survival (**B**) (c-indexes of the models were provided in brackets). Additional collation with our model was presented with the respective *p*-Values.

## 4. Discussion

In the current paper, we revisited the idea of using prognostic models in ccRCC with the incorporation of easily obtainable clinical factors that increase the prognostic properties to be used in a localized setting. Thus, the predictive value of tumor stage, size and grade was exploited, with the inclusion of CCI and novel hematological biomarkers, i.e., either SIRI or SII, depending on the end-point assessed. These features were incorporated into four-feature models, predicting either OS or CSS in localized ccRCC with increased accuracy when compared with three well-recognized models used in non-metastatic disease.

The constant search for an optimal tool to determine the scheme of follow-up after radical treatment, taking into consideration the risk of recurrence and survival, is just one perspective. The schedule includes risk, timing and the site of recurrence, which, in turn, imposes close monitoring in high-risk disease [9]. In the light of growing evidence on the efficacy of adjuvant treatment, the personalization of therapy using models for localized disease is the other side of the coin [10]. Clinical tools to assess patients may be even more sought after in order to determine possible high-risk candidates for future adjuvant treatment, e.g., in the paper by Choueiri et al. summarizing the results of the KEYNOTE-564 trial, adjuvant immunotherapy resulted in a remarkable increase in disease-free survival in high-risk patients [17].

There is no consensus established regarding the optimal risk stratification policy in localized RCC, although a variety of prognostic models are available [9–11,14,18,19]. While awaiting results of clinical trials on the role of perioperative systemic therapy, the appropriate selection of candidates may be vital. Taking into consideration the side effects and costs of this approach, validation and application of the risk-based hierarchy will be necessary to optimize and simplify inclusion criteria [18].

The question that arises is as follows: what is the true value of additional features that are included in the already established prognostic models in the light of 'overfitting' phenomenon during model creation? Only after providing the answer can one justify their everyday clinical application [20]. Furthermore, none of the existing models is routinely recommended based on its approved accuracy [14,19]. As a consequence, there is a need for balance between predictive accuracy and simplicity in practice: incorporating additional features may not result in better prognostic value, while it may make the tool too complicated.

Although it is obviously included in all the models, TNM staging proved to have limited accuracy if selected as a single prognostic factor [2]. Additional information has been routinely gathered from pathological examination, i.e., grading or presence of tumor necrosis or sarcomatoid features [2]. Here, we introduced a novel prognostic model developed in the contemporary ccRCC cohort with a stress on both overall and cancer-specific survival using easily approachable features. Firstly, we established significant predictors for CSS in multivariate analysis to be used in a future model. Apart from tumor stage, grade and size, we observed statistical significance for a single hematological marker, i.e., SII. On the other hand, in the multivariate analysis of OS we determined that next to tumor grade and size CCI and SIRI were significant predictors of survival. Berger et al. pinpointed that coexisting chronic diseases remain significant prognostic factors for overall survival after nephrectomy [21]. Collecting the relevant information and translating it into a validated score may increase the efficacy of perioperative evaluation of the candidates for surgery, as discussed by Charlson et al. [16]. It seems reasonable then to opt for the incorporation of the Charlson Comorbidity Index into the prognostic tools in the hope of achieving more personalized approaches [22]. We determined that CCI (>4 vs. ≤4) was a significant predictor in both univariate and multivariate analyses of OS but not CSS. Although a detailed description of patient comorbidities is a routine preoperative work-up to establish both perioperative risk and to define the benefits of invasive treatment, it is rarely taken into consideration, when survival after the nephrectomy is analyzed [3]. Santos Arrontes et al. found that a significant predictor of OS was not only stage but also CCI (discrimination ≤ 2 and >2) [23], while Ather et al. observed a feature of >5 CCI to be an independent predictor of OS in cases treated with either radical or partial nephrectomy for RCC [3]. On the other hand, one should be familiar with another finding i.e., Gettman et al. failed to confirm a similar association between CCI and CSS in a cohort of selected patients with venous tumor thrombus and emphasized the TNM of the primary lesion as of greatest importance [24]. It seems, however, that OS in RCC is not only tumor-dependent but also patient-dependent, as relevant factors including individuals' comorbidities, gender and age should be acknowledged. Here, we found that age but not gender was significantly associated with survival in univariate analyses of both endpoints. However, we failed to incorporate it into the further multivariate analyses. It is consistent with the nationwide cohort study (n = 7894 participants) that pinpointed the relationship between survival of patients with RCC and comorbidities (cases with CCIs of 1–2 and ≥3 were found to have increased mortality rates when compared with patients with no defined comorbidity), regardless of age [25].

Recently, we found that the highest c-indexes were found when including SIRI or, alternatively, SII and NLR in the prognosis of localized RCC [13]. However, in the present population of ccRCC patients with a longer follow-up, only SIRI and SII reached statistical significance. In a recent paper by Mao et al., elevated SIRI was a better predictor of worse OS and CSS than LMR and hemoglobin [12]. Then, based on their own results, Lv et al. claimed that enforcing prognostic models with preoperative SIRI results in increased accuracy for RCC with tumor thrombus [26]. Hu et al. observed that high SII was found in cases with worse OS and CSS in a non-metastatic RCC cohort post-nephrectomy (n = 646) [27]. Ozbek et al. reported that elevated SII was found in patients with poor OS, but no association was revealed for disease-specific survival, despite the use of different thresholds [28]. Finally, in a meta-analysis that included 3180 RCC cases, Jin et al. reported that elevated SII was a strong indicator of poor OS (and aggressive disease) but not progression-free survival/disease-free survival or CSS [29]. These findings may shed some light on the associations of SIRI with OS and SII with CSS.

Interestingly, we failed to confirm associations with uptake of common drugs, including statins. This is consistent with recent papers, including a nationwide case–control study from Denmark (n = 4606 participants) [30]. Pottegard et al. did not confirm the hypothesis of a chemopreventive effect of long-term statin use on the development of RCC. On the other hand, Berquist reported that statin use resulted in improved CSS and OS [31].

Here, we validated three well-recognized models (VENUSS, GRANT and Leibovich) in our cohort and subsequently proceeded with the preparation of our own predictive tool based on clinicopathological features, including CCI and single inflammatory markers. Clearly, there is no single best model for all the populations of RCC that could be used in the assessment of all outcomes, i.e., OS, CSS and RFS [5]. In our model, we focused on localized ccRCC cases in the hope that we might determine other features that would have better discriminative properties when compared with TNM staging only. In the light of the multivariate analyses presented above, we described four-feature models for OS and CSS, respectively. Using ROC analyses we found that our model outperformed Leibovich and GRANT with respect to OS prognosis and GRANT with respect to CSS. On the other hand, we confirmed the non-inferiority of our model when compared with VENUSS. Therefore, external validation of the model would allow us to incorporate it into clinical applications, e.g., in enrollment for clinical trials purposes. Importantly, we discriminated between $\leq$T2 and $\geq$T3, high- vs. low-grade tumors and tumor sizes <7 or $\geq$7 cm, so Tumor characteristics were considered not only through T stage, while no additional pathological assessment was necessary (e.g., sarcomatoid features). The strength of the model may also lie with the incorporation of hematological biomarkers of established accuracy in the prognosis of RCC. Our model is not based on subjective clinical variables such as performance status but on intuitive calculations of CCI. Its validation in terms of predictive accuracy will enable its application in the adjuvant setting for high-risk patients treated with radical surgery to estimate the inclusion criteria for individuals that would gain benefit from systemic treatment. Finally, novel models and risk calculators can find their place in the field of transplantology, both during recipient qualification and the acceptance of organs with small renal lesions frequently found during donor assessment [32]. Our model may be of special interest to transplant clinicians due to the incorporation of blood count derivatives.

A principal limitation of our model establishment is the retrospective nature of the data from a single tertiary center. However, we focused on records that were complete for all patients and used a single pathological laboratory, a single laboratory for blood-count analyses and a single tool for CCI calculations. Additionally, the TNM classification that we used was based on the 2017 consensus [15], yet we included pathological grading according to Fuhrman and/or WHO/ISUP when adequate. Moreover, although the sample size was relatively small, we managed to obtain a satisfactory duration of follow-up with a standardized scheme. Our model, similar to other predictive models, is characterized by a significant deterioration in its performance over time. Furthermore, the outcome data were mainly based on intermediate- and low-risk patients. Finally, without external validation, we cannot exclude the possibility of model overfitting because of variable and threshold selections. Therefore, the prospective evaluation of our model in a larger population would enable its clinical application.

## 5. Conclusions

In conclusion, four different features were included in a model predicting the CSS (grade, size, stage and SII) and OS (grade, size, CCI and SIRI) of patients with localized non-metastatic ccRCC, characterized by adequate or even superior accuracy when compared with the VENUSS [9], Grant [10] and Leibovich [11] prognostic tools. The described scoring system for the risk of cancer-specific death and overall mortality can be used to stratify patients into respective risk groups for follow-up establishment or enrollment into clinical trials after prospective validation in a large population.

**Author Contributions:** Conceptualization, Ł.Z. and A.Ś.; methodology, Ł.Z. and A.Ś.; software, A.Ś.; validation, Ł.Z., A.Ś. and P.Z.; formal analysis, Ł.Z. and A.Ś.; investigation, Ł.Z. and A.Ś.; resources, Ł.Z., A.Ś., R.W., P.K., K.G. and P.Z.; data curation, A.Ś.; writing, Ł.Z. and A.Ś.; writing and re-editing, Ł.Z. and A.Ś.; visualization, Ł.Z. and A.Ś.; supervision, P.R.; project administration, Ł.Z. and A.Ś.; funding acquisition, N/A. All authors contributed to editorial changes to the manuscript. All authors have read and agreed to the published version of the manuscript.

**Funding:** This research received no external funding.

**Institutional Review Board Statement:** The study was conducted under the Ethics Committee vote AKBE/72/2021 of the Medical University of Warsaw.

**Informed Consent Statement:** Informed consent was obtained from all subjects involved in the study.

**Data Availability Statement:** The data presented in this study are available on request from the corresponding authors.

**Conflicts of Interest:** The authors declare no conflict of interest.

## References

1. Velis, J.M.; Ancizu, F.J.; Hevia, M.; Merino, I.; Garcia, A.; Domenech, P.; Algarra, R.; Tienza, A.; Pascual, J.I.; Robles, J.E. Risk models for patients with localised renal cell carcinoma. *Actas Urol. Esp.* **2017**, *41*, 564–570. [CrossRef] [PubMed]
2. Sun, M.; Shariat, S.F.; Cheng, C.; Ficarra, V.; Murai, M.; Oudard, S.; Pantuck, A.J.; Zigeuner, R.; Karakiewicz, P.I. Prognostic factors and predictive models in renal cell carcinoma: A contemporary review. *Eur. Urol.* **2011**, *60*, 644–661. [CrossRef] [PubMed]
3. Ather, M.H.; Nazim, S.M. Impact of Charlson's comorbidity index on overall survival following tumor nephrectomy for renal cell carcinoma. *Int. Urol. Nephrol.* **2010**, *42*, 299–303. [CrossRef] [PubMed]
4. Campbell, S.; Uzzo, R.G.; Allaf, M.E.; Bass, E.B.; Cadeddu, J.A.; Chang, A.; Clark, P.E.; Davis, B.J.; Derweesh, I.H.; Giambarresi, L.; et al. Renal Mass and Localized Renal Cancer: AUA Guideline. *J. Urol.* **2017**, *198*, 520–529. [CrossRef]
5. Usher-Smith, J.A.; Li, L.; Roberts, L.; Harrison, H.; Rossi, S.H.; Sharp, S.J.; Coupland, C.; Hippisley-Cox, J.; Griffin, S.J.; Klatte, T.; et al. Risk models for recurrence and survival after kidney cancer: A systematic review. *BJU Int.* **2021**, *online ahead of print*. [CrossRef]
6. Mickisch, G.; Carballido, J.; Hellsten, S.; Schulze, H.; Mensink, H.; European Association of Urology. Guidelines on renal cell cancer. *Eur. Urol.* **2001**, *40*, 252–255. [CrossRef]
7. Aron, M.; Nguyen, M.M.; Stein, R.J.; Gill, I.S. Impact of gender in renal cell carcinoma: An analysis of the SEER database. *Eur. Urol.* **2008**, *54*, 133–140. [CrossRef]
8. Hollingsworth, J.M.; Miller, D.C.; Daignault, S.; Hollenbeck, B.K. Five-year survival after surgical treatment for kidney cancer: A population-based competing risk analysis. *Cancer* **2007**, *109*, 1763–1768. [CrossRef]
9. Klatte, T.; Gallagher, K.M.; Afferi, L.; Volpe, A.; Kroeger, N.; Ribback, S.; McNeill, A.; Riddick, A.C.P.; Armitage, J.N.; Aho, T.F.; et al. The VENUSS prognostic model to predict disease recurrence following surgery for non-metastatic papillary renal cell carcinoma: Development and evaluation using the ASSURE prospective clinical trial cohort. *BMC Med.* **2019**, *17*, 182. [CrossRef]
10. Buti, S.; Puligandla, M.; Bersanelli, M.; DiPaola, R.S.; Manola, J.; Taguchi, S.; Haas, N.B. Validation of a new prognostic model to easily predict outcome in renal cell carcinoma: The GRANT score applied to the ASSURE trial population. *Ann. Oncol.* **2017**, *28*, 2747–2753. [CrossRef]
11. Leibovich, B.C.; Blute, M.L.; Cheville, J.C.; Lohse, C.M.; Frank, I.; Kwon, E.D.; Weaver, A.L.; Parker, A.S.; Zincke, H. Prediction of progression after radical nephrectomy for patients with clear cell renal cell carcinoma: A stratification tool for prospective clinical trials. *Cancer* **2003**, *97*, 1663–1671. [CrossRef] [PubMed]
12. Mao, W.; Sun, S.; He, T.; Jin, X.; Wu, J.; Xu, B.; Zhang, G.; Wang, K.; Chen, M. Systemic Inflammation Response Index is an Independent Prognostic Indicator for Patients with Renal Cell Carcinoma Undergoing Laparoscopic Nephrectomy: A Multi-Institutional Cohort Study. *Cancer Manag. Res.* **2021**, *13*, 6437–6450. [CrossRef] [PubMed]
13. Zapała, Ł.; Ślusarczyk, A.; Garbas, K.; Mielczarek, Ł.; Ślusarczyk, C.; Zapała, P.; Radziszewski, P. Complete blood count-derived inflammatory markers and survival in patients with localized renal cell cancer treated with partial or radical nephrectomy: A retrospective single-tertiary-center study. *Front. Biosci.* **2022**, *14*, 5. [CrossRef] [PubMed]
14. Correa, A.F.; Jegede, O.A.; Haas, N.B.; Flaherty, K.T.; Pins, M.R.; Adeniran, A.; Messing, E.M.; Manola, J.; Wood, C.G.; Kane, C.J.; et al. Predicting Disease Recurrence, Early Progression, and Overall Survival Following Surgical Resection for High-risk Localized and Locally Advanced Renal Cell Carcinoma. *Eur. Urol.* **2021**, *80*, 20–31. [CrossRef]
15. Sobin, L.; Gospodarowicz, M.K.; Wittekind, C. *TNM Classification of Malignant Tumors*; John Wiley & Sons: Hoboken, NJ, USA, 2009; Volume 7, pp. 1–5.
16. Charlson, M.E.; Pompei, P.; Ales, K.L.; MacKenzie, C.R. A new method of classifying prognostic comorbidity in longitudinal studies: Development and validation. *J. Chronic. Dis.* **1987**, *40*, 373–383. [CrossRef]

17. Choueiri, T.K.; Tomczak, P.; Park, S.H.; Venugopal, B.; Ferguson, T.; Chang, Y.H.; Hajek, J.; Symeonides, S.N.; Lee, J.L.; Sarwar, N.; et al. Adjuvant Pembrolizumab after Nephrectomy in Renal-Cell Carcinoma. *N. Engl. J. Med.* **2021**, *385*, 683–694. [CrossRef]
18. Graham, J.; Dudani, S.; Heng, D.Y.C. Prognostication in Kidney Cancer: Recent Advances and Future Directions. *J. Clin. Oncol.* **2018**, *36*, 3567–3573. [CrossRef]
19. Correa, A.F.; Jegede, O.; Haas, N.B.; Flaherty, K.T.; Pins, M.R.; Messing, E.M.; Manola, J.; Wood, C.G.; Kane, C.J.; Jewett, M.A.S.; et al. Predicting Renal Cancer Recurrence: Defining Limitations of Existing Prognostic Models With Prospective Trial-Based Validation. *J. Clin. Oncol.* **2019**, *37*, 2062–2071. [CrossRef]
20. Retel Helmrich, I.R.; van Klaveren, D.; Steyerberg, E.W. Research Note: Prognostic model research: Overfitting, validation and application. *J. Physiother.* **2019**, *65*, 243–245. [CrossRef]
21. Berger, D.A.; Megwalu, I.I.; Vlahiotis, A.; Radwan, M.H.; Serrano, M.F.; Humphrey, P.A.; Piccirillo, J.F.; Kibel, A.S. Impact of comorbidity on overall survival in patients surgically treated for renal cell carcinoma. *Urology* **2008**, *72*, 359–363. [CrossRef] [PubMed]
22. Kang, H.W.; Kim, S.M.; Kim, W.T.; Yun, S.J.; Lee, S.C.; Kim, W.J.; Hwang, E.C.; Kang, S.H.; Hong, S.H.; Chung, J.; et al. The age-adjusted Charlson comorbidity index as a predictor of overall survival of surgically treated non-metastatic clear cell renal cell carcinoma. *J. Cancer Res. Clin. Oncol.* **2020**, *146*, 187–196. [CrossRef] [PubMed]
23. Santos Arrontes, D.; Fernandez Acenero, M.J.; Garcia Gonzalez, J.I.; Martin Munoz, M.; Paniagua Andres, P. Survival analysis of clear cell renal carcinoma according to the Charlson comorbidity index. *J. Urol.* **2008**, *179*, 857–861. [CrossRef] [PubMed]
24. Gettman, M.T.; Boelter, C.W.; Cheville, J.C.; Zincke, H.; Bryant, S.C.; Blute, M.L. Charlson co-morbidity index as a predictor of outcome after surgery for renal cell carcinoma with renal vein, vena cava or right atrium extension. *J. Urol.* **2003**, *169*, 1282–1286. [CrossRef] [PubMed]
25. Horsbol, T.A.; Dalton, S.O.; Christensen, J.; Petersen, A.C.; Azawi, N.; Donskov, F.; Holm, M.L.; Norgaard, M.; Lund, L. Impact of comorbidity on renal cell carcinoma prognosis: A nationwide cohort study. *Acta Oncol.* **2022**, *61*, 58–63. [CrossRef]
26. Lv, Z.; Feng, H.Y.; Wang, T.; Ma, X.; Zhang, X. Preoperative systemic inflammation response index indicates poor prognosis in patients treated with resection of renal cell carcinoma with inferior vena cava tumor thrombus. *Urol. Oncol.* **2022**, *40*, 167.e9–167.e19. [CrossRef]
27. Hu, X.; Shao, Y.X.; Yang, Z.Q.; Dou, W.C.; Xiong, S.C.; Li, X. Preoperative systemic immune-inflammation index predicts prognosis of patients with non-metastatic renal cell carcinoma: A propensity score-matched analysis. *Cancer Cell Int.* **2020**, *20*, 222. [CrossRef]
28. Ozbek, E.; Besiroglu, H.; Ozer, K.; Horsanali, M.O.; Gorgel, S.N. Systemic immune inflammation index is a promising non-invasive marker for the prognosis of the patients with localized renal cell carcinoma. *Int. Urol. Nephrol.* **2020**, *52*, 1455–1463. [CrossRef]
29. Jin, M.; Yuan, S.; Yuan, Y.; Yi, L. Prognostic and Clinicopathological Significance of the Systemic Immune-Inflammation Index in Patients With Renal Cell Carcinoma: A Meta-Analysis. *Front. Oncol.* **2021**, *11*, 735803. [CrossRef]
30. Pottegard, A.; Clark, P.; Friis, S.; Hallas, J.; Lund, L. Long-term Use of Statins and Risk of Renal Cell Carcinoma: A Population-based Case-Control Study. *Eur. Urol.* **2016**, *69*, 877–882. [CrossRef]
31. Berquist, S.W.; Lee, H.J.; Hamilton, Z.; Bagrodia, A.; Hassan, A.E.; Beksac, A.T.; Dufour, C.A.; Wang, S.; Mehrazin, R.; Patterson, A.; et al. Statin utilization improves oncologic and survival outcomes in patients with dyslipidemia and surgically treated renal cell carcinoma. *Minerva Urol. Nefrol.* **2017**, *69*, 501–508. [CrossRef] [PubMed]
32. Eccher, A.; Girolami, I.; Motter, J.D.; Marletta, S.; Gambaro, G.; Momo, R.; Nacchia, F.; Donato, P.; Boschiero, L.; Boggi, U.; et al. Donor-transmitted cancer in kidney transplant recipients: A systematic review. *J. Nephrol.* **2020**, *33*, 1321–1332. [CrossRef] [PubMed]

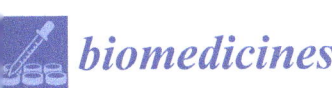

*Review*

# Prostate Cancer in Transplant Receivers—A Narrative Review on Oncological Outcomes

Karolina Hanusz, Piotr Domański, Kacper Strojec, Piotr Zapała *, Łukasz Zapała and Piotr Radziszewski

Department of General, Oncological and Functional Urology, Medical University of Warsaw, Poland Lindleya 4, 02-005 Warsaw, Poland; hanuszkarolina@gmail.com (K.H.); piotrek.dom12@wp.pl (P.D.); kstrojec1@gmail.com (K.S.); lukasz.zapala@wum.edu.pl (Ł.Z.); pradziszewski@wum.edu.pl (P.R.)
* Correspondence: zapala.piotrek@gmail.com

**Abstract:** Prostate cancer (PCa) is a low tumor mutational burden (TMB) cancer with a poor response to immunotherapy. Nonetheless, immunotherapy can be useful, especially in metastatic castration-resistant PCa (mCRPC). Increased cytotoxic T lymphocytes (CTLs) density is correlated with a shorter overall survival (OS), an early biochemical relapse, and a generally poor PCa prognosis. An increased number of CCR4+ regulatory T cells (CCR4 + Tregs) relates to a higher Gleason score or earlier progression. The same therapeutic options are available for renal transplant recipients (RTRs) as for the population, with a comparable functional and oncological outcome. Radical retropubic prostatectomy (RRP) is the most common method of radical treatment in RTRs. Brachytherapy and robot-assisted radical prostatectomy (RARP) seem to be promising therapies. Further studies are needed to assess the need for prostatectomy in low-risk patients before transplantation. The rate of adverse pathological features in RTRs does not seem to differ from those observed in the non-transplant population and the achieved cancer control seems comparable. The association between PCa and transplantation is not entirely clear. Some researchers indicate a possible association between a more frequent occurrence of PCa and a worse prognosis in advanced or metastatic PCa. However, others claim that the risk and survival prognosis is comparable to the non-transplant population.

**Keywords:** prostate cancer; transplant; immunosuppression; progression; metastatic prostate cancer

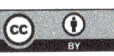

## 1. Introduction

### 1.1. Prostate Cancer in Immunocompromised Patients—Pathophysiology and Mechanisms of Development

The mechanism lying behind the increased risk of cancer development and progression in immunocompromised individuals has been described as a result of the cross-talk between the host immune system and the tumor microenvironment (TME).

The TME consist of many different types of cells that can be found within the tumor margins and distant tumor locations. Although it is believed to bear poor immunogenicity, prostate cancer develops a unique TME with an improper amount and/or function of immune cells compared to normal prostate tissue [1]. The most potent effectors in the immune response against cancer are CD8+ cytotoxic T lymphocytes (CTLs) [2]. It is important to note that the increased presence of CTLs within tumor margins is an optimistic prognostic factor in many solid tumors, and a number of studies show a correlation between elevated CD8+ CTLs and better prognosis [3,4]. However, the TME of typical PCa features decreased CTL infiltration [5]. Furthermore, PCa is an interesting example in which an increased CTL density correlates with a shorter overall survival (OS), early biochemical relapse, and generally poor prognosis [6,7]. The causes of this dysfunctional activity of CTLs are not clear at this time and requires further research. Another T lymphocyte subpopulation which is a part of the TME is regulatory T lymphocytes (Tregs). In normal tissue, these cells suppress the immune system response and prevent its overactivity. Furthermore, Tregs show immunosuppressive activity also in tumor tissue, limiting the anti-tumor response of other immune cells, including CTLs [8]. FOXP3+ Tregs are present within tumor margins in most PCa cases, with a significantly higher burden when compared to healthy tissue [9]. Additionally, there is a correlation between a higher infiltration of FOXP3+ Tregs and shorter progression-free survival (PFS) and shorter OS [10]. Another report shows that an increased number of CCR4+ Tregs correlates with a poor prognosis, more advanced clinical stage of PCa, higher Gleason score, earlier progression, and shorter survival time [11]. B cell infiltration and density are also increased in the typical PCa TME [5]. Noteworthy, although the B cell density does not correlate with the baseline PCa characteristics, it becomes significantly higher in patients experiencing recurrence or progression [12]. One of the most noticeable innate immune cell types infiltrating PCa is the macrophage. Macrophages can present with two different types of activity—classic, proinflammatory activity (M1) or immunosuppressive activity (M2), with M2 macrophages expressing various immunosuppressive chemokines and cytokines (e.g., TGF-β, CCL17, CCL22, CCL24, IL-10) resulting in the recruitment of Tregs and inhibition of CTLs [13]. Some studies show increased numbers of both M1 and M2 macrophages in tumor tissue compared to normal tissue [5]. However, another report suggests that in PCa, the majority of tumor-infiltrating macrophages are M2 macrophages [14]. This study also shows that high infiltration of M2 macrophages correlates with a worse prognosis. Additionally, other reports present similar results showing that in general, the increased infiltration of macrophages within the PCa tissue is associated with a poor prognosis [15,16]. Another group of cells participating in creating the TME of PCa are cancer-associated fibroblasts (CAFs). Chronic inflammation within the tumor tissue activates CAFs, which leads to monocyte recruitment and promotes their differentiation into immunosuppressive M2 macrophages [17]. Interestingly, M2 macrophages can affect CAFs leading to their increased reactivity, which creates positive feedback and results in suppressing the anti-tumor response and CTL activity [17].

Immunosuppression can interact with the immune aspects of PCa pathophysiology and its natural history in a large spectrum of patterns. As shown in the previous part, the interactions between the immune system and PCa are complex and it is hard to determine how immunosuppression impacts PCa development. The main agents used for pharmacological immunosuppression are calcineurin inhibitors (CNIs, e.g., cyclosporine A, tacrolimus), mammalian target of rapamycin (mTOR) inhibitors (e.g., sirolimus and everolimus), antimetabolites (e.g., azathioprine and mycophenolate), and glucocorticoids [18].

Immunosuppressive therapy affects mainly cell-mediated immunity, decreasing the activity of T cells. It is especially important in cancer with immunosuppressive TME, such as PCa. Studies show that immunosuppression may affect the incidence of post-transplant neoplasms [19]. However, there is no unambiguous evidence of an increased incidence of PCa in the immunocompromised population. CNIs suppress the immune system function by inhibiting the interleukin 2 production, leading to reduced CTL activity [20]. Azathioprine and mycophenolate inhibit de novo purine synthesis, blocking B and T lymphocyte proliferation, including CTL proliferation [20]. Decreased CTL activity and proliferation may lead to the decreased CTL infiltration of PCa tissue and potentially exacerbate the immunosuppressive character of the PCa TME. The improper function of CTLs may potentially lead to the faster loss of immune surveillance and faster progression of PCa. However, as was highlighted in previous section, CTLs' influence on the PCa prognosis is inconclusive. Thus, it is hard to define the impact of decreased CTL activity on PCa development. It has been speculated that PCa carcinogenesis can be associated with chronic inflammation [21]. Based on that, immunosuppressive agents might theoretically prevent PCa carcinogenesis in some individuals by inhibiting the inflammatory response. Also, some immunosuppressive drugs demonstrate anti-tumor activity. Cyclosporine A and tacrolimus can potentially inhibit PCa cell proliferation, migration and invasion in both hormone-naïve and castration-resistant PCa [22]. Everolimus can sensitize PCa cells to docetaxel, and combined with docetaxel can decrease the production of vascular endothelial growth factor (VEGF) by PCa cells [23,24]. Glucocorticoids, on that matter, can potentially reduce tumor growth by blocking angiogenesis due to VEGF gene inhibition [25,26]. The reduction in VEGF production potentially inhibits tumor angiogenesis in PCa. Finally, it has been suggested that mycophenolate mofetil might reduce the invasive behavior of PCa cells [27]. These data suggest that definite conclusions on the influence of immunosuppression on the development of PCa are still hard to draw.

It is also worth mentioning that the post-COVID era has yielded several observational reports providing a significant amount of evidence of its impact on the RTR population. The presence of ACE2 receptors in the kidneys allows the binding of SARS-CoV-2's spike proteins, leading to endocytosis [28]. The resulting cytokine storm, triggered by the body's exaggerated response to the virus, can affect not only the lungs but also the kidneys [29,30]. Studies have indicated that RTRs face an elevated risk of acute kidney injury (AKI) and often require dose adjustments for immunosuppressive medications [31–34].

### 1.1.1. PCa as "Immunologically Cold" Neoplasm

Along with advances in immunotherapy, PCa has been initially described as an "immunologically cold" neoplasm based on its modest immunoreactivity and poor response to immune checkpoint inhibitors (ICIs) [35]. Possible biological mechanisms that make PCa unresponsive to immunotherapies are the immunosuppressive TME, low tumor mutational burden, loss of MHC class I expression, mutations in specific genes, and low PD-L1 expression [36,37]. Low CTL infiltration combined with the high infiltration and activity of M2 macrophages and Tregs create a highly immunosuppressive TME, resulting in the inhibition of anti-tumor CTL activity. The tumor mutational burden (TMB), defined as the number of somatic nonsynonymous mutations per megabase, has been shown to differ among different types of cancer. A high TMB is associated with a high cancer neoantigen expression, while a low TMB correlates with a low cancer neoantigen expression [36]. A low neoantigen expression on tumor cells results in a poorly immunogenic cancer [38]. The TMB is also a prognostic factor for the clinical response to ICI treatment and there is a correlation between a higher TMB and better OS among cancer patients treated with ICIs [39]. PCa is a low TMB cancer [40]. In comparison to PCa, high TMB cancers, such as melanoma or bladder cancer, have a good response to ICIs [39,40]. Consequently, clinical samples and metastatic PCa cell lines both exhibit a decrease in MHC Class I expression, which may indicate that this mechanism participates in creating the cold TME of PCa [41,42]. Finally, regarding the checkpoint inhibition of PD-1/PD-L1, which strongly correlates with the expression of target antigens, PCa cells present with a low expression of PD-L1 [43].

### 1.1.2. Immunotherapy in PCa—Defining the Subset of Immunoreactive PCa Patients

Several immunotherapies have been developed and successfully implemented in PCa, in particular in the metastatic, castration-resistant setting. For instance, sipuleucel-T is a therapeutic cancer vaccine, consisting of autologous peripheral dendritic cells collected from blood by leukapheresis. These cells are then incubated ex vivo with a recombinant fusion protein (PA2024) composed of prostatic acid phosphatase (PAP) and GM-CSF, allowing them to activate PAP-specific CTLs. This therapy was registered by the Food and Drug Administration (FDA) as a treatment of metastatic castration-resistant PCa (mCRPC). A double-blind, placebo-controlled, multicenter, phase III trial (IMPACT) of mCRPC treatment showed that the median OS was 4.1 months longer in the sipuleucel-T group compared to the placebo group (25.8 month vs. 21.7 months; hazard ratio (HR), 0.77; $p = 0.02$) and the 36-month survival probability was also better in the sipuleucel-T group than in the placebo group (31.7% vs. 23.0%) [44]. Moreover, a further analysis of these data showed that the best effects of the treatment were associated with lower PSA serum levels. According to researchers, it suggests that patients with less advanced mCRPC may be better targets for sipuleucel-T treatment [45]. In another review, researchers suggest that it might be due to a more active immune system and less immunosuppressive TME in the early stage mCRPC [46].

Another cancer vaccine that could be potentially used for PCa treatment is PROSTVAC. PROSTVAC is a drug composed of two live poxviral-based vectors that contain the PSA gene and three costimulatory molecules for T cells (TRICOM): B7.1, ICAM-1, and LFA-3. A phase II randomized, controlled, and blinded clinical trial for the treatment of mCRPC with PROSTVAC showed promising results. In this trial, 82 patients received PROSTVAC with GM-CSF and 40 received empty vectors (control group). Although there was no significant difference in the PFS, there was a better median survival (25.1 vs. 16.6 months), OS at 3 years post-treatment (30.5% vs. 17.5%) and the estimated hazard ratio was 0.56 (95% CI, 0.37 to 0.85; $p$ = 0.0061) compared to the control group [47]. However, further randomized, double-blind, placebo-controlled phase III trials for the mCRPC treatment did not confirm the previous results. There was no significant difference in the primary and secondary endpoints between the PROSTVAC and placebo groups [48].

In the phase II trial, another vaccine consisting of myeloid and plasmocytic dendritic cells (mDCs, pDCs) was administered to the group of 21 patients with asymptomatic/minimally symptomatic, chemotherapy-naïve, castration-resistant prostate cancer (CRPC). DCs present in vaccines were loaded with tumor-associated antigens: NY-ESO-1, MAGE-C2, and MUC1. Patients were randomly assigned to three groups treated with the mDCs vaccine, pDCs vaccine, and mDCs-pDCs combined vaccine, respectively. No significant difference in the radiological PFS (rPFS) between the treatment groups was found. Tumor antigen-specific (dm+) and IFN-γ expressing (IFN-γ+) T cells were detected in 5 of 13 (38%) radiological non-progressive patients and in 0 of 8 (0%) radiological progressive patients. Moreover, the dm+ and IFN-γ+ patients presented with a better rPFS compared to the dm- or IFN-γ- patients (18.8 months vs. 5.1 months, $p$ = 0.02) [49].

DCVAC/PCa is an immunotherapy based on dendritic cells that activate an anti-tumor immune response. A phase I/II trial of DCVAC/PCa treatment of mCRPC presented promising results, with an improved OS and the increased presence of PSA-specific T cells [50]. However, the phase III trial did not meet previous outcomes and no significant differences in any primary or secondary endpoints were found [51].

ICIs are a group of monoclonal antibodies targeting and blocking immune checkpoint proteins (CTLA-4, PD-1, PD-L1) which increase CTLs' cytotoxic response against tumor cells. Ipilimumab, a CTLA-4 inhibitor, was used in several phase III trials of mCRPC treatment. In one trial, ipilimumab following radiotherapy was administered to patients with mCRPC after the failure of previous docetaxel therapy. Although there was no significant difference in the OS between ipilimumab plus radiotherapy and placebo plus radiotherapy groups, the PFS was significantly higher in the ipilimumab group [52]. However, the prolonged observation of these patients and further analysis of this trial showed a significant improvement in the OS in the ipilimumab group [53]. In another trial, ipilimumab was administered to patients with asymptomatic/minimally symptomatic, chemotherapy-naïve mCRPC. Similar to the previous study, there was no significant difference in the OS but the median PFS was higher in the ipilimumab group (5.6 months vs. 3.8 months) [54]. In the phase II trial, pembrolizumab (PD-1 inhibitor) was used as a monotherapy in mCRPC patients treated previously with docetaxel and targeted endocrine therapy. There were three cohorts in this study: PD-L1+ with measurable disease, PD-L1- with measurable disease, and bone-predominant, respectively. The best OS, disease control rate, and the most satisfying anti-tumor activity were found in the bone-predominant cohort. Additionally, the objective response rate (5% vs. 3%) and OS (9.5 months vs. 7.9 months) were higher in the PD-L1+ cohort when compared to the PD-L1- cohort [55]. Moreover, a retrospective study assessing the correlation between the TMB and pembrolizumab treatment efficiency showed that a TMB $\geq$ 175 mutations/exome is associated with a greater efficiency of pembrolizumab monotherapy and better outcomes compared to chemotherapy in many advanced solid tumor types, including mCRPC [56]. Another phase II trial checked the efficiency of avelumab (PD-L1 inhibitor) as a treatment for progressive neuroendocrine or aggressive-variant metastatic prostate cancer (NEPC/AVPC). Out of the 15 patients enrolled on this trial, only one (6.7%) experienced complete remission. Importantly, this patient had an *MSH2* somatic mutation, a high TMB (73 mut/Mb) and a high microsatellite instability status. Additionally, the flow cytometry results from this patient with complete remission presented qualitatively increased levels of NKT cells, PD-1+ helper T-cells, CXCR2+ CTLs, and decreased levels of CXCR2+ monocytes, which suggest enhanced CXCR2-dependent myeloid and T-cell responses in this exceptional responder. Except for this unique individual, the rest of the patients (microsatellite stable) experienced stable or progressive disease with a poor efficacy of the treatment [57].

In the phase II clinical trial, sipuleucel-T combined with ipilimumab (CTLA-4 inhibitor) was used as a treatment for asymptomatic/minimally symptomatic, chemotherapy-naïve mCRPC patients. Fifty patients initially received three doses of sipuleucel-T and then were divided with randomization into two groups. The first group (26 patients) received ipilimumab immediately after the last dose of sipuleucel-T, and in the second group (24 patients), ipilimumab treatment was delayed by 3 weeks. Six patients responded to the treatment, with a reduction in serum PSA levels of at least >30%. The median OS was 31.9 months, the median rPFS was 5.72 months, and there were no significant differences between these groups in these parameters. Interestingly, the patients that responded to the treatment presented with a significantly decreased expression of CTLA-4+ on T-cells, compared to other patients. This difference was present even prior to the treatment. Moreover, this lower CTLA-4 expression correlated with prior radiotherapy of the prostate or prostatic fossa. Prior radiotherapy also correlated with a better rPFS [58]. However, in another phase II trial, 51 patients with mCRPC received sipuleucel-T treatment with or without prior radiotherapy and there was no significant difference in any parameter between those groups. Radiotherapy did not enhance the immunological response to sipuleucel-T treatment in this trial [59].

In another trial, patients with mCRPC treated with sipuleucel-T were randomly assigned to two groups: the observation group and the IL-7 group that received recombinant human IL-7 (rhIL-7). Although, there was no significant difference in the clinical outcomes (rPFS, OS) between those groups, rhIL-7 treatment caused the increased expansion of CD4+ and CD8+ T cells, and CD56bright natural killer cells [60].

Cetuximab is a monoclonal antibody that inhibits epidermal growth factor receptor (EGFR). It is used in the immunotherapy of colorectal cancer and squamous cell carcinoma of the head and neck. In the phase II trial of mCRPC treatment based on cetuximab and docetaxel, 34% of the patients achieved a confirmed PFS at 12 weeks and 20% achieved it at 24 weeks. Additionally, the median PFS was 2.8 months and the median OS was 13.3 months. Importantly, a better PFS significantly correlated with the overexpression of EGFR and the persistent expression of the *PTEN* gene, which may indicate the better efficiency of cetuximab treatment in this specific group of patients [61].

The population of patients with immunoreactive PCa is not easy to define. Many factors could potentially affect PCa immunological reactivity, such as the progression of PCa, specific gene mutations, TMB, expression of cellular proteins, type of immunotherapy, and accompanying treatments. The sipuleucel-T treatment efficiency may depend on the PAP expression on PCa cells and lesser disease progression. Simultaneously, ICI treatment efficiency depends on the target protein expression (PD-1, PD-L1, CTLA-4) and potentially is associated with a high TMB. Patients with the overexpression of EGFR and persistent expression of *PTEN* may be potentially good targets for cetuximab therapy.

## 2. Prostate Cancer Treatment in Transplant Receivers

### 2.1. Radical Treatment in Transplant Receivers

Systemic reviews from 2018 have shown that the most frequent therapy for patients with localized PCa after kidney transplantation is radical prostatectomy (RP) (82%), followed by external beam radiotherapy (ERBT) (12%) and brachytherapy (6%) [62]. All surgical approaches seem feasible but retropubic radical prostatectomy (RRP) remains the most common surgical choice [62,63]. Intraoperative difficulties are usually associated with the typical location of the graft and the transplanted ureter in the iliac fossa. Previous operations in this area also disrupt the normal anatomy and result in the formation of numerous adhesions.

A transperineal approach to RP has been suggested to provide better exposure to the bladder neck and prostate. Yiou et al. [64] implied that it prevents the potential risk of graft damage as well as provides a wider feasibility of kidney transplants in the further track, which is advantageous, especially for young people [64–66]. Unfortunately, the major limitation of this approach is poor access to the regional lymph nodes, which limits the candidates for transperineal RP to rare low-risk individuals detected in the post-transplantation setting in whom lymphadenectomy might be spared. Among the advances in minimally invasive techniques, laparoscopic radical prostatectomy (LRP) has also been confirmed as technically feasible and safe [67–70], with a robot-assisted approach (RARP) as the emerging surgical standard. Currently, RARP is the second most frequent technique in renal transplant recipients (RTRs) [71] because it seems to be a safe and minimally invasive method.

Radiotherapy is relatively rarely used to avoid potential radiation nephritis and graft ureteric stricture [72]. The majority of patients scheduled for RT will be treated with adjuvant androgen deprivation therapy (ADT). However, in recent years, brachytherapy has gained more popularity and some studies have shown very positive oncological and non-oncological outcomes [73–75]. This technique enables limiting the range of radiation and thus reducing the risk of the above-mentioned complications.

It should be mentioned that active surveillance (AS) can also be considered a viable option in selected individuals, including elderly transplant recipients and those with multiple comorbidities, who are at a potentially low risk of cancer progression. A recent case–control study has evaluated the difference in the active surveillance of renal transplant recipients and the general population [76,77]. Soeterik et al. [76], respectively matched (13) RTRs to (24) non-transplant PCa patients. The median total follow-up exceeded 5 years in both groups. The median AS duration was longer in the RTRs group 4.5 vs. 3.3 ($p = 0.223$) and discontinuation due to tumor progression was reported more commonly after transplant than in controls (47 vs. 34%). The five-year survival of the RTR and non-RTR patients was 39 vs. 76% ($p = 0.067$) for the progression-free survival, 59 vs. 76% ($p = 0.29$) for the retreatment-free survival and 88 vs. 100% ($p = 0.046$) for the overall survival. That might suggest that severe chronic diseases and problems related to organ transplantation are associated with a higher risk of death than prostate cancer itself. It should be noted, however, that the non-randomized character of the existing evidence bears an inevitable selection bias. Delaying transplantation until the eradication of prostate cancer remains the standard in the majority of cases, including low-risk individuals. The guidelines for kidney transplantation as well as other organ transplants assume that the recipient does not have any active malignancies [78,79]. Along with the increasing awareness of the natural history of PCa, the "cancer-free" rule in patients diagnosed with low-risk prostate cancer becomes more frequently contested [77]. It has been recently suggested that the course of PCa after transplantation remains similar to the general population and surgical treatment for low-risk cases can be considered overtreatment as in a standard setting [80]. Based on a survey study, 2/3 of transplantologists would consider AS oncologically safe among treatment-naïve candidates for transplantation [81]. Bieri et al. [80] conducted a simulated study which was developed based on a systemic literature search, clinical guidelines, and expert opinion. The simulation included 400,000 men aged 50–75 with stage 4 or 5 CKD and prostate cancer managed with AS. Four treatment strategies were considered and the primary outcomes included quality-adjusted life years (QALYs). Active surveillance and immediate listing proved to provide the best summaric health outcomes (6.97 QALYs), while definitive treatment and listing after a waiting period of 2 years were associated with significantly lower survival benefits (6.32 QALYs). However, due to the simulative character of the study, its results should be interpreted with caution.

In addition, immunosuppression does not appear to promote prostate cancer progression, but research on this topic remains inconsistent [82]. The time that should pass from radical treatment to transplantation is also a matter of dispute. The decision to transplant should be made by a multidisciplinary team consisting of a urologist and a transplantologist. It should depend on the biochemical response and adverse pathological features. Until high-level evidence emerges, the decision on active treatment in low-risk transplant receivers should be made on an individual basis [62,63].

Beyond individual patients, the COVID-19 pandemic has put a strain on the healthcare system. The waiting period for organ transplantation has increased and the number of procedures performed, including oncological surgeries, has decreased [83,84]. Interestingly, researchers have discovered that SARS-CoV-2's spike proteins can exert antiproliferative effects in vitro by downregulating cyclin-dependent kinase 4 (CDK4). Furthermore, they can enhance apoptosis by upregulating the expression of FAS ligand (FasL) [85]. However, further in vivo research is essential to establish the actual correlation between SARS-CoV-2 infection and PCa.

*2.2. Functional Outcomes and Complications following Radical Treatment*

2.2.1. Surgery

Heidenreich et al. [86] delivered a series of open approach (retropubic and transperineal) radical prostatectomies and reported no major complications during the operation and postoperative track. Blood loss, operative duration, and postoperative recovery also did not differ significantly between the RTRs and non-transplant group [86], although, some previous series [87] found a longer RRP operating time in RTRs (108 vs. 89 min). Among the RTRs, impaired wound healing and perioperative wound infections were observed significantly more frequently (29% vs. 7%, $p < 0.05$) [88]. The functional outcomes remained maintained with only two (9%) patients requiring one safety pad per day at 1 year after surgery [86]. The corresponding results were delivered by Kleinclauss et al. [65]. Noteworthily, erectile function with or without 5-phosphodiesterase inhibitors could be preserved in as much as 60% of the patients utilizing a nerve-sparing approach [86], which becomes a major point considering erectile dysfunction in patients after kidney transplantation is significantly less common than among dialysis patients [89]. Finally, graft function was maintained in all patients analyzed [65,86,87,89].

The choice of approach (minimally invasive vs. open) is currently an issue of shifting dogma. It has been suggested that laparoscopic radical prostatectomy in RTRs might bear an increased risk of rectal injury due to technical difficulties [70], although, no need for temporal colostomy or fistula was recorded in the available series [90–92]. The majority of the series was, however, carried out on patients treated with a robotic approach. The mean estimated blood loss (EBL) in open surgery seems to be higher than in RARP (404 vs. 300 mL) [63,90]. In fact, some studies have shown that in RARP, EBL may be much less than 200 mL [87,93,94]. In a contemporary series of patients treated with RARP by Marra et al. [90], no complications scored as Clavien 4 or 5 were recorded. The authors point out that, similarly to the open-approach series [86], the most common complications remain infections. On the contrary, Felber et al. [92] reported a significantly higher number of complications in RTRs matched for age, PSA level, and clinical stage in a case–control study. Postoperative complications were encountered in 51.2 vs. 8.2% and 10.2% of patients experiencing a Clavien–Dindo classification graded 3 or higher [64,95].

Lymphadenectomy (LND) in post-transplant settings remains a controversial topic. Although feasible, LND carries a particular risk of complications and impedes access to a potential second kidney transplantation. Furthermore, even normally low-grade complications such as hematoma or lymphocele in the area of the graft can carry serious consequences [90]. Although previously reported DVT-related graft loss reported in the literature did not follow lymphadenectomy [96], it should be emphasized that LND increases the risk of DVT, which eventually can lead to graft loss. The aforementioned risks discourage surgeons from performing lymphadenectomy; therefore, about 2/3 of patients are estimated to be spared an LND [63], with bilateral lymphadenectomy being performed even less frequently (in 5% of patients) [63,90]. The nodal staging remains the only rationale of LND and increasing the access to PET-PSMA might facilitate a more conservative approach, especially considering that the majority of patients will be staged pN0 [62,90].

The risk cutoff set for the general population should be reconsidered for recipients, so that the risk of progression and the risk of severe complications can be balanced [97].

2.2.2. Radiotherapy

Evidence regarding the utility of RT in RTRs remains limited and a consecutive post-transplant dedicated complication reporting system is lacking [62,98]. In all available studies to date [74,75,98,99], graft function was maintained and glomerular filtration remained satisfying after irradiation. Based on the limited existing evidence, the prevalence of the most common complications does not differ from the standard post-radiation track and includes diarrhea and cystitis as the most common early complication (67.5%) [100], and urethral strictures as late complications (13–38%) (3/23 = 13%) [75,101].

*2.3. Oncological Outcomes and Prognosis*

All curative modalities seem feasible in post-transplant settings, although RP—both RRP and minimally invasive—is the most frequently chosen method of radical treatment in RTRs. The rate of adverse pathological features in RTRs does not seem to differ from those observed in the standard post-RP population [63,90,92,95], with positive surgical margins (PSM) estimated to be present in 17–32% of individuals. The cancer control achieved in the post-transplant setting also seems comparable [90]. In the PCa cohort recruited from RTRs and treated with RARP delivered by Marra et al., the majority of patients remained free of PCa and no patients experienced systemic progression. During the follow-up of 42 months (22–64), out of 41 patients, four underwent adjuvant RT, two experienced biochemical recurrence (BCR) and two PSA persistence, one had localized disease persistence and one had local recurrence after RARP [90].

A multicenter study by Felber et al. enrolled 321 patients, including RTRs (group 1, n = 39) and non-transplant patients (group 2, n = 282). After a mean follow-up of 47.9 months, a total of 3 (7%) and 24 (8.5%) patients experienced BCR in group 1 and 2, respectively. The RTRs had a 96.4% progression-free survival rate at 4 years, while the non-transplant group had a rate of 90.6% [92].

The systematic review by Hevia et al. included 41 studies, with 319 patients with localized PCa after KTx. The patients were stratified according to the curative intent strategy, and the outcomes were compared after a mean follow-up of 33 (1–240) months. The recurrence of PCa after RP and EBR at 5 years, respectively was 12.3% and 50%. There were no recurrences of PCa after brachytherapy, but it was utilized only in 6% of the patients, so the heterogeneity analysis could have been biased. The cancer-specific survival (CSS) at 5 years after RP, EBR, and brachytherapy was 97.5%, 87.5%, and 94.4%, respectively, whereas the OS at 5 years was 85.3%, 75.9%, and 94.4%, respectively [63].

From the clinical point of view, many surgeons would go for open-approach surgery, bearing in mind the potential risk of the laparoscopic approach in RTRs. Smaller contemporary series have introduced RRP as a safe and oncologically efficient modality in RTRs [71,86]. Kleinclauss et al. evaluated the oncological outcomes of RRP in RTRs (n = 20) and compared it with the non-transplant group (n = 40). In fact, a tendency towards a lower rate of PSM in RTRs was observed, although it failed the conventional level of significance (10% vs. 37.5%; $p = 0.06$). The PCa recurrence rate was 10% (n = 2) in the RTRs and 25% (n = 10) in the non-recipients ($p = 0.3$) [65].

## 3. Metastatic and Progressive Prostate Cancer in Transplant Receivers

*3.1. Metastatic Prostate Cancer in Transplant Receivers*

The a priori aggressive screening in the transplant recipient population is very likely to constitute one of the main reasons for the more frequent PCa detection in this population [102,103]. This could also be the cause of TRs being diagnosed with PCa at a younger age than in the general non-transplant population [62,63,102,104,105]. Regarding the mean age of PCa diagnosis, RTRs were diagnosed around the age of 63 while the general population was around 70 years [102]; TRs vs. the general non-transplant population age at PCa diagnosis were 62 and 67 years, respectively [105]; and the RTR age at diagnosis was younger that in the general population (mean age 61.8 years) [63].

The largest group of studies was conducted on patients after kidney transplant (KTx), however, the association between PCa and transplantation is not entirely clear. Some previous research indicate a connection with a more frequent occurrence of PCa in patients after KTx [106–110]. The incidence ratio for PCa in RTRs is estimated to range from 0.88 to 1.70 [107]. Another analysis noticed that for 18 RTRs diagnosed with PCa, the standardized incidence ratio (SIR) was 4.47 (95% CI 2.64–7.06) [108]. A multicenter French study shows 1680 RTRs with 11 (0.65%) cases of PCa and after a follow-up, 1,2% of cases of PCa (n = 28/2338), which meant a higher incidence than expected [109]. Likewise, the study by Haroon et al. indicates a more frequent incidence of PCa—the RTR vs. non-transplant population was 1126/100,000 and 160/100,000 ($p = 0.01$), respectively [110]. However, others claim that the risk was not increased and is comparable to the risk in the non-transplant population [19,103,111,112]. According to Bratt et al., RTRs were not more likely to be diagnosed with PCa than the non-transplant population (OR 0.84, 95% CI 0.70–0.99) [100]. Another study compares the observed cases and expected cases of PCa, with the result of 1039 vs. 1126.9, respectively (95% CI 0.87–0.98, $p = 0.009$) [19].

There is a significant lack of well-established studies evaluating the treatment options available for mCRPC in RTRs. Despite this limitation, the existing reports seem promising, indicating that these patients can access contemporary therapies such as Lutetium-177 and abiraterone. Lutetium-177 targeted therapy, highlighted in both a prospective study and a case report, underscores the importance of dose reduction in minimizing the nephrotoxicity risk. These studies show the therapy's effectiveness while maintaining an acceptable adverse event profile [113,114]. There are several cases in the literature describing the possibility of using drugs in the treatment of PCa during immunosuppression caused by liver or renal transplantation [115,116]. A noteworthy case involved the use of abiraterone alongside dexamethasone, achieving notable efficacy in an mCRPC patient. Interestingly, the treatment strategy adapted by switching from dexamethasone to prednisone when the PSA levels constantly increased in the subsequent measurements. In addition to new anti-androgen drugs, the patient received denosumab for bone metastases. This diverse array of treatment options illustrates a very wide range of possibilities in the treatment of mCRPC. Importantly, the effectiveness and safety profiles of these treatments appear comparable to those observed in the general population. Further exploration is essential to confirm these observations and improve our knowledge regarding treatment approaches specifically for this group of patients.

### 3.2. Progression to mPCa in Organ-Confined or Locally Advanced Patients after Transplant

The most commonly diagnosed form of PCa is localized disease. Pettenati et al. show that cT1-T2 Pca was diagnosed in 87.5% (n = 21) of patients whereas T3 was found in 12.75% of patients (n = 3) [117].

Retrospective analyses by Haroon and Hevia yielded similar results—76% (n = 26/34) and 89% (n = 8/9) of patients were reported with localized PCa in both studies, respectively [110,118]. Cormier et al. indicate that clinical stage T1 and T2 were diagnosed in 50% and 25% of patients, respectively [109]. On the other hand, a higher incidence of advanced/metastatic PCa in TRs has been recently raised [102,105]. More recent observational studies report that 11–36% and 19.3–40% of PCa patients in the TR population are a priori staged as locally advanced and metastatic, respectively [102,105].

The increased prevalence of mPCa has been questioned recently [108,111,119]. The case–control study by Bratt et al. shows that patients with high-risk organ-confined or metastatic PCa were less likely to be diagnosed with PCa than the control group (OR 0.84, 95% CI 0.62–1.13). The authors concluded that the probability of developing advanced PCa over time in RTRs, even on immunosuppression, is not significantly higher than in the general population [111,119].

Furthermore, it is not entirely clear whether TRs have a worse prognosis in advanced or metastatic PCa. It has been speculated that biochemical recurrence in TRs can have a more aggressive track, and survival outcomes can be significantly compromised in post-transplant individuals with metastatic progression [103–105,107,109]. Konety et al. show that advanced or metastatic PCa can progress more rapidly in TRs and it is correlated with poor prognosis—33% mortality after a mean follow-up of 32 (1–79) months [104]. Sherer et al. noticed that in RTRs, after diagnosis, PCa progresses more rapidly and the disease-specific survival for stages II, III, and IV is shorter [107]. Miao et al. observed that PCa stage III was diagnosed more frequently in the general population than in TRs (24% vs. 11%; $p = 0.043$). However, stage IV occurred more often in RTs than in the non-transplant population (30% vs. 24%; $p = 0.043$) [105].

On the other hand, some studies suggest that the survival prognosis in TRs is comparable to that of non-transplant recipients. In the cross-sectional study by D'Arcy et al., there were 30 cancer-specific deaths (7.3 cancer-specific mortality rate) and 36.891 cancer-specific deaths (7.9 cancer-specific mortality rate) among TRs and non-recipients, respectively [120]. Likewise, Bratt et al. noticed that RTRs were not more likely to be diagnosed with PCa than the non-transplant population (OR 0.84, 95% CI 0.70–0.99), and no significant difference in the survival between RTRs with PCa and without KTx (PCa-related death—HR 0.87, 95% CI 0.47–1.62) was observed [111].

A consecutive review on transplant and non-transplant patients stratified by baseline, pathological, and clinical characteristics is depicted in Table 1.

Table 1. PCa characteristics in RTRs and non-RTRs.

| Author, Year | Accrual Period | RTR | Patients, n | Local T Stage, n (%) | Gleason Score, n (%) | Mean (Range) Age of the RTRs, Years | Mean PSA at PCa Presentation, ng/mL | Mean (Range) Follow-Up, Months | Time from KTx to PCa Detection, Months |
|---|---|---|---|---|---|---|---|---|---|
| Cormier et al., 2003 [109] | 1998 | YES | 28 | T1 n = 12 (43)<br>T2 n = 10 (36)<br>T3 n = 5 (18)<br>T4 n = 1 (3) | <7 n = 18 (64.3)<br>≥7 n = 10 (35.7) | 63.0 (54–74) | 8.0 (1.9–318) | 18 (6–30) | 60 (1–156) |
| Hafron et al., 2004 [66] | 1991–2004 | YES | 7 | T1 n = 5 (71.4)<br>T2 n = 2 (28.6) | <7 n = 5 (71.4)<br>≥7 n = 2 (28.6) | 62.3 (2.5, 55–74) | 7.9 (5.6–10) | 22 (2–130) | 86.5 (25.25, 24–192) |
| Kleinclauss et al., 2008 [102] | 1983–2005 | YES | 62 | T1 n = 19 (30.6)<br>T2 n = 21 (33.9)<br>T3 n = 21 (33.9)<br>T4 n = 1 (1.6) | <7 n = 42 (67.7)<br>≥7 n = 20 (32.3) | 69.2 (50.8–75.1) | 7.6 (1.6–597) | 24.7 ±24 | 67 ±42 |
| Hoda et al., 2010 [87] | 2001–2007 | YES | 16 | T2 n = 16 (100) | <7 n = 14 (87)<br>≥7 n = 2 (13) | 61.8 (51–66) | 4.7 ±1.4 | 25 | 81.2 ±19.1 |
|  |  | NO | 294 | T2 n = 194 (66)<br>T3 n = 100 (34) | <7 n = 248 (84.4)<br>≥7 n = 46 (15.6) | 64.4 ±9.3 | 6.32 ±1.7 | 34 | - |
| Heidenreich et al., 2014 [86] | 2000–2011 | YES | 23 | T2 n = 16 (69.6)<br>T3 n = 7 (30.4) | <7 n = 14 (60.9)<br>≥7 n = 9 (39.1) | 64 (59–67) | 4.5 (3–17.5) | 42.5 (10–141) | 95 (24–206) |
| Hevia et al., 2014 [118] | 1977–2010 | YES | 9 | NA | NA | 59 (56–65.5) | NA | 31 (15.8–34.0) | 57 (39–76) |
| Pettenati et al., 2016 [117] | 2000–2013 | YES | 24 | T1 n = 7 (29.2)<br>T2 n = 14 (58.3)<br>T3 n = 3 (12.5) | <7 n = 10 (41.7)<br>≥n = 14 (58.3) | 63.5 (51–78) | 7.5 (3.8–11.2) | 46 ±29 | 55 (1–402) |
|  |  | NO | 64 | ≤T2c n = 55 (86)<br>T3 n = 9 (14) | <7 n = 30 (46.9)<br>≥7 n = 34 (53.1) | 63.9 ±5.1 | 7.5 ±3.3 | 34.1 ±25 | - |
| Bratt et al., 2020 [111] | 1998–2016 | YES | 133 | T1 n = 73 (55)<br>T2 n = 39 (29)<br>T3 n = 11 (8)<br>T4 n = 3 (2)<br>Missing n = 7 (5) | <7 n = 67 (50)<br>≥7 n = 63 (48)<br>Missing n = 3 (2) | 56 (47–63) | NA | NA | 120 (72–216) |
|  |  | NO | 665 | T1 n = 360 (54)<br>T2 n = 182 (27)<br>T3 n = 93 (14)<br>T4 n = 18 (3)<br>Missing n = 12 (2) | <7 n = 307 (46)<br>≥7 n = 350 (53)<br>Missing n = 8 (1) | 66 (61–72) | NA | NA | - |
| Marra et al., 2022 [90] | 2009–2019 | YES | 41 | T2 n = 29 (70.7)<br>T3 n = 11 (26.8)<br>Missing n = 1 (2.5) | <7 n = 9 (22)<br>≥7 n = 32 (78) | 60 (57–64) | 6.5 (5.2–10.2) | 42 (22–64) | 118 (57–184) |

**Author Contributions:** Conceptualization, P.Z., Ł.Z. and P.R.; methodology, P.Z.; software, P.Z.; resources, P.R., Ł.Z. and P.Z.; writing—original draft preparation, K.H., P.D., K.S., P.Z., Ł.Z. and P.R.; writing—review and editing, P.Z., Ł.Z. and P.R.; supervision, P.Z., Ł.Z. and P.R.; project administration, P.Z., Ł.Z. and P.R.; funding acquisition, Ł.Z. All authors have read and agreed to the published version of the manuscript.

**Funding:** This research received no external funding.

**Institutional Review Board Statement:** Not applicable.

**Informed Consent Statement:** Not applicable.

**Conflicts of Interest:** The authors declare no conflict of interest.

## References

1. Kwon, J.T.W.; Bryant, R.J.; Parkes, E.E. The tumor microenvironment and immune responses in prostate cancer patients. *Endocr. Relat. Cancer* **2021**, *28*, T95–T107. [CrossRef] [PubMed]
2. Raskov, H.; Orhan, A.; Christensen, J.P.; Gögenur, I. Cytotoxic CD8+ T cells in cancer and cancer immunotherapy. *Br. J. Cancer* **2021**, *124*, 359–367. [CrossRef]
3. Fridman, W.H.; Zitvogel, L.; Sautès–Fridman, C.; Kroemer, G. The immune contexture in cancer prognosis and treatment. *Nat. Rev. Clin. Oncol.* **2017**, *14*, 717–734. [CrossRef]
4. Bruni, D.; Angell, H.K.; Galon, J. The immune contexture and Immunoscore in cancer prognosis and therapeutic efficacy. *Nat. Rev. Cancer* **2020**, *20*, 662–680. [CrossRef]
5. Wu, Z.; Chen, H.; Luo, W.; Zhang, H.; Li, G.; Zeng, F.; Deng, F. The Landscape of Immune Cells Infiltrating in Prostate Cancer. *Front. Oncol.* **2020**, *10*, 517637. [CrossRef]
6. Ness, N.; Andersen, S.; Valkov, A.; Nordby, Y.; Donnem, T.; Al-Saad, S.; Busund, L.-T.; Bremnes, R.M.; Richardsen, E. Infiltration of CD8+ lymphocytes is an independent prognostic factor of biochemical failure-free survival in prostate cancer: CD8+ Lymphocytes in Prostate Cancer. *Prostate* **2014**, *74*, 1452–1461. [CrossRef]
7. Kaur, H.B.; Guedes, L.B.; Lu, J.; Maldonado, L.; Reitz, L.; Barber, J.R.; De Marzo, A.M.; Tosoian, J.J.; Tomlins, S.A.; Schaeffer, E.M.; et al. Association of tumor-infiltrating T-cell density with molecular subtype, racial ancestry and clinical outcomes in prostate cancer. *Mod. Pathol.* **2018**, *31*, 1539–1552. [CrossRef]
8. Tanaka, A.; Sakaguchi, S. Regulatory T cells in cancer immunotherapy. *Cell Res.* **2017**, *27*, 109–118. [CrossRef] [PubMed]
9. Kiniwa, Y.; Miyahara, Y.; Wang, H.Y.; Peng, W.; Peng, G.; Wheeler, T.M.; Thompson, T.C.; Old, L.J.; Wang, R.-F. CD8+ Foxp3+ Regulatory T Cells Mediate Immunosuppression in Prostate Cancer. *Clin. Cancer Res.* **2007**, *13*, 6947–6958. [CrossRef]
10. Nardone, V.; Botta, C.; Caraglia, M.; Martino, E.C.; Ambrosio, M.R.; Carfagno, T.; Tini, P.; Semeraro, L.; Misso, G.; Grimaldi, A.; et al. Tumor infiltrating T lymphocytes expressing FoxP3, CCR7 or PD-1 predict the outcome of prostate cancer patients subjected to salvage radiotherapy after biochemical relapse. *Cancer Biol. Ther.* **2016**, *17*, 1213–1220. [CrossRef]
11. Watanabe, M.; Kanao, K.; Suzuki, S.; Muramatsu, H.; Morinaga, S.; Kajikawa, K.; Kobayashi, I.; Nishikawa, G.; Kato, Y.; Zennami, K.; et al. Increased infiltration of CCR4-positive regulatory T cells in prostate cancer tissue is associated with a poor prognosis. *Prostate* **2019**, *79*, 1658–1665. [CrossRef]
12. Woo, J.R.; Liss, M.A.; Muldong, M.T.; Palazzi, K.; Strasner, A.; Ammirante, M.; Varki, N.; Shabaik, A.; Howell, S.; Kane, C.J.; et al. Tumor infiltrating B-cells are increased in prostate cancer tissue. *J. Transl. Med.* **2014**, *12*, 30. [CrossRef]
13. Biswas, S.K.; Mantovani, A. Macrophage plasticity and interaction with lymphocyte subsets: Cancer as a paradigm. *Nat. Immunol.* **2010**, *11*, 889–896. [CrossRef]
14. Lundholm, M.; Hägglöf, C.; Wikberg, M.L.; Stattin, P.; Egevad, L.; Bergh, A.; Wikström, P.; Palmqvist, R.; Edin, S. Secreted Factors from Colorectal and Prostate Cancer Cells Skew the Immune Response in Opposite Directions. *Sci. Rep.* **2015**, *5*, 15651. [CrossRef]
15. Lanciotti, M.; Masieri, L.; Raspollini, M.R.; Minervini, A.; Mari, A.; Comito, G.; Giannoni, E.; Carini, M.; Chiarugi, P.; Serni, S. The Role of M1 and M2 Macrophages in Prostate Cancer in relation to Extracapsular Tumor Extension and Biochemical Recurrence after Radical Prostatectomy. *BioMed Res. Int.* **2014**, *2014*, 486798. [CrossRef]
16. Nonomura, N.; Takayama, H.; Nakayama, M.; Nakai, Y.; Kawashima, A.; Mukai, M.; Nagahara, A.; Aozasa, K.; Tsujimura, A. Infiltration of tumour-associated macrophages in prostate biopsy specimens is predictive of disease progression after hormonal therapy for prostate cancer: Tumour-associated macrophages predicts the efficacy of hormonal therapy. *BJU Int.* **2011**, *107*, 1918–1922. [CrossRef]
17. Comito, G.; Giannoni, E.; Segura, C.P.; Barcellos-de-Souza, P.; Raspollini, M.R.; Baroni, G.; Lanciotti, M.; Serni, S.; Chiarugi, P. Cancer-associated fibroblasts and M2-polarized macrophages synergize during prostate carcinoma progression. *Oncogene* **2014**, *33*, 2423–2431. [CrossRef]
18. Malat, G.; Culkin, C. The ABCs of Immunosuppression. *Med. Clin. N. Am.* **2016**, *100*, 505–518. [CrossRef]
19. Engels, E.A.; Pfeiffer, R.M.; Fraumeni, J.F.; Kasiske, B.L.; Israni, A.K.; Snyder, J.J.; Wolfe, R.A.; Goodrich, N.P.; Bayakly, A.R.; Clarke, C.A.; et al. Spectrum of Cancer Risk Among US Solid Organ Transplant Recipients. *JAMA* **2011**, *306*, 1891. [CrossRef]
20. Barshes, N.R.; Goodpastor, S.E.; Goss, J.A. Pharmacologic immunosuppression. *Front. Biosci.* **2004**, *9*, 411–420. [CrossRef]

21. Tewari, A.K.; Stockert, J.A.; Yadav, S.S.; Yadav, K.K.; Khan, I. Inflammation and Prostate Cancer. In *Cell & Molecular Biology of Prostate Cancer*; Schatten, H., Ed.; Springer International Publishing: Cham, Switzerland, 2018; Volume 1095, pp. 41–65, (Advances in Experimental Medicine and Biology). [CrossRef]
22. Kawahara, T.; Kashiwagi, E.; Ide, H.; Li, Y.; Zheng, Y.; Ishiguro, H.; Miyamoto, H. The role of NFATc1 in prostate cancer progression: Cyclosporine A and tacrolimus inhibit cell proliferation, migration, and invasion: NFAT in Prostate Cancer. *Prostate* **2015**, *75*, 573–584. [CrossRef] [PubMed]
23. Alshaker, H.; Wang, Q.; Kawano, Y.; Arafat, T.; Böhler, T.; Winkler, M.; Cooper, C.; Pchejetski, D. Everolimus (RAD001) sensitizes prostate cancer cells to docetaxel by down-regulation of HIF-1α and sphingosine kinase 1. *Oncotarget* **2016**, *7*, 80943–80956. [CrossRef] [PubMed]
24. Alshaker, H.; Wang, Q.; Böhler, T.; Mills, R.; Winkler, M.; Arafat, T.; Kawano, Y.; Pchejetski, D. Combination of RAD001 (everolimus) and docetaxel reduces prostate and breast cancer cell VEGF production and tumour vascularisation independently of sphingosine-kinase-1. *Sci. Rep.* **2017**, *7*, 3493. [CrossRef] [PubMed]
25. Yano, A.; Fujii, Y.; Iwai, A.; Kageyama, Y.; Kihara, K. Glucocorticoids Suppress Tumor Angiogenesis and In vivo Growth of Prostate Cancer Cells. *Clin. Cancer Res.* **2006**, *12*, 3003–3009. [CrossRef]
26. Yano, A.; Fujii, Y.; Iwai, A.; Kawakami, S.; Kageyama, Y.; Kihara, K. Glucocorticoids Suppress Tumor Lymphangiogenesis of Prostate Cancer Cells. *Clin. Cancer Res.* **2006**, *12*, 6012–6017. [CrossRef]
27. Engl, T.; Makarević, J.; Relja, B.; Natsheh, I.; Müller, I.; Beecken, W.-D.; Jonas, D.; Blaheta, R.A. Mycophenolate mofetil modulates adhesion receptors of the beta1 integrin family on tumor cells: Impact on tumor recurrence and malignancy. *BMC Cancer* **2005**, *5*, 4. [CrossRef]
28. Sagnelli, C.; Sica, A.; Gallo, M.; Peluso, G.; Varlese, F.; D'Alessandro, V.; Ciccozzi, M.; Crocetto, F.; Garofalo, C.; Fiorelli, A.; et al. Renal involvement in COVID-19: Focus on kidney transplant sector. *Infection* **2021**, *49*, 1265–1275. [CrossRef]
29. Farkash, E.A.; Wilson, A.M.; Jentzen, J.M. Ultrastructural Evidence for Direct Renal Infection with SARS-CoV-2. *J. Am. Soc. Nephrol.* **2020**, *31*, 1683–1687. [CrossRef]
30. Hassanein, M.; Radhakrishnan, Y.; Sedor, J.; Vachharajani, T.; Vachharajani, V.T.; Augustine, J.; Demirjian, S.; Thomas, G. COVID-19 and the kidney. *Cleve. Clin. J. Med.* **2020**, *87*, 619–631. [CrossRef]
31. Yang, X.; Tian, S.; Guo, H. Acute kidney injury and renal replacement therapy in COVID-19 patients: A systematic review and meta-analysis. *Int. Immunopharmacol.* **2021**, *90*, 107159. [CrossRef]
32. Hirsch, J.S.; Ng, J.H.; Ross, D.W.; Sharma, P.; Shah, H.H.; Barnett, R.L.; Hazzan, A.D.; Fishbane, S.; Jhaveri, K.D. Acute kidney injury in patients hospitalized with COVID-19. *Kidney Int.* **2020**, *98*, 209–218. [CrossRef] [PubMed]
33. Coates, P.T.; Wong, G.; Drueke, T.; Rovin, B.; Ronco, P. Early experience with COVID-19 in kidney transplantation. *Kidney Int.* **2020**, *97*, 1074–1075. [CrossRef] [PubMed]
34. Banerjee, D.; Popoola, J.; Shah, S.; Ster, I.C.; Quan, V.; Phanish, M. COVID-19 infection in kidney transplant recipients. *Kidney Int.* **2020**, *97*, 1076–1082. [CrossRef] [PubMed]
35. Venkatachalam, S.; McFarland, T.R.; Agarwal, N.; Swami, U. Immune Checkpoint Inhibitors in Prostate Cancer. *Cancers* **2021**, *13*, 2187. [CrossRef]
36. Vitkin, N.; Nersesian, S.; Siemens, D.R.; Koti, M. The Tumor Immune Contexture of Prostate Cancer. *Front. Immunol.* **2019**, *10*, 603. [CrossRef]
37. Wang, I.; Song, L.; Wang, B.Y.; Rezazadeh Kalebasty, A.; Uchio, E.; Zi, X. Prostate cancer immunotherapy: A review of recent advancements with novel treatment methods and efficacy. *Am. J. Clin. Exp. Urol.* **2022**, *10*, 210–233.
38. Schreiber, R.D.; Old, L.J.; Smyth, M.J. Cancer Immunoediting: Integrating Immunity's Roles in Cancer Suppression and Promotion. *Science* **2011**, *331*, 1565–1570. [CrossRef]
39. Samstein, R.M.; Lee, C.-H.; Shoushtari, A.N.; Hellmann, M.D.; Shen, R.; Janjigian, Y.Y.; Barron, D.A.; Zehir, A.; Jordan, E.J.; Omuro, A.; et al. Tumor mutational load predicts survival after immunotherapy across multiple cancer types. *Nat. Genet.* **2019**, *51*, 202–206. [CrossRef]
40. Lawrence, M.S.; Stojanov, P.; Polak, P.; Kryukov, G.V.; Cibulskis, K.; Sivachenko, A.; Carter, S.L.; Stewart, C.; Mermel, C.H.; Roberts, S.A.; et al. Mutational heterogeneity in cancer and the search for new cancer-associated genes. *Nature* **2013**, *499*, 214–218. [CrossRef]
41. Sanda, M.G.; Restifo, N.P.; Walsh, J.C.; Kawakami, Y.; Nelson, W.G.; Pardoll, D.M.; Simons, J.W. Molecular Characterization of Defective Antigen Processing in Human Prostate Cancer. *JNCI J. Natl. Cancer Inst.* **1995**, *87*, 280–285. [CrossRef]
42. Bander, N.H.; Yao, D.; Liu, H.; Chen, Y.-T.; Steiner, M.; Zuccaro, W.; Moy, P. MHC class I and II expression in prostate carcinoma and modulation by interferon-alpha and -gamma. *Prostate* **1997**, *33*, 233–239. [CrossRef]
43. Martin, A.M.; Nirschl, T.R.; Nirschl, C.J.; Francica, B.J.; Kochel, C.M.; Van Bokhoven, A.; Meeker, A.K.; Lucia, M.S.; Anders, R.A.; DeMarzo, A.M.; et al. Paucity of PD-L1 expression in prostate cancer: Innate and adaptive immune resistance. *Prostate Cancer Prostatic Dis.* **2015**, *18*, 325–332. [CrossRef] [PubMed]
44. Kantoff, P.W.; Higano, C.S.; Shore, N.D.; Berger, E.R.; Small, E.J.; Penson, D.F.; Redfern, C.H.; Ferrari, A.C.; Dreicer, R.; Sims, R.B.; et al. Sipuleucel-T Immunotherapy for Castration-Resistant Prostate Cancer. *N. Engl. J. Med.* **2010**, *363*, 411–422. [CrossRef]
45. Schellhammer, P.F.; Chodak, G.; Whitmore, J.B.; Sims, R.; Frohlich, M.W.; Kantoff, P.W. Lower Baseline Prostate-specific Antigen Is Associated With a Greater Overall Survival Benefit From Sipuleucel-T in the Immunotherapy for Prostate Adenocarcinoma Treatment (IMPACT) Trial. *Urology* **2013**, *81*, 1297–1302. [CrossRef]

46. Crawford, E.D.; Petrylak, D.P.; Higano, C.S.; Kibel, A.S.; Kantoff, P.W.; Small, E.J.; Shore, N.D.; Ferrari, A. Optimal timing of sipuleucel-T treatment in metastatic castration-resistant prostate cancer. *Can. J. Urol.* **2015**, *22*, 8048–8055.
47. Kantoff, P.W.; Schuetz, T.J.; Blumenstein, B.A.; Glode, L.M.; Bilhartz, D.L.; Wyand, M.; Manson, K.; Panicali, D.L.; Laus, R.; Schlom, J.; et al. Overall Survival Analysis of a Phase II Randomized Controlled Trial of a Poxviral-Based PSA-Targeted Immunotherapy in Metastatic Castration-Resistant Prostate Cancer. *J. Clin. Oncol.* **2010**, *28*, 1099–1105. [CrossRef] [PubMed]
48. Gulley, J.L.; Borre, M.; Vogelzang, N.J.; Ng, S.; Agarwal, N.; Parker, C.C.; Pook, D.W.; Rathenborg, P.; Flaig, T.W.; Carles, J.; et al. Phase III Trial of PROSTVAC in Asymptomatic or Minimally Symptomatic Metastatic Castration-Resistant Prostate Cancer. *J. Clin. Oncol.* **2019**, *37*, 1051–1061. [CrossRef]
49. Westdorp, H.; Creemers, J.H.A.; Van Oort, I.M.; Schreibelt, G.; Gorris, M.A.J.; Mehra, N.; Simons, M.; De Goede, A.L.; Van Rossum, M.M.; Croockewit, A.J.; et al. Blood-derived dendritic cell vaccinations induce immune responses that correlate with clinical outcome in patients with chemo-naive castration-resistant prostate cancer. *J. Immunother. Cancer* **2019**, *7*, 302. [CrossRef] [PubMed]
50. Podrazil, M.; Horvath, R.; Becht, E.; Rozkova, D.; Bilkova, P.; Sochorova, K.; Hromadkova, H.; Kayserova, J.; Vavrova, K.; Lastovicka, J.; et al. Phase I/II clinical trial of dendritic-cell based immunotherapy (DCVAC/PCa) combined with chemotherapy in patients with metastatic, castration-resistant prostate cancer. *Oncotarget* **2015**, *6*, 18192–18205. [CrossRef]
51. Vogelzang, N.J.; Beer, T.M.; Gerritsen, W.; Oudard, S.; Wiechno, P.; Kukielka-Budny, B.; Samal, V.; Hajek, J.; Feyerabend, S.; Khoo, V.; et al. Efficacy and Safety of Autologous Dendritic Cell–Based Immunotherapy, Docetaxel, and Prednisone vs Placebo in Patients With Metastatic Castration-Resistant Prostate Cancer: The VIABLE Phase 3 Randomized Clinical Trial. *JAMA Oncol.* **2022**, *8*, 546. [CrossRef]
52. Kwon, E.D.; Drake, C.G.; Scher, H.I.; Fizazi, K.; Bossi, A.; Van Den Eertwegh, A.J.M.; Krainer, M.; Houede, N.; Santos, R.; Mahammedi, H.; et al. Ipilimumab versus placebo after radiotherapy in patients with metastatic castration-resistant prostate cancer that had progressed after docetaxel chemotherapy (CA184-043): A multicentre, randomised, double-blind, phase 3 trial. *Lancet Oncol.* **2014**, *15*, 700–712. [CrossRef] [PubMed]
53. Fizazi, K.; Drake, C.G.; Beer, T.M.; Kwon, E.D.; Scher, H.I.; Gerritsen, W.R.; Bossi, A.; Den Eertwegh, A.J.M.V.; Krainer, M.; Houede, N.; et al. Final Analysis of the Ipilimumab Versus Placebo Following Radiotherapy Phase III Trial in Postdocetaxel Metastatic Castration-resistant Prostate Cancer Identifies an Excess of Long-term Survivors. *Eur. Urol.* **2020**, *78*, 822–830. [CrossRef] [PubMed]
54. Beer, T.M.; Kwon, E.D.; Drake, C.G.; Fizazi, K.; Logothetis, C.; Gravis, G.; Ganju, V.; Polikoff, J.; Saad, F.; Humanski, P.; et al. Randomized, Double-Blind, Phase III Trial of Ipilimumab Versus Placebo in Asymptomatic or Minimally Symptomatic Patients With Metastatic Chemotherapy-Naive Castration-Resistant Prostate Cancer. *J. Clin. Oncol.* **2017**, *35*, 40–47. [CrossRef] [PubMed]
55. Antonarakis, E.S.; Piulats, J.M.; Gross-Goupil, M.; Goh, J.; Ojamaa, K.; Hoimes, C.J.; Vaishampayan, U.; Berger, R.; Sezer, A.; Alanko, T.; et al. Pembrolizumab for Treatment-Refractory Metastatic Castration-Resistant Prostate Cancer: Multicohort, Open-Label Phase II KEYNOTE-199 Study. *J. Clin. Oncol.* **2020**, *38*, 395–405. [CrossRef]
56. Cristescu, R.; Aurora-Garg, D.; Albright, A.; Xu, L.; Liu, X.Q.; Loboda, A.; Lang, L.; Jin, F.; Rubin, E.H.; Snyder, A.; et al. Tumor mutational burden predicts the efficacy of pembrolizumab monotherapy: A pan-tumor retrospective analysis of participants with advanced solid tumors. *J. Immunother. Cancer* **2022**, *10*, e003091. [CrossRef] [PubMed]
57. Brown, L.C.; Halabi, S.; Somarelli, J.A.; Humeniuk, M.; Wu, Y.; Oyekunle, T.; Howard, L.; Huang, J.; Anand, M.; Davies, C.; et al. A phase 2 trial of avelumab in men with aggressive-variant or neuroendocrine prostate cancer. *Prostate Cancer Prostatic Dis.* **2022**, *25*, 762–769. [CrossRef]
58. Sinha, M.; Zhang, L.; Subudhi, S.; Chen, B.; Marquez, J.; Liu, E.V.; Allaire, K.; Cheung, A.; Ng, S.; Nguyen, C.; et al. Pre-existing immune status associated with response to combination of sipuleucel-T and ipilimumab in patients with metastatic castration-resistant prostate cancer. *J. Immunother. Cancer* **2021**, *9*, e002254. [CrossRef]
59. Twardowski, P.; Wong, J.Y.C.; Pal, S.K.; Maughan, B.L.; Frankel, P.H.; Franklin, K.; Junqueira, M.; Prajapati, M.R.; Nachaegari, G.; Harwood, D.; et al. Randomized phase II trial of sipuleucel-T immunotherapy preceded by sensitizing radiation therapy and sipuleucel-T alone in patients with metastatic castrate resistant prostate cancer. *Cancer Treat. Res. Commun.* **2019**, *19*, 100116. [CrossRef]
60. Pachynski, R.K.; Morishima, C.; Szmulewitz, R.; Harshman, L.; Appleman, L.; Monk, P.; Bitting, R.L.; Kucuk, O.; Millard, F.; Seigne, J.D.; et al. IL-7 expands lymphocyte populations and enhances immune responses to sipuleucel-T in patients with metastatic castration-resistant prostate cancer (mCRPC). *J. Immunother. Cancer* **2021**, *9*, e002903. [CrossRef]
61. Cathomas, R.; Rothermundt, C.; Klingbiel, D.; Bubendorf, L.; Jaggi, R.; Betticher, D.C.; Brauchli, P.; Cotting, D.; Droege, C.; Winterhalder, R.; et al. Efficacy of Cetuximab in Metastatic Castration-Resistant Prostate Cancer Might Depend on EGFR and PTEN Expression: Results from a Phase II Trial (SAKK 08/07). *Clin. Cancer Res.* **2012**, *18*, 6049–6057. [CrossRef]
62. Marra, G.; Dalmasso, E.; Agnello, M.; Munegato, S.; Bosio, A.; Sedigh, O.; Biancone, L.; Gontero, P. Prostate cancer treatment in renal transplant recipients: A systematic review. *BJU Int.* **2018**, *121*, 327–344. [CrossRef] [PubMed]
63. Hevia, V.; Boissier, R.; Rodríguez-Faba, Ó.; Fraser-Taylor, C.; Hassan-Zakri, R.; Lledo, E.; Regele, H.; Buddde, K.; Figueiredo, A.; Olsburgh, J.; et al. Management of Localised Prostate Cancer in Kidney Transplant Patients: A Systematic Review from the EAU Guidelines on Renal Transplantation Panel. *Eur. Urol. Focus* **2018**, *4*, 153–162. [CrossRef] [PubMed]
64. Yiou, R.; Salomon, L.; Colombel, M.; Patard, J.-J.; Chopin, D.; Abbou, C.-C. Perineal approach to radical prostatectomy in kidney transplant recipients with localized prostate cancer. *Urology* **1999**, *53*, 822–824. [CrossRef] [PubMed]

65. Kleinclauss, F.M.; Neuzillet, Y.; Tillou, X.; Terrier, N.; Guichard, G.; Petit, J.; Lechevallier, E. Renal Transplantation Committee of French Urological Association. Morbidity of retropubic radical prostatectomy for prostate cancer in renal transplant recipients: Multicenter study from Renal Transplantation Committee of French Urological Association. *Urology* **2008**, *72*, 1366–1370. [CrossRef]
66. Hafron, J.; Fogarty, J.D.; Wiesen, A.; Melman, A. Surgery for localized prostate cancer after renal transplantation. *BJU Int.* **2005**, *95*, 319–322. [CrossRef]
67. Shah, K.K.; Ko, D.S.C.; Mercer, J.; Dahl, D.M. Laparoscopic radical prostatectomy in a renal allograft recipient. *Urology* **2006**, *68*, 672.e5–672.e7. [CrossRef]
68. Thomas, A.A.; Nguyen, M.M.; Gill, I.S. Laparoscopic Transperitoneal Radical Prostatectomy in Renal Transplant Recipients: A Review of Three Cases. *Urology* **2008**, *71*, 205–208. [CrossRef]
69. Maestro, M.Á.; Gómez, A.T.; Alonso, Y.; Gregorio, S.; Ledo, J.C.; De La Peña Barthel, J.; Martínez-Piñeiro, L. Laparoscopic transperitoneal radical prostatectomy in renal transplant recipients. A review of the literature. *BJU Int.* **2010**, *105*, 844–848. [CrossRef]
70. Robert, G.; Elkentaoui, H.; Pasticier, G.; Couzi, L.; Merville, P.; Ravaud, A.; Ballanger, P.; Ferrière, J.-M.; Wallerand, H. Laparoscopic Radical Prostatectomy in Renal Transplant Recipients. *Urology* **2009**, *74*, 683–687. [CrossRef]
71. Narváez, A.; Suarez, J.; Riera, L.; Castells-Esteve, M.; Cocera, R.; Vigués, F. Nuestra experiencia en el manejo del cáncer de próstata en pacientes trasplantados renales. *Actas Urológicas Españolas* **2018**, *42*, 249–255. [CrossRef]
72. Marks, L.B.; Yorke, E.D.; Jackson, A.; Ten Haken, R.K.; Constine, L.S.; Eisbruch, A.; Bentzen, S.M.; Nam, J.; Deasy, J.O. Use of Normal Tissue Complication Probability Models in the Clinic. *Int. J. Radiat. Oncol. Biol. Phys.* **2010**, *76*, S10–S19. [CrossRef] [PubMed]
73. Beydoun, N.; Bucci, J.; Malouf, D. Iodine-125 prostate seed brachytherapy in renal transplant recipients: An analysis of oncological outcomes and toxicity profile. *J. Contemp. Brachytherapy* **2014**, *1*, 15–20. [CrossRef] [PubMed]
74. Coombs, C.C.; Hertzfeld, K.; Barrett, W. Outcomes in transplant patients undergoing brachytherapy for prostate cancer. *Am. J. Clin. Oncol.* **2012**, *35*, 40–44. [CrossRef] [PubMed]
75. Tasaki, M.; Kasahara, T.; Kaidu, M.; Kawaguchi, G.; Hara, N.; Yamana, K.; Maruyama, R.; Takizawa, I.; Ishizaki, F.; Saito, K.; et al. Low-Dose-Rate and High-Dose-Rate Brachytherapy for Localized Prostate Cancer in ABO-Incompatible Renal Transplant Recipients. *Transplant. Proc.* **2019**, *51*, 774–778. [CrossRef]
76. Soeterik, T.F.W.; Van Den Bergh, R.C.N.; Van Melick, H.H.E.; Kelder, H.; Peretti, F.; Dariane, C.; Timsit, M.-O.; Branchereau, J.; Mesnard, B.; Tilki, D.; et al. Active surveillance in renal transplant patients with prostate cancer: A multicentre analysis. *World J. Urol.* **2023**, *41*, 725–732. [CrossRef]
77. Liauw, S.L.; Ham, S.A.; Das, L.C.; Rudra, S.; Packiam, V.T.; Koshy, M.; Weichselbaum, R.R.; Becker, Y.T.; Bodzin, A.S.; Eggener, S.E. Prostate Cancer Outcomes Following Solid-Organ Transplantation: A SEER-Medicare Analysis. *JNCI J. Natl. Cancer Inst.* **2020**, *112*, 847–854. [CrossRef]
78. Kälble, T.; Lucan, M.; Nicita, G.; Sells, R.; Revilla, F.J.B.; Wiesel, M. Eau Guidelines on Renal Transplantation. *Eur. Urol.* **2005**, *47*, 156–166. [CrossRef]
79. EASL Clinical Practice Guidelines: Liver transplantation. *J. Hepatol.* **2016**, *64*, 433–485. [CrossRef]
80. Bieri, U.; Hübel, K.; Seeger, H.; Kulkarni, G.S.; Sulser, T.; Hermanns, T.; Wettstein, M.S. Management of Active Surveillance-Eligible Prostate Cancer during Pretransplantation Workup of Patients with Kidney Failure: A Simulation Study. *Clin. J. Am. Soc. Nephrol.* **2020**, *15*, 822–829. [CrossRef]
81. Gin, G.E.; Pereira, J.F.; Weinberg, A.D.; Mehrazin, R.; Lerner, S.M.; Sfakianos, J.P.; Phillips, C.K. Prostate-specific antigen screening and prostate cancer treatment in renal transplantation candidates: A survey of U.S. transplantation centers. *Urol. Oncol. Semin. Orig. Investig.* **2016**, *34*, 57.e9–57.e13. [CrossRef]
82. Stöckle, M.; Junker, K.; Fornara, P. Low-risk Prostate Cancer Prior to or After Kidney Transplantation. *Eur. Urol. Focus* **2018**, *4*, 148–152. [CrossRef] [PubMed]
83. Craig-Schapiro, R.; Salinas, T.; Lubetzky, M.; Abel, B.T.; Sultan, S.; Lee, J.R.; Kapur, S.; Aull, M.J.; Dadhania, D.M. COVID-19 outcomes in patients waitlisted for kidney transplantation and kidney transplant recipients. *Am. J. Transpl.* **2021**, *21*, 16351. [CrossRef]
84. Zapała, P.; Ślusarczyk, A.; Rajwa, P.; Przydacz, M.; Krajewski, W.; Dybowski, B.; Kubik, P.; Kuffel, B.; Przudzik, M.; Osiecki, R.; et al. Not as black as it is painted? The impact of the first wave of COVID-19 pandemic on surgical treatment of urological cancer patients in Poland-a cross-country experience. *Arch. Med. Sci.* **2023**, *19*, 107–115. [CrossRef] [PubMed]
85. Johnson, B.D.; Zhu, Z.; Lequio, M.; Powers, C.G.D.; Bai, Q.; Xiao, H.; Fajardo, E.; Wakefield, M.R.; Fang, Y. SARS-CoV-2 spike protein inhibits growth of prostate cancer: A potential role of the COVID-19 vaccine killing two birds with one stone. *Med. Oncol.* **2022**, *39*, 32. [CrossRef] [PubMed]
86. Heidenreich, A.; Pfister, D.; Thissen, A.; Piper, C.; Porres, D. Radical retropubic and perineal prostatectomy for clinically localised prostate cancer in renal transplant recipients. *Arab J. Urol.* **2014**, *12*, 142–148. [CrossRef]
87. Hoda, M.R.; Hamza, A.; Greco, F.; Wagner, S.; Reichelt, O.; Heynemann, H.; Fischer, K.; Fornara, P. Management of localized prostate cancer by retropubic radical prostatectomy in patients after renal transplantation. *Nephrol. Dial. Transplant.* **2010**, *25*, 3416–3420. [CrossRef]

88. Iizuka, J.; Hashimoto, Y.; Kondo, T.; Takagi, T.; Inui, M.; Nozaki, T.; Omoto, K.; Shimizu, T.; Ishida, H.; Tanabe, K. Robot-Assisted Radical Prostatectomy for Localized Prostate Cancer in Asian Renal Transplant Recipients. *Transplant. Proc.* **2016**, *48*, 905–909. [CrossRef]
89. Rahman, I.A.; Rasyid, N.; Birowo, P.; Atmoko, W. Effects of renal transplantation on erectile dysfunction: A systematic review and meta-analysis. *Int. J. Impot. Res.* **2022**, *34*, 456–466. [CrossRef]
90. Marra, G.; Agnello, M.; Giordano, A.; Soria, F.; Oderda, M.; Dariane, C.; Timsit, M.-O.; Branchereau, J.; Hedli, O.; Mesnard, B.; et al. Robotic Radical Prostatectomy for Prostate Cancer in Renal Transplant Recipients: Results from a Multicenter Series. *Eur. Urol.* **2022**, *82*, 639–645. [CrossRef]
91. Moreno Sierra, J.; Ciappara Paniagua, M.; Galante Romo, M.I.; Senovilla Pérez, J.L.; Redondo González, E.; Galindo Herrero, M.I.; Novo Gómez, N.; Blázquez Izquierdo, J. Robot Assisted Radical Prostatectomy in Kidney Transplant Recipients. *Our Clin. Exp. A Syst. Rev. Urol. Int.* **2016**, *97*, 440–444. [CrossRef]
92. Felber, M.; Drouin, S.J.; Grande, P.; Vaessen, C.; Parra, J.; Barrou, B.; Matillon, X.; Crouzet, S.; Leclerc, Q.; Rigaud, J.; et al. Morbidity, perioperative outcomes and complications of robot-assisted radical prostatectomy in kidney transplant patients: A French multicentre study. *Urol. Oncol. Semin. Orig. Investig.* **2020**, *38*, 599.e15–599.e21. [CrossRef] [PubMed]
93. Plagakis, S.; Foreman, D.; Sutherland, P.; Fuller, A. Transperitoneal Robot-Assisted Radical Prostatectomy Should Be Considered in Prostate Cancer Patients with Pelvic Kidneys. *J. Endourol. Case Rep.* **2016**, *2*, 38–40. [CrossRef] [PubMed]
94. Smith, D.L.; Jellison, F.C.; Heldt, J.P.; Tenggardjaja, C.; Bowman, R.J.; Jin, D.H.; Chamberlin, J.; Lui, P.D.; Baldwin, D.D. Robot-Assisted Radical Prostatectomy in Patients with Previous Renal Transplantation. *J. Endourol.* **2011**, *25*, 1643–1647. [CrossRef]
95. Zeng, J.; Christiansen, A.; Pooli, A.; Qiu, F.; LaGrange, C.A. Safety and Clinical Outcomes of Robot-Assisted Radical Prostatectomy in Kidney Transplant Patients: A Systematic Review. *J. Endourol.* **2018**, *32*, 935–943. [CrossRef] [PubMed]
96. Tyritzis, S.I.; Wallerstedt, A.; Steineck, G.; Nyberg, T.; Hugosson, J.; Bjartell, A.; Wilderäng, U.; Thorsteinsdottir, T.; Carlsson, S.; Stranne, J.; et al. Thromboembolic Complications in 3,544 Patients Undergoing Radical Prostatectomy with or without Lymph Node Dissection. *J. Urol.* **2015**, *193*, 117–125. [CrossRef]
97. Heidenreich, A. Still Unanswered: The Role of Extended Pelvic Lymphadenectomy in Improving Oncological Outcomes in Prostate Cancer. *Eur. Urol.* **2021**, *79*, 605–606. [CrossRef]
98. Detti, B.; Scoccianti, S.; Franceschini, D.; Villari, D.; Greto, D.; Cipressi, S.; Sardaro, A.; Zanassi, M.; Cai, T.; Biti, G. Adjuvant Radiotherapy for a Prostate Cancer After Renal Transplantation and Review of the Literature. *Jpn. J. Clin. Oncol.* **2011**, *41*, 1282–1286. [CrossRef]
99. Gojdic, M.; Zilinska, Z.; Krajcovicova, I.; Lukacko, P.; Grezdo, J.; Obsitnik, B.; Sr, J.B.; Trebaticky, B. Radiotherapy of prostate cancer in renal transplant recipients: Single-center experience. *Neoplasma* **2019**, *66*, 155–159. [CrossRef]
100. Mouzin, M.; Bachaud, J.-M.; Kamar, N.; Gamé, X.; Vaessen, C.; Rischmann, P.; Rostaing, L.; Malavaud, B. Three-Dimensional Conformal Radiotherapy for Localized Prostate Cancer in Kidney Transplant Recipients. *Transplantation* **2004**, *78*, 1496–1500. [CrossRef]
101. Ileana, P.Á.S.; Rubi, R.P.; Javier, L.R.F.; Sagrario, M.G.M.D.; Haydeé, F.B.C. Pelvic radiation therapy with volumetric modulated arc therapy and intensity-modulated radiotherapy after renal transplant: A report of 3 cases. *Rep. Pract. Oncol. Radiother.* **2020**, *25*, 548–555. [CrossRef]
102. Kleinclauss, F.; Gigante, M.; Neuzillet, Y.; Mouzin, M.; Terrier, N.; Salomon, L.; Iborra, F.; Petit, J.; Cormier, L.; Lechevallier, E.; et al. Prostate cancer in renal transplant recipients. *Nephrol. Dial. Transplant.* **2008**, *23*, 2374–2380. [CrossRef] [PubMed]
103. Breyer, B.N.; Whitson, J.M.; Freise, C.E.; Meng, M.V. Prostate Cancer Screening and Treatment in the Transplant Population: Current Status and Recommendations. *J. Urol.* **2009**, *181*, 2018–2026. [CrossRef] [PubMed]
104. Konety, B.R.; Tewari, A.; Howard, R.J.; Barry, J.M.; Hodge, E.E.; Taylor, R.; Jordan, M.L. Prostate cancer in the post-transplant population. *Urology* **1998**, *52*, 428–432. [CrossRef] [PubMed]
105. Miao, Y.; Everly, J.J.; Gross, T.G.; Tevar, A.D.; First, M.R.; Alloway, R.R.; Woodle, E.S. De Novo Cancers Arising in Organ Transplant Recipients are Associated With Adverse Outcomes Compared With the General Population. *Transplantation* **2009**, *87*, 1347–1359. [CrossRef]
106. Melchior, S.; Franzaring, L.; Shardan, A.; Schwenke, C.; Plümpe, A.; Schnell, R.; Dreikorn, K. Urological De Novo Malignancy After Kidney Transplantation: A Case for the Urologist. *J. Urol.* **2011**, *185*, 428–432. [CrossRef]
107. Sherer, B.A.; Warrior, K.; Godlewski, K.; Hertl, M.; Olaitan, O.; Nehra, A.; Deane, L.A. Prostate cancer in renal transplant recipients. *Int. Braz. J. Urol.* **2017**, *43*, 1021–1032. [CrossRef]
108. Lengwiler, E.; Stampf, S.; Zippelius, A.; Salati, E.; Zaman, K.; Schfer, N.; Schardt, J.; Siano, M.; Hofbauer, G. Solid cancer development in solid organ transplant recipients within the Swiss Transplant Cohort Study. *Swiss Med. Wkly.* **2019**, *149*, w20078. [CrossRef]
109. Cormier, L.; Lechevallier, E.; Barrou, B.; Benoit, G.; Bensadoun, H.; Boudjema, K.; Descottes, J.-L.; Doré, B.; Guy, L.; Malavaud, B.; et al. Diagnosis and treatment of prostate cancers in renal-transplant recipients. *Transplantation* **2003**, *75*, 237–239. [CrossRef]
110. From the Department of Urology and Transplant Surgery, Beaumont Hospital, Dublin, Ireland; Haroon, U.H.; Davis, N.F.; Mohan, P.; Little, D.M.; Smyth, G.; Forde, J.C.; Power, R.E. Incidence, Management, and Clinical Outcomes of Prostate Cancer in Kidney Transplant Recipients. *Exp. Clin. Transplant.* **2019**, *17*, 298–303. [CrossRef]
111. Bratt, O.; Drevin, L.; Prütz, K.-G.; Carlsson, S.; Wennberg, L.; Stattin, P. Prostate cancer in kidney transplant recipients-a nationwide register study: Kidney transplants and prostate cancer. *BJU Int.* **2020**, *125*, 679–685. [CrossRef]

12. Hall, E.C.; Pfeiffer, R.M.; Segev, D.L.; Engels, E.A. Cumulative incidence of cancer after solid organ transplantation: Cancer Incidence After Transplantation. *Cancer* **2013**, *119*, 2300–2308. [CrossRef] [PubMed]
13. Aghdam, R.; Amoui, M.; Ghodsirad, M.; Khoshbakht, S.; Mofid, B.; Kaghazchi, F.; Tavakoli, M.; Pirayesh, E.; Ahmadzadehfar, H. Efficacy and safety of 177Lutetium-prostate-specific membrane antigen therapy in metastatic castration-resistant prostate cancer patients: First experience in West Asia–A prospective study. *World J. Nucl. Med.* **2019**, *18*, 258–265. [CrossRef] [PubMed]
14. Mahdi, R.A.; Aggarwal, P.; Kumar, S.; Sood, A.; Paul, D.; Mittal, B.R. Excellent Response to Full-Dose 177 Lu-PSMA-617 RLT in Metastatic Castration-Resistant Prostate Cancer With Transplant Kidney: A Step Ahead. *Clin. Nucl. Med.* **2023**, *48*, e470–e471. [CrossRef] [PubMed]
15. Norouzi, G.; Aghdam, R.A.; Hashemifard, H.; Pirayesh, E. Excellent Response to Lower Dose of 177Lu-PSMA-617 in a Metastatic Castration-Resistant Prostate Cancer Patient with a Transplanted Kidney. *Clin. Nucl. Med.* **2019**, *44*, 483–484. [CrossRef]
16. Tapper, A.; Marin, M.; Samarapungavan, D.; Pam Jones, R.N.; Hafron, J. Management of metastatic castrate-resistant prostate cancer following renal transplantation. *Case Rep. Images Surg.* **2018**, *1*, 1–4. [CrossRef]
17. Pettenati, C.; Jannot, A.-S.; Hurel, S.; Verkarre, V.; Kreis, H.; Housset, M.; Legendre, C.; Méjean, A.; Timsit, M.-O. Prostate cancer characteristics and outcome in renal transplant recipients: Results from a contemporary single center study. *Clin. Transplant.* **2016**, *30*, 964–971. [CrossRef]
18. Hevia, V.; Gómez, V.; Díez Nicolás, V.; Álvarez, S.; Gómez Del Cañizo, C.; Galeano, C.; Gomis, A.; García-Sagredo, J.M.; Marcen, R.; Burgos, F.J. Development of Urologic de Novo Malignancies after Renal Transplantation. *Transplant. Proc.* **2014**, *46*, 170–175. [CrossRef]
19. Haeuser, L.; Nguyen, D.-D.; Trinh, Q.-D. Prostate cancer and kidney transplantation-exclusion or co-existence? *BJU Int.* **2020**, *125*, 628–629. [CrossRef]
20. D'Arcy, M.E.; Coghill, A.E.; Lynch, C.F.; Koch, L.A.; Li, J.; Pawlish, K.S.; Morris, C.R.; Rao, C.; Engels, E.A. Survival after a cancer diagnosis among solid organ transplant recipients in the United States. *Cancer* **2019**, *125*, 933–942. [CrossRef]

**Disclaimer/Publisher's Note:** The statements, opinions and data contained in all publications are solely those of the individual author(s) and contributor(s) and not of MDPI and/or the editor(s). MDPI and/or the editor(s) disclaim responsibility for any injury to people or property resulting from any ideas, methods, instructions or products referred to in the content.

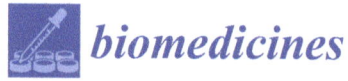 

*Review*

# The Role of Focal Therapy and Active Surveillance for Small Renal Mass Therapy

Milena Matuszczak, Adam Kiljańczyk and Maciej Salagierski *

Department of Urology, Collegium Medicum, University of Zielona Góra, 65-046 Zielona Góra, Poland
* Correspondence: m.salagierski@cm.uz.zgora.pl

**Abstract:** Small and low-grade renal cell carcinomas have little potential for metastasis and disease-related mortality. As a consequence, the main problem remains the use of appropriately tailored treatment for each individual patient. Surgery still remains the gold standard, but many clinicians are questioning this approach and present the advantages of focal therapy. The choice of treatment regimen remains a matter of debate. This article summarizes the current treatment options in the management of small renal masses.

**Keywords:** focal therapy; kidney cancer; thermal ablation

## 1. Introduction

The detection rate of small renal masses (SRMs) is increasing every year. This is mainly due to improvements in diagnostic methods, as well as increased life expectancy, which contributes to the possibility of recurrence. In 2020, there were 431,288 kidney cancer cases and 179,368 deaths worldwide [1]. The estimated number of cases in the United States in 2022 is 79,000, and that of deaths is 13,920 [2]. Kidney cancer is most often detected incidentally when imaging is performed for other reasons and occurs about 2 times more often in men than in women. More than half of currently diagnosed renal masses are detected incidentally [3]. SRMs are defined by most of the literature as smaller than 4 cm, which is usually synonymous with grade T1a of the TNM classification of renal cell carcinoma (RCC) [4]. The typical triad of symptoms (hematuria/abdominal mass/flank pain) is rarely seen nowadays, as it is associated with advanced RCC, which is diagnosed less and less frequently. The specific survival rate for T1-T2 stage RCC is as high as 80–90% after 5 years [3]. Scientific data prove that small and low-grade renal cell carcinomas have little potential for metastasis and disease-related mortality. The main problem in their therapy is the use of appropriately tailored treatment for the patient. Among the therapeutic approaches, we distinguish active surveillance (AS), partial nephrectomy (PN), radical nephrectomy (RN), focal therapy (FT) in which cryoablation, radiofrequency ablation (RFA), microwave ablation (MWA), and irreversible electroporation (IRE) are included. Surgery still remains the gold standard, but many clinicians are questioning it and presenting the advantages of alternative methods such as FT or AS. Which method to choose and what treatment regimen to use still remain matters to consider and question. This manuscript, which analyzes data from the last 4 years in this area, aims to answer at least briefly the above-mentioned questions, pointing out the advantages and disadvantages of each solution.

## 2. Methods

A literature review was performed by searching PubMed/MEDLINE database from August 2018 to July 2022 to identify studies on the role of the focal therapy (FT) and active surveillance (AS) of small renal masses (SRM). The search terms included small renal masses; renal cell carcinoma; renal cancer; kidney neoplasm; focal therapy; active surveillance; cryoablation; thermoablation; microwave ablation; radiofrequency using search terms database = specific—medical subject headings terms in various combinations appropriate to the research objective.

Papers presenting data in the form of reviews, letters to the editor, editorials, research protocols, case reports, brief correspondence and articles not published in English were excluded. Co-workers checked the literature of all included papers for additional studies of interest. On this basis, articles published before April 2018 were also included (17 articles).

Publications based on tissue, blood, cell lines and animals were excluded. Articles concerning more than one cancer, e.g., additional prostate or bladder were omitted. In addition, papers focusing on technical feasibility and specifications of measurement methods rather than method and clinical utility were excluded. Publications based on small cohorts, i.e., including fewer than five patients, were also excluded.

Researchers independently extracted the following information from the included articles: author name, year of publication, number of patients, stage and/or grade of cancer, tumor size (mean and/or median), follow-up time (mean and/or median) as well as OS, RFS, DSS, MFS, DFS, PFS, PE, SE to assess oncological outcomes. All data extraction discrepancies were resolved by consensus with the co-authors.

## 3. Results

### 3.1. Thermal Ablation

Thermal ablation (TA) involves the destruction of tumor cancer cells using extreme temperatures (both high and low) by one or more applicators. This method includes RFA, MWA, IRE and CA. Of these, RFA and CA appear to be the most studied [5]. These approaches are the most widely used, have the best long-term results and similar oncologic efficacy with no significant differences in OS, CSS and RFS [6].

The European Association of Urology (EAU) [7] gives a (weak) recommendation that this technique should be offered on an equal basis with AS to SRM patients with poor health and/or comorbidities, but stresses that one should always remember to discuss the potential benefits and risks, as well as the possible complications and oncologic effect of the chosen therapeutic option (strong recommendation). The publications prove that there is no significant difference between 5-year CSS with AS or TA [8].

The American Urological Association (AUA) and the National Comprehensive Cancer Network (NCCN) [5,9] recommend TA as an alternative treatment option for cT1a tumors <3 cm in size. RFA as well as CA provide similar oncologic outcomes and can therefore be used as an option when choosing TA. These interventions can also be used for larger lesions however, recommendations [9] mention that this approach is associated with higher recurrence rates and more frequent complications.

In addition, the NCCN authors based on AUA 2017 [10] and Pierorazio et al. [11] warn that ablative techniques may require multiple approaches to achieve an oncologic outcome similar to conventional surgery. They recommend using a percutaneous technique whenever possible because of the reduced mortality rate.

### 3.1.1. Cryoablation

Cryoablation can be performed either laparoscopically or percutaneously, both techniques have a success rate of over 95%. Despite this, recommendations advise (NCCN) to use the percutaneous approach. Although cryoablation is classified as a thermal ablation method, the EAU guidelines [7] in contrast to the group-wide restriction against using TA for tumors over 3 cm, set a slightly higher limit for CA—for tumors over 4 cm.

Compared to standard surgery, CA provides similar performance in terms of disease-free survival (DFS), in addition, it is associated with lower complication rates, but carries the risk of more frequent tumor recurrence [12,13]. His trend increases with clinical stage as demonstrated by a cohort of 308 patients [14]. For cT1a tumors, the recurrence rate was 7.7% compared to cT1b where the rate rose as high as 34.5%. Other publications have reported values for cT1: RFS = 93.9%, MFS = 94.4% [15] and 10-year DFS = 94% [16].

It was indicated that laparoscopic CA was significantly associated with better preservation of renal function at month 6 compared to PN [17]. The authors [18] suggest that there is no significant difference between RFA and cryoablation in recurrence rate, metastatic progression, incidence of complications or length of CSS. In addition, a more recent publication [19] reported that recurrence occurs less frequently after cryoablation than after RFA. The method is also safe and effective for senior patients. A publication [20] proved that the procedure is easy to perform, has a low complication rate and is well tolerated by the elderly.

A recently published paper [13] confirms previous reports that this method preserves renal function and does not lead to a significant decline in its function after treatment. Their conclusions are based not only on the available literature but also on the basis of the cohort studied. In addition, the authors remind us that this method is performed percutaneously and very rarely requires general anesthesia, which saves time, money, as well as prevents potential side effects of anesthesiology. It is worth mentioning that possible reports of complications may be related to the eligibility of patients who are disqualified from more invasive methods due to high ASA score.

A publication [12] reported that repeat cryoablation has a significantly lower success rate compared to the original procedure. In most cases, failure after CA can be repaired with re-cryoablation, but this is the point at which it is worth considering other alternatives. Re-cryoablation unfortunately achieves poor results and only 45% of patients have a 2-year DFS. In terms of cryoablation, CT shows a significant advantage over laparoscopic or navigated ultrasound approaches.

In summary, we can mention the unfavorable risk of recurrence compared to standard surgery, as well as the poor results of re-cryoablation, but this method has many advantages in terms of 3- and 5-year OS, low complication rate and avoids general anesthesia. The potential disadvantage of what may be the appearance of recurrence is not significant, and the technique provides good MFS.

3.1.2. Radiofrequency Ablation

RFA is a technique that uses radiofrequency energy delivered through a needle inserted into a cancerous tumor, causing necrosis of the tissue. The method was first described in 1997 [21], and for many years has ranked as a recommended method in therapy for those who are not in sufficient condition for surgery, and the tumor appears to be able to be completely cured by ablation.

The US FDA has approved a method of high-temperature ablation of soft tissue tumors such as SRM of the kidney. The effectiveness of this method has been described in extensive research [22].

RFA is a safe and effective method for the treatment of SRM less than 3 cm in diameter, with therapeutic success in up to 97% of patients. Patients with such tumors as reported in the study [22] had relatively good oncologic outcomes and a 10-year survival rate, with DFS of 82%, CSS of 94% and OS of 49%. No recurrences developed at 5 years after intervention, but patients with tumors larger than 3 cm had worse outcomes (10-year DFS = 68%).

RFA, like cryoablation, is associated with more frequent recurrences than surgical procedures. The technique offers satisfactory results, especially in an aging population due to the reduction in mortality, recovery time, and risks that classical surgery poses.

3.1.3. Microwave Ablation

This technique is categorized among other alternatives. The EAU has not made any recommendations.

In an article [23], researchers described the effectiveness of using percutaneous microwave ablation (MWA) in renal cell carcinoma (RCC) of T1 stage. It is worth mentioning that their cohort included not only SRM, but also larger tumors, but smaller than 7 cm (with an average tumor size of 3.2 cm). They analyzed populations of 100 patients (108 tumors) undergoing treatment over 6 years. Unsurprisingly, the group of patients with T1a tumors achieved better results from treatment compared to T1b. Primary efficacy was 89% and 52%, for T1a and T1b, respectively. Fifteen lesions (including 7 T1a) underwent MWA reablation for residual disease in one ($n = 13$) and two ($n = 2$, both T1b) sessions, achieving secondary efficacy rates of 99% (T1a) and 95% (T1b). Local tumor recurrence (LTR) was equally frequent in both groups (2 each for T1a and T1b). Adverse effects (clinically significant ones were included—grade 3–5 of the Clavien–Dindo classification) were 2 times more frequent in the T1b group than in T1a (2 T1a and 4 T1b were described). Based on the above results, it can be concluded that MWA is a safe treatment option for RCC in both T1a and T1b stages (however, this approach is less effective in more advanced tumor).

A report [24] based on the observation of 48 patients with RCC (with a mean size of 3.1 cm) showed that this method achieves satisfactory OS (95.8%) with few non-significant (observation of hematomas in 4% of patients) complications. One of the disadvantages of this method reported in the literature is the frequency of recurrence, however, nowadays more and more publications show the low severity of the magnitude of this problem (6.25% described here) with increasingly better clinical successes (97.9% overall). Therefore, the authors of the study concluded that this method is an effective technique for SRM and medium-sized tumors.

In addition, the 2021 paper [25] based on a cohort of 101 patients confirms these reports—MWA is a safe and effective (Table 1) treatment for SRM, with a low relapse rate and minimal side effects. However, the authors note the need to observe long-term outcomes.

3.1.4. Irreversible Electroporation

Irreversible electroporation (IRE) is a new non-thermal focal ablation technique that uses a series of short but intense electrical pulses delivered through paired electrodes to the targeted tissue area, killing cells by irreversibly disrupting the integrity of the cell membrane. The effect of IRE is not uniform and depends on the internal conductivity of the tissue, the number of pulses delivered, the current flow achieved and the total treatment time. In clinical practice, it can be performed both percutaneously under imaging guidance (e.g., CT) and during open surgery under direct visual guidance. IRE is a less invasive method for the patient than other ablations, due to its low impact on nerves or connective tissue. This makes the method more suitable for tumors located in the area of vital large vessels, as it allows the lesion to be removed without damaging them. Its low invasiveness also argues for performing procedures using it in patients in severe general condition, with comorbidities or during treatment with chemotherapeutic agents.

Table 1. Comparison of results for thermal ablation methods.

| Method | Study | Study Group | Stage | Mean/Median Tumor Size (cm) | Mean/Median Follow-Up (Months) | Results | |
|---|---|---|---|---|---|---|---|
| | Morkos et al., 2020 [16] | 134 patients | cT1a (115/134) | Median 2.8 | Median 88.8 | 5 y<br>OS = 87%,<br>RFS = 85%,<br>DSS = 94% | 10 y<br>OS = 72%,<br>RFS = 69%,<br>DSS = 94%, |
| | | | cT1b (19/134) | | | OS = 88%<br>RFS = 89%,<br>DSS = 94% | OS = 88%<br>RFS = 89%,<br>DSS = 94% |
| | Zangiacomo et al., 2021 [26] | 69 patients | cT1a | Median 2.3 | Mean 56 | 1 y<br>OS = 100%<br>PFS = 98.8%<br>MFS = 100%<br>DSS = 100% | 5 y<br>OS = 98.4%,<br>PFS = 93%<br>MFS = 100%<br>DSS = 100% PE= 95.7% |
| | Andrews et al., 2019 [27] | 226 patients | cT1a (178/226) | Median 2.8 | Median 75.6 | 5 y<br>OS = 77%<br>DSS = 100%<br>RFS = 95.9%<br>MFS = 100% | |
| Cryoablation | | | cT1b (48/226) | Median 4.8 | Median 72 | OS = 56%<br>DSS = 91%<br>RFS = 95%<br>MFS = 90% | |
| | Spiliopoulos et al., 2021 [28] | 53 patients (54 tumors) | cT1a (49/54) | Mean 2.8 | Mean 46.7 | 1 y<br>OS = 98%<br>DFS = 100%<br>PFS = 100%<br>DSS = 100% | 3 y<br>OS = 90.3%<br>DFS = 95.5%<br>PFS = 94.3%<br>DSS = 100% 5 y<br>OS = 71.6%<br>DFS = 88.6%<br>PFS = 91%<br>DSS = 95.8% |
| | | | cT1b (5/54) | | | | |
| | Breen et al., 2018 [15] | 220 patients (221 tumors) | cT1a (166/221)<br>cT1b (55/221) | Mean 3.4/<br>Median 3.4 | Median 31 | 3 y<br>OS = 93.2%<br>RFS = 97.2%<br>MFS = 97.7% | 5 y<br>OS = 84.8%<br>RFS = 93.9%<br>MFS = 94.4% |
| | Gunn et al., 2019 [29] | 37 patients (37 tumors) | cT1b | Median 4.73 | Mean 26.4 | 1 y<br>RFS = 96.5%<br>OS = 96.7%<br>DSS = 100% | 2 y<br>RFS = 86.1%<br>OS = 91.8%<br>DSS = 100% 3 y<br>RFS = 62.6%<br>OS = 77.6%<br>DSS = 100% |

Table 1. Cont.

| Method | Study | Study Group | Stage | Mean/Median Tumor Size (cm) | Mean/Median Follow-Up (Months) | Results |
|---|---|---|---|---|---|---|
| | Zhou et al., 2019 [30] | 26 patients | cT1a | Mean 2.4 | No data | 2 y<br>DFS = 100%<br>PFS = 100%<br>DSS = 100% | PE = 88% |
| | Grange et al., 2019 [31] | 23 patients | cT1b | Mean 4.56 | Mean 13.9 /Median 11 | 1 y<br>PFS = 66.7%<br>DSS = 100% | 2 y<br>PFS = 66.7%<br>DSS = 85.7% | PE = 86.3%<br>SE = 100% |
| | Shimizu et al., 2021 [32] | 28 patients | cT1b | Mean 4.6 | Mean 42 | 1 y<br>OS = 96.3%<br>DFS = 89.1%<br>RFS = 92.7% | 3 y<br>OS = 92.3%<br>DFS = 85.4%<br>RFS = 92.7% | 5 y<br>OS = 89.1%<br>DFS = 85.4%<br>RFS = 92.7% |
| | UEMURA et al., 2021 [33] | 48 patients | cT1a (46/48)<br>cT1b (2/48) | Median 2.6 | Median 12 | 3 y<br>RFS = 90.3%<br>OS = 97.4% | |
| | Chan et al., 2022 [34] | 103 patients | cT1a (72/103) | Median 2.85 | Median 75.6 | 5 y<br>DSS = 100%<br>OS = 90.3%<br>RFS = 98.5%<br>MFS = 100% | 10 y<br>DSS = 100%<br>OS = 73.9%<br>RFS = 92.3%<br>MFS = 100% |
| | | | cT1b (31/103) | Median 4.5 | Median 72.5 | 5 y<br>DSS = 96.4%<br>OS = 71%<br>RFS = 92.8%<br>MFS = 96.7% | 10 y<br>DSS = 96.4%<br>OS = 43.5%<br>RFS = 86.4%<br>MFS = 96.7% |
| | B. A. Johnson et al., 2019 [22] | 106 patients (112 tumors) | cT1a | Mean 2.5 | Median 79 | 10 y<br>DFS = 81.5%,<br>DSS = 94%<br>MFS = 94%<br>OS = 49% | |
| Radiofrequency ablation | Zangiacomo et al., 2021 [26] | 16 patients | cT1a | Median 2.3 | Mean 56 | 1 y<br>OS = 100%<br>PFS = 98.8%<br>MFS = 100%<br>DSS = 100% | 5 y<br>OS = 98.4%,<br>PFS = 93%<br>MFS = 100%<br>DSS = 100% | PE = 95.7% |

Table 1. Cont.

| Method | Study | Study Group | Stage | Mean/Median Tumor Size (cm) | Mean/Median Follow-Up (Months) | Results | |
|---|---|---|---|---|---|---|---|
| | Andrews et al., 2019 [27] | 175 patients | cT1a | Median 1.9 | Median 90 | 5 y<br>OS = 72%<br>DSS = 95.6%<br>RFS = 95.9%<br>MFS = 93.9% | |
| | Zhou et al., 2019 [30] | 244 patients | cT1a | Mean 2.4 | No data | 2 y<br>DFS = 100%<br>PFS = 100%<br>DSS = 100% | PE = 95% |
| | Chan et al., 2022 [34] | 100 patients | cT1a (87/100) | Median 2.8 | Median 106 | 5 y<br>DSS = 98.8%<br>OS = 93%<br>RFS = 95.7%<br>MFS = 97.3% | 10 y<br>DSS = 98.8%<br>OS = 89%<br>RFS = 91.4%<br>MFS = 97.3% |
| | | | cT1b (13/100) | Median 4.5 | Median 59.5 | 5 y<br>DSS = 92.3%<br>OS = 61.5%<br>RFS = 87.5%<br>MFS = 92.3% | 10 y<br>DSS = 92.3%<br>OS = 52.8%<br>RFS = 87.5%<br>MFS = 92.3% |
| | Aarts et al., 2020 [23] | 100 patients (108 tumors) | cT1a (77/100) | Median 2.8 | Median 19 | PE = 89%<br>SE = 99% | |
| | | | cT1b (23/100) | Median 4.5 | | PE = 52%<br>SE = 95% | |
| | Zhou et al., 2019 [30] | 27 patients | cT1a | Mean 2.2 | No data | 2 y<br>DFS = 100%<br>PFS = 100%<br>DSS = 100% | PE = 96% |
| Microwave ablation | Wilcox Vanden Berg et al., 2021 [25] | 101 patients (110 tumors) | cT1a | Median 2.0 | Median 12.5 | 1 y<br>RFS = 97.3%<br>OS = 100%<br>DSS = 100%<br>MFS = 100% | 2 y<br>RFS = 97.3%<br>OS = 100%<br>DSS = 100%<br>MFS = 100% |
| | Filippiadis et al., 2018 [24] | 48 patients | cT1a (44/48) | Mean 3.1 | Mean 43 | 3 year survival<br>OS = 95.8% | PE = 98.2%<br>SE = 100% |
| | | | cT1b (4/48) | | | RFS = 73.75% | |

Table 1. Cont.

| Method | Study | Study Group | Stage | Mean/Median Tumor Size (cm) | Mean/Median Follow-Up (Months) | Results | | |
|---|---|---|---|---|---|---|---|---|
| | Guo and Arellano, 2021 [35] | 106 patients (119 tumors) | cT1a | Mean 2.4 | Median 24 | 1 y<br>PFS = 100%<br>OS = 99%<br>DSS = 100% | 2 y<br>PFS = 92.8%<br>OS = 97.7%<br>DSS = 100% | 3 y<br>PFS = 90.6%<br>OS = 94.6%<br>DSS = 100% |
| | John et al., 2021 [36] | 113 patients | cT1a (102/113)<br>cT1b (11/113) | Median 2.5 | Median 12 | 1 y<br>RFS = 97.3%<br>MFS = 98.2%<br>OS = 100% | | |
| Irreversible electroporation | Wah et al., 2021 [37] | 26 patients (30 tumors) | cT1a | Mean 2.5 | Median 37 | 2 y<br>RFS = 91%<br>MFS = 87%<br>DSS = 96%<br>OS = 89% | 3 y<br>RFS = 91%<br>MFS = 87%<br>DSS = 96%<br>OS = 89% | |
| | Canvasser et al., 2017 [38] | 41 patients (42 tumors) | cT1a | Mean 2 | Mean 22 | 2 y<br>RFS = 83%<br>OS = 100% | | |

DFS—disease-free survival, DSS—disease-specific survival, MFS—metastasis free survival, OS—overall survival, PE—primary efficacy, PFS—progression-free survival, RFS—recurrence-free survival, SE—secondary efficacy. 1 y—1-year survival, 2 y—2-year survival, 3 y—3-year survival, 5 y—5-year survival, 10 y—10-year survival.

We prospectively evaluated CT [37]—it navigated IRE and showed suboptimal results and acceptable complications (Table 1). Thirty RCC tumors with an average size of 2.5 cm were treated with this method and achieved a primary technique success rate of 73.3%, which improved to 97% after performing CA-7 residual disease. However, it should be mentioned that so far this method is insufficiently studied and carries a high risk of complications (one patient had a complication of Clavien–Dindo III—damage to the proximal ureter and five patients had a decrease in eGFR of more than 25% immediately after IRE). However, all patients had sufficiently well-preserved renal function that they did not require dialysis. One patient did not have a repeat procedure, as he died of an unexpected stroke at 4 months after IRE.

*3.2. Active Surveillance*

Over the past few years, active surveillance has been the recommended treatment option for patients with tumors less than 2 cm in diameter. Such management is based on studies showing that many tumors less than 2 cm required no intervention, and that the delayed interventions used did not differ in terms of metastasis or mortality [6].

To verify which patients with SRM will benefit more from Robot-assisted laparoscopic partial nephrectomy (partial nephrectomy is currently the preferred surgical strategy due to preservation of renal function and excellent oncologic outcomes) vs. AS, a review was conducted [39] of the Delayed Intervention and Surveillance of Small Kidney Masses (DISSRM) Registry data collected over 10 years. This registry includes patients with cT1a tumors <4 cm (in the axial dimension of imaging), after exclusion of familial RCC syndromes and metastases. This work was created with the idea of eliminating unnecessary surgeries, as data show that approximately 5624 needless resections of benign SRMs are performed annually in the US [40].

The risk of using AS is the appearance of metastases, however, their incidence is less than 1% for tumors <3 cm in diameter and about 2% for tumors <4 cm [41,42]. The low rates of metastatic progression (1–6% of literature reports) and SRM-related mortality (0–18%) for untreated small RCC support the choice of this treatment modality.

AS currently has various recommendations from medical societies:

NCCN recommends AS as an option for selected asymptomatic T1 patients:

- with SRM < 2 cm,
- with T1a tumors ($\leq$4 cm) with a predominantly cystic component.
- with cT1 SRM and significant competing risks of death or morbidity associated with the intervention.

According to the NCCN definition, AS includes:

- serial abdominal imaging studies
- periodic blood tests and chest imaging (verification of possible metastases)
- interventions in a timely manner if the mass shows changes indicative of progression (e.g., increasing tumor size, rapid growth, infiltration) indicating increasing metastatic potential.

The American Society of Clinical Oncology (ASCO) recommends its use as an initial treatment for populations with significant comorbidities and poor predicted survival [4].

AUA, on the other hand, suggests the initial use of this method, for any patient with a tumor less than 2 cm or for larger lesions in an elderly and ailing population, [5] as well as for those at high risk of complications from surgical intervention. AS is an option that requires careful clinical risk assessment, patient and physician co-decision-making, and periodic reevaluation (reassessment). Post-intervention follow-up allows identification of potential implications of treatment and local or systemic recurrence. No consensus has been established on the exact timing of imaging study surveillance.

EAU guidelines [7] recommend AS as an initial method of monitoring SRM, which can always be changed to another therapeutic method. The recommendations for this strategy are mainly for the aged and sickly, who could suffer more losses from more invasive methods, and those whose life expectancy is low. Besides, this method can also be considered in other patients, due to the fact that the 5-year follow-up showed no significant difference in CSS between the AS group and surgical patients [43]. Based on the results of the biopsy and the determination of its histological specification, it is possible to assess the risk of progression and whether the tumor can be safely overseen or whether more invasive methods should be undertaken [39].

Factors triggering intervention in the DISSRM registry include tumor size (>4 cm), growth rate (>0.5 cm/year) [44], symptom development (hematuria with no other cause), elective change (change in patient preference or improvement in patient health), or metastatic disease.

In addition, Mir et al. [45] showed that the linear growth rate of patients who developed metastases was not significantly different from the overall growth rate of clinically localized renal masses. Moreover, because both benign and malignant lesions can grow at similar or non-zero rates, growth rate thresholds alone should not be used as a predictor of mass histology or malignancy potential.

Cancer-specific death and progression of metastatic disease do not appear to be related to the rate of tumor growth [46]. Post-treatment based on overall tumor size is now recommended, as it has been shown to be the best predictor of malignant histology, aggressive pathology and oncologic outcomes [47].

## 4. Discussion

In our review paper, we collected results from 24 papers on SRM ablative techniques. In total, the data cover 2150 patients at stage cT1a or cT1b, and includes more advanced tumors than previous reports [48].

Considering the characteristics of radicality with which surgical treatment is associated, and because it is undeniably the longest follow-up (period of observation for this method), it remains the standard of care (SOC) for SRM and localized RCC. An alternative is FA, which for several years now has been an officially accepted method of treating SRM with efficacy similar to PN (for tumors <3 cm). The results achieved with FT are satisfactory, and moreover, percutaneous TA carries a lower risk of serious complications than even minimally invasive surgery.

Among TA, the available literature suggests the superiority of CA over RFA in terms of local tumor control and less frequent reoperations (retreatments). However, there are skeptical voices from researchers who question the necessity of intervention due to the low malignancy and risks that are associated with the natural course of SRM. Due to the development of accessibility and the possibility of regular imaging studies, it is increasingly recommended that AS be undertaken in (high-risk) patients with contraindications to surgery. However, all agree that before making a decision, it is important to consider all variables that may affect the patient's health and also to assess whether the intervention is beneficial to the patient. Published data in the literature indicate that AS is a safe intervention, and TA in the elderly should only be undertaken when outweighed by the gains made during AS.

Mean results for CA, RFA, MWA and IRE procedures are summarized in Table 2.

The average 5-year survival results for CA were 87.97%, 94.08%, 97.96%, 98.6% for OS, RFS, DSS and MFS for cT1a tumors, respectively. For cT1b, the results were: 77.78%, 92.68%, 93.8%, 93.7% for OS, RFS, DSS and MFS, respectively. Which, when compared to the work of Aron et al. 2010 [49] with OS, RFS, DSS and MFS results of 84%, 87%, 89% and 89% for cT1a, presents results in favor of the more recent work [15,16,26–28,34], presented in our review.

Wośkowiak et al. [48] pointed out that data on long term follow-up of CA and RFA are limited. We managed to find results [16,34] on 10 year survival with mean OS, RFS, DSS, MFS of 72.95%, 80.65%, 97%, 100%, respectively for CA and 5 year [26,27,34] for RFA with mean OS, RFS, DSS, MFS of 87.8%, 95.8%, 98.13% and 97.07%, respectively, which are superior to the OS, RFS, DSS and MFS results of 75.8%, 93.5%, 97.9% and 87.7% in a study [50] mentioned in an earlier review [48].

Table 2. Overview of mean results for ablative methods.

| Method | No. of Studies | Study Group | Stage (Tumors) | Tumor Size (cm) Mean | Tumor Size (cm) Median | Follow-Up (Months) Mean | Follow-Up (Months) Median | Follow-Up Time | Mean Results (%) [No. of Studies with Included Results] OS | RFS | DSS | MFS | DFS | PFS | PE | SE |
|---|---|---|---|---|---|---|---|---|---|---|---|---|---|---|---|---|
| Cryoablation | 11 | 967 patients (969 tumors) | cT1a (721) | 2.87 [3] | 2.79 [6] | 37 [5] | 40.37 [6] | 1 year | 99 [2] | n/a | 100 [2] | 100 [1] | 100 [1] | 99.4 [2] | | |
| | | | | | | | | 2 years | n/a | n/a | 100 [1] | n/a | 100 [1] | 100 [1] | | |
| | | | | | | | | 3 years | 93.63 [3] | 93.75 [2] | 100 [1] | 97.7 [1] | 95.5 [1] | 94.3 [1] | 91.85 [2] | n/a |
| | | | | | | | | 5 years | 87.97 [6] | 94.08 [4] | 97.96 [5] | 98.6 [4] | 88.6 [1] | 92 [2] | | |
| | | | | | | | | 10 years | 72.95 [2] | 80.65 [2] | 97 [2] | 100 [1] | n/a | n/a | | |
| | | | cT1b (248) | 3.84 [4] | 3.8 [6] | | | 1 year | 97 [3] | 94.6 [2] | 100 [3] | n/a | 94.55 [2] | 83.35 [2] | | |
| | | | | | | | | 2 years | 91.8 [1] | 86.1 [1] | 92.85 [2] | n/a | n/a | 66.7 [1] | | |
| | | | | | | | | 3 years | 90.16 [5] | 85.7 [4] | 100 [2] | 97.7 [1] | 90.45 [2] | 94.3 [1] | 86.3 [1] | 100 [1] |
| | | | | | | | | 5 years | 77.78 [5] | 92.68 [5] | 93.8 [3] | 93.7 [3] | 85.4 [1] | n/a | | |
| | | | | | | | | 10 years | 65.75 [2] | 87.7 [2] | 95.2 [2] | 96.7 [1] | n/a | n/a | | |
| Radiofrequency ablation | 5 | 621 patients (627 tumors) | cT1a (614) | 2.5 [1] | 2.35 [4] | 56 [1] | 83.92 [3] | 1 year | 100 [1] | n/a | 100 [1] | 100 [1] | 100 [1] | 98.8 [1] | | |
| | | | | | | | | 2 years | n/a | n/a | 100 [1] | n/a | 100 [1] | 100 [1] | | |
| | | | | | | | | 5 years | 87.8 [3] | 95.8 [2] | 98.13 [3] | 97.07 [3] | n/a | 93 [1] | 95.35 [2] | n/a |
| | | | | | | | | 10 years | 69 [2] | 91.4 [1] | 96.4 [2] | 95.65 [2] | 81.5 [1] | n/a | | |
| | | | cT1b (13) | n/a | 4.5 [1] | | | 5 years | 61.5 [1] | 87.5 [1] | 92.3 [1] | 92.3 [1] | n/a | n/a | | |
| | | | | | | | | 10 years | 52.8 [1] | 87.5 [1] | 92.3 [1] | 92.3 [1] | n/a | n/a | n/a | n/a |
| Microwave ablation | 6 | 495 patients (525 tumors) | cT1a (479) | 2.57 [3] | 2.43 [3] | 43 [1] | 16.88 [4] | 1 year | 96.67 [2] | 97.3 [2] | 100 [2] | 99.1 [2] | n/a | 100 [1] | | |
| | | | | | | | | 2 years | 98.85 [2] | 97.3 [1] | 100 [3] | 100 [1] | 100 [1] | 96.4 [2] | 94.4 [3] | 99.5 [2] |
| | | | | | | | | 3 years | 96.8 [3] | 85.53 [2] | 100 [2] | 100 [1] | n/a | 90.6 [1] | | |
| | | | cT1b (38) | 3.1 [1] | 3.5 [2] | | | 1 year | 100 [1] | 97.3 [1] | n/a | 98.2 [1] | n/a | n/a | 52 [1] | 95 [1] |
| | | | | | | | | 3 years | 95.8 [1] | 73.75 [1] | n/a | n/a | n/a | n/a | | |
| Irreversible electroporation | 2 | 67 (72 tumors) | cT1a (72) | 2.25 [2] | n/a | 22 [1] | 37 [1] | 2 years | 94.5 [2] | 87 [2] | 96 [1] | 87 [1] | n/a | n/a | n/a | n/a |

DFS—disease-free survival, DSS—disease-specific survival, MFS—metastasis-free survival, OS—overall survival, PE—primary efficacy, PFS—progression-free survival, RFS—recurrence-free survival, SE—secondary efficacy.

The average MWA results for 1-year and 3-year survival, respectively, were: 96.67% and 96.8% for OS, 99.1 and 100% for MFS, 97.3% and 85.53% for RFS, 100% for DSS. Which compares with the 1 and 3 year results of older publications: Yu et al., 2014 [51], respectively OS = 97.9% and 89.7%, MFS = 97.9% and 87.4%, and Guan et al., 2012 [52], RFS = 100% and 95.1%, and for each group DSS = 100%, yielded similar results.

The least studied method is IRE, which despite being available for more than 20 years is still not very popular. The average results in our comparison were, respectively: 94.5%, 87%, 96%, 87% for 2-year OS, RFS, DSS and MFS. These results look worse than the 2-year OS, RFS, DSS, MFS at: 98.85%, 97.3%, 100%, 100% for MWA.

According to our findings CA seems to be the most studied method, followed by RFA and MWA, with a total cohort of 967, 621 and 495 patients, respectively. Also in the case of CA, we noted a large group of cT1b patients, which may indicate the use of this method in patients with more advanced cancer.

The new long-term data we compiled in the tables show a similarly favorable oncological outcome for RFA and CA. Which confirms the conclusions of Wośkowiak et al., regarding the efficacy of these methods.

In the case of MWA, the survival data from 6 articles mentioned in our review are limited to 3 years, therefore it seems difficult to compare this method to more extensively studied ones, as more long-term data are needed.

A clinical study [30] that retrospectively evaluated 297 patients with T1a RCC who underwent percutaneous ablation (navigated CT), performed with RF (82%), MWA (9%) or cryoablation (9%), was referenced to compare all thermoablative methods presented (excluding IRE). The average size of the tumor undergoing surgery was 2.4 cm, and the study cohort included populations that had been treated at the clinic over a 10-year period. The results showed that the success rate of the techniques was similar for all three methods, but primary efficacy at 1 month postablation was more likely to be achieved in the RF and MWA groups than cryoablation. Other values such as 2-year follow-up, RCC-related mortality, metastatic progression or local recurrence were equally common for each group. Also, eGFR did not differ between them. Thus, the authors concluded that both RF ablation, cryoablation and MWA after 2 years in the treatment of T1a RCC yield good (and equivalent between them) results in terms of therapeutic outcome, renal function and low rates of adverse events. For this reason, each modality can be used in patients who may benefit from their treatment.

Having compared the 2017 AUA guidelines [53] with the latest 2021 ones [54], no changes were published regarding TA. For AS, we also found no significant changes in the recommendations.

For the EAU, the 2018 [55] and 2022 [7] guidelines for AS are no different except for the mention of a published paper [56]. In addition, they found no significant differences in 5-year CSS between AS and TA. In the case of TA, there is a lack of high-quality evidence to support the superiority of TA over PN. This method can only be recommended for ailing patients.

Changes to the NCCN guidelines between the 2018 [57] and 2022 [9] editions include more specific criteria for the use of TA and AS, while mentioning the possibility of needing repeat TA procedures to achieve a similar oncologic effect as with conventional surgery.

The latest ASCO guidelines were published in 2017 and there has been no update since then [4].

It seems that the progress achieved in terms of clinical results can be attributed to greater experience of operators, as well as the development of technology.

The selection bias of retrospective work, although significant, should be borne in mind that randomized prospective studies involve much greater costs and time required. The goal for the next few years should be to establish diagnostic methods on comparable, large cohorts and also to establish predictors to help make the most tailored options for patients. And the collection of this information on a long-term scale, since the published data are promising but mostly based on short-term oncology studies.

## 5. Conclusions

According to current AUA guidelines, patients with SRM < 2 cm may undergo AS, TA and PN, and tailored treatment should take into account patient preference and the potential risks each method carries [5]. Despite the advances that have been made over the past few years in focal methods, the NCCN still recommends PN as the preferred method in patients with stage T1a tumors. The guidelines also recommend RN in selected patients, and leave active surveillance along with ablative techniques as available primary treatments [9]. AS is still recommended in sicker patients, especially the elderly, where surgery is high risk.

Several articles with long-term survival data (5–10 years) were collected, which can help evaluate the effectiveness of TA methods. We suppose that more long-term and larger cohort-based studies will help confirm the clinical utility of these methods and demonstrate their advantages over classical surgery.

In this article, we have updated the publication of Wośkowiak et al. [48], the data of TA procedures presented in our paper present results similar or better than the articles published before 2018. These conclusions were made on the basis of summary tables (Tables 1 and 2), as well as analyzed guidelines and other reports from recent years.

**Author Contributions:** All authors made substantial contributions to this work; acquisition and interpretation of data by online search, M.M. and A.K.; design of tables and graphic, M.M. and A.K.; draft and supervision of the work, M.S.; revision of the work, M.S. All authors have read and agreed to the published version of the manuscript.

**Funding:** This research received no external funding.

**Institutional Review Board Statement:** Not applicable.

**Informed Consent Statement:** Not applicable.

**Data Availability Statement:** Not applicable.

**Conflicts of Interest:** The authors declare no conflict of interest.

## Abbreviations

| | |
|---|---|
| AS | Active surveillance |
| ASA | American Society of Anesthesiology |
| ASCO | American Society of Clinical Oncology |
| AUA | American Urological Association |
| CA | Cryoablation |
| CT | Computed tomography |
| DFS | Disease-free survival |
| DISSRM | Delayed Intervention and Surveillance of Small Kidney Masses |
| DSS | Disease-specific survival |
| EAU | European Association of Urology |
| eGFR | Estimated glomer |
| FDA | Food and Drug Administration |
| FT | Focal therapy |
| IRE | Irreversible electroporation |
| MFS | Metastasis-free survival |
| MWA | Microwave ablation |
| NCCN | National Comprehensive Cancer Network |
| OS | Overall survival |
| PE | Primary efficacy |
| PFS | Progression-free survival |

| | |
|---|---|
| PN | Partial nephrectomy |
| RCC | Renal cell carcinoma |
| RFA | Radiofrequency ablation |
| RFS | Recurrence-free survival |
| RN | Radical nephrectomy |
| SE | Secondary efficacy |
| SOC | Standard of care |
| SRM | Small renal masses |
| TA | Thermal ablation |

## References

1. Sung, H.; Ferlay, J.; Siegel, R.L.; Laversanne, M.; Soerjomataram, I.; Jemal, A.; Bray, F. Global Cancer Statistics 2020: GLOBOCAN Estimates of Incidence and Mortality Worldwide for 36 Cancers in 185 Countries. *CA Cancer J. Clin.* **2021**, *71*, 209–249. [CrossRef] [PubMed]
2. Siegel, R.L.; Miller, K.D.; Fuchs, H.E.; Jemal, A. Cancer statistics, 2022. *CA: A Cancer J. Clin.* **2022**, *72*, 7–33. [CrossRef] [PubMed]
3. Campbell, S.C.; Wein, A.J. Malignant renal tumors. In *Campbell-Walsh Wein-Urology*, 12th ed.; Partin, A.W., Pe-ters, C.A., Kavoussi, L.R., Dmochowski, R.R., Wein, A.J., Eds.; Elsevier: Philadelphia, PA, USA, 2019.
4. Finelli, A.; Ismaila, N.; Bro, B.; Durack, J.; Eggener, S.; Evans, A.; Gill, I.; Graham, D.; Huang, W.; Jewett, M.A.; et al. Management of Small Renal Masses: American Society of Clinical Oncology Clinical Practice Guideline. *J. Clin. Oncol.* **2017**, *35*, 668–680. [CrossRef] [PubMed]
5. Campbell, S.C.; Clark, P.E.; Chang, S.S.; Karam, J.A.; Souter, L.; Uzzo, R.G. Renal Mass and Localized Renal Cancer: Evaluation, Management, and Follow-Up: AUA Guideline: Part I. *J. Urol.* **2021**, *206*, 199–208. [CrossRef] [PubMed]
6. Tang, Y.; Liu, F.; Mao, X.; Li, P.; Mumin, M.A.; Li, J.; Hou, Y.; Song, H.; Lin, H.; Tan, L.; et al. The impact of tumor size on the survival of patients with small renal masses: A population–based study. *Cancer Med.* **2022**, *11*, 2377–2385. [CrossRef] [PubMed]
7. Ljungberg, B.; Albiges, L.; Abu-Ghanem, Y.; Bedke, J.; Capitanio, U.; Dabestani, S.; Fernández-Pello, S.; Giles, R.H.; Hofmann, F.; Hora, M.; et al. European Association of Urology Guidelines on Renal Cell Carcinoma: The 2022 Update. *Eur. Urol.* **2022**, *82*, 399–410. [CrossRef]
8. Xing, M.; Kokabi, N.; Zhang, D.; Ludwig, J.M.; Kim, H.S. Comparative Effectiveness of Thermal Ablation, Surgical Resection, and Active Surveillance for T1a Renal Cell Carcinoma: A Surveillance, Epidemiology, and End Results (SEER)–Medicare-linked Population Study. *Radiology* **2018**, *288*, 81–90. [CrossRef]
9. Motzer, R.J.; Jonasch, E.; Agarwal, N.; Alva, A.; Baine, M.; Beckermann, K.; Carlo, M.I.; Choueiri, T.K.; Costello, B.A.; Derweesh, I.H.; et al. Kidney Cancer, Version 2.2023, NCCN Clinical Practice Guidelines in Oncology. *J. Natl. Compr. Cancer Netw.* **2022**, *20*, 71–90. Available online: https://www.nccn.org/login?ReturnURL=https://www.nccn.org/professionals/physician%20gls/pdf/kidney.pdf (accessed on 21 August 2022). [CrossRef]
10. Campbell, S.; Uzzo, R.G.; Allaf, M.E.; Bass, E.; Cadeddu, J.A.; Chang, A.; Clark, P.E.; Davis, B.; Derweesh, I.H.; Giambarresi, L.; et al. Renal Mass and Localized Renal Cancer: AUA Guideline. *J. Urol.* **2017**, *198*, 520–529. [CrossRef]
11. Pierorazio, P.M.; Johnson, M.H.; Patel, H.D.; Sozio, S.; Sharma, R.; Iyoha, E.; Bass, E.; Allaf, M.E. Management of Renal Masses and Localized Renal Cancer: Systematic Review and Meta-Analysis. *J. Urol.* **2016**, *196*, 989–999. [CrossRef]
12. Sundelin, M.O.; Lagerveld, B.; Ismail, M.; Keeley, F.X.; Nielsen, T.K. Repeated Cryoablation as Treatment Modality after Failure of Primary Renal Cryoablation: A European Registry for Renal Cryoablation Multinational Analysis. *J. Endourol.* **2019**, *33*, 909–913. [CrossRef] [PubMed]
13. Stacul, F.; Sachs, C.; Giudici, F.; Bertolotto, M.; Rizzo, M.; Pavan, N.; Balestreri, L.; Lenardon, O.; Pinzani, A.; Pola, L.; et al. Cryoablation of renal tumors: Long-term follow-up from a multicenter experience. *Abdom. Radiol.* **2021**, *46*, 4476–4488. [CrossRef] [PubMed]
14. Pickersgill, N.A.; Vetter, J.M.; Kim, E.H.; Cope, S.J.; Du, K.; Venkatesh, R.J.; Giardina, J.D.; Saad, N.E.; Bhayani, S.B.; Figenshau, R.S. Ten-Year Experience with Percutaneous Cryoablation of Renal Tumors: Tumor Size Predicts Disease Progression. *J. Endourol.* **2020**, *34*, 1211–1217. [CrossRef]
15. Breen, D.J.; King, A.J.; Patel, N.; Lockyer, R.; Hayes, M. Image-guided Cryoablation for Sporadic Renal Cell Carcinoma: Three- and 5-year Outcomes in 220 Patients with Biopsy-proven Renal Cell Carcinoma. *Radiology* **2018**, *289*, 554–561. [CrossRef]
16. Morkos, J.; Rodriguez, K.A.P.; Zhou, A.; Kolarich, A.R.; Frangakis, C.; Rodriguez, R.; Georgiades, C.S. Percutaneous Cryoablation for Stage 1 Renal Cell Carcinoma: Outcomes from a 10-year Prospective Study and Comparison with Matched Cohorts from the National Cancer Database. *Radiology* **2020**, *296*, 452–459. [CrossRef] [PubMed]
17. Hu, X.; Shao, Y.-X.; Wang, Y.; Yang, Z.-Q.; Yang, W.-X.; Li, X. Partial nephrectomy versus ablative therapies for cT1a renal masses: A Systematic Review and meta-analysis. *Eur. J. Surg. Oncol. EJSO* **2019**, *45*, 1527–1535. [CrossRef] [PubMed]
18. Sanchez, A.; Feldman, A.S.; Hakimi, A.A. Current Management of Small Renal Masses, Including Patient Selection, Renal Tumor Biopsy, Active Surveillance, and Thermal Ablation. *J. Clin. Oncol.* **2018**, *36*, 3591–3600. [CrossRef] [PubMed]
19. Wang, Y.; Shao, J.; Lü, Y.; Li, X. Thulium Laser-Assisted Versus Conventional Laparoscopic Partial Nephrectomy for the Small Renal Mass. *Lasers Surg. Med.* **2019**, *52*, 402–407. [CrossRef] [PubMed]

20. Selvaggio, O.; Silecchia, G.; Gravina, M.; Falagario, U.G.; Stallone, G.; Macarini, L.; Carrieri, G.; Cormio, L. Mini invasive approaches in the treatment of small renal masses: TC-guided renal cryoablation in elderly. *Arch. Ital. Urol. Androl.* **2020**, *92*, 4. [CrossRef] [PubMed]
21. Zlotta, A.R.; Wildschutz, T.; Raviv, G.; Peny, M.-O.; van Gansbeke, D.; Noel, J.-C.; Schulman, C.C. Radiofrequency Interstitial Tumor Ablation (RITA) Is a Possible New Modality for Treatment of Renal Cancer: Ex Vivo and in Vivo Experience. *J. Endourol.* **1997**, *11*, 251–258. [CrossRef] [PubMed]
22. Johnson, B.A.; Sorokin, I.; Cadeddu, J.A. Ten-Year Outcomes of Renal Tumor Radio Frequency Ablation. *J. Urol.* **2018**, *201*, 251–258. [CrossRef]
23. Aarts, B.M.; Prevoo, W.; Meier, M.A.J.; Bex, A.; Beets-Tan, R.G.H.; Klompenhouwer, E.G.; Gómez, F.M. Percutaneous Microwave Ablation of Histologically Proven T1 Renal Cell Carcinoma. *Cardiovasc. Interv. Radiol.* **2020**, *43*, 1025–1033. [CrossRef]
24. Filippiadis, D.K.; Gkizas, C.; Chrysofos, M.; Siatelis, A.; Velonakis, G.; Alexopoulou, E.; Kelekis, A.; Brountzos, E. Percutaneous microwave ablation of renal cell carcinoma using a high power microwave system: Focus upon safety and efficacy. *Int. J. Hyperth.* **2017**, *34*, 1077–1081. [CrossRef] [PubMed]
25. Berg, R.N.W.V.; Calderon, L.P.; LaRussa, S.; Enobakhare, O.; Craig, K.; Del Pizzo, J.; McClure, T.D. Microwave ablation of cT1a renal cell carcinoma: Oncologic and functional outcomes at a single center. *Clin. Imaging* **2021**, *76*, 199–204. [CrossRef]
26. Zangiacomo, R.N.; Martins, G.L.P.; Viana, P.C.C.; Horvat, N.; Arap, M.A.; Nahas, W.C.; Srougi, M.; Cerri, G.G.; Menezes, M.R. Percutaneous thermoablation of small renal masses (T1a) in surgical candidate patients: Oncologic outcomes. *Eur. Radiol.* **2021**, *31*, 5370–5378. [CrossRef] [PubMed]
27. Andrews, J.R.; Atwell, T.; Schmit, G.; Lohse, C.M.; Kurup, A.N.; Weisbrod, A.; Callstrom, M.R.; Cheville, J.C.; Boorjian, S.A.; Leibovich, B.C.; et al. Oncologic Outcomes Following Partial Nephrectomy and Percutaneous Ablation for cT1 Renal Masses. *Eur. Urol.* **2019**, *76*, 244–251. [CrossRef]
28. Spiliopoulos, S.; Marzoug, A.; Ra, H.; Ragupathy, S.K.A. Long-term outcomes of CT-guided percutaneous cryoablation of T1a and T1b renal cell carcinoma. *Diagn. Interv. Radiol.* **2021**, *27*, 524–528. [CrossRef]
29. Gunn, A.J.; Joe, W.B.; Salei, A.; El Khudari, H.; Mahmoud, K.H.; Bready, E.; Keasler, E.M.; Patten, P.P.; Gordetsky, J.B.; Rais-Bahrami, S.; et al. Percutaneous Cryoablation of Stage T1b Renal Cell Carcinoma: Safety, Technical Results, and Clinical Outcomes. *Cardiovasc. Interv. Radiol.* **2019**, *42*, 970–978. [CrossRef]
30. Zhou, W.; Herwald, S.E.; McCarthy, C.; Uppot, R.N.; Arellano, R.S. Radiofrequency Ablation, Cryoablation, and Microwave Ablation for T1a Renal Cell Carcinoma: A Comparative Evaluation of Therapeutic and Renal Function Outcomes. *J. Vasc. Interv. Radiol.* **2019**, *30*, 1035–1042. [CrossRef] [PubMed]
31. Grange, R.; Tradi, F.; Izaaryene, J.; Daidj, N.; Brunelle, S.; Walz, J.; Gravis, G.; Piana, G. Computed tomography-guided percutaneous cryoablation of T1b renal tumors: Safety, functional and oncological outcomes. *Int. J. Hyperth.* **2019**, *36*, 1064–1070. [CrossRef] [PubMed]
32. Shimizu, K.; Enoki, K.; Kameoka, Y.; Motohashi, K.; Yanagisawa, T.; Miki, J.; Baba, A.; Sekiguchi, H.; Sadaoka, S. Image-guided percutaneous cryoablation of T1b renal cell carcinomas in patients with comorbidities. *Jpn. J. Radiol.* **2021**, *39*, 1213–1222. [CrossRef]
33. Uemura, T.; Kato, T.; Nagahara, A.; Kawashima, A.; Hatano, K.; Ujike, T.; Ono, Y.; Higashihara, H.; Fujita, K.; Fukuhara, S.; et al. Therapeutic and Clinical Outcomes of Robot-assisted Partial Nephrectomy Versus Cryoablation for T1 Renal Cell Carcinoma. *Vivo* **2021**, *35*, 1573–1579. [CrossRef] [PubMed]
34. Chan, V.W.-S.; Osman, F.H.; Cartledge, J.; Gregory, W.; Kimuli, M.; Vasudev, N.S.; Ralph, C.; Jagdev, S.; Bhattarai, S.; Smith, J.; et al. Long-term outcomes of image-guided ablation and laparoscopic partial nephrectomy for T1 renal cell carcinoma. *Eur. Radiol.* **2022**, *32*, 1–10. [CrossRef] [PubMed]
35. Guo, J.; Arellano, R.S. Percutaneous Microwave Ablation of Category T1a Renal Cell Carcinoma: Intermediate Results on Safety, Technical Feasibility, and Clinical Outcomes of 119 Tumors. *Am. J. Roentgenol.* **2021**, *216*, 117–124. [CrossRef]
36. John, J.B.; Anderson, M.; Dutton, T.; Stott, M.; Crundwell, M.; Llewelyn, R.; Gemmell, A.; Bufacchi, R.; Spiers, A.; Campain, N. Percutaneous microwave ablation of renal masses in a UK cohort. *Br. J. Urol.* **2020**, *127*, 486–494. [CrossRef] [PubMed]
37. Wah, T.M.; Lenton, J.; Smith, J.; Bassett, P.; Jagdev, S.; Ralph, C.; Vasudev, N.; Bhattarai, S.; Kimuli, M.; Cartledge, J. Irreversible electroporation (IRE) in renal cell carcinoma (RCC): A mid-term clinical experience. *Eur. Radiol.* **2021**, *31*, 7491–7499. [CrossRef] [PubMed]
38. Canvasser, N.E.; Lay, A.H.; Morgan, M.S.C.; Ozayar, A.; Trimmer, C.; Sorokin, I.; Cadeddu, J.A. Irreversible electroporation of small renal masses: Suboptimal oncologic efficacy in an early series. *World J. Urol.* **2017**, *35*, 1549–1555. [CrossRef] [PubMed]
39. Ray, S.; Cheaib, J.G.; Pierorazio, P.M. Active Surveillance for Small Renal Masses. *Rev. Urol.* **2020**, *22*, 9–16.
40. Johnson, D.C.; Vukina, J.; Smith, A.B.; Meyer, A.-M.; Wheeler, S.B.; Kuo, T.-M.; Tan, H.-J.; Woods, M.E.; Raynor, M.C.; Wallen, E.M.; et al. Preoperatively Misclassified, Surgically Removed Benign Renal Masses: A Systematic Review of Surgical Series and United States Population Level Burden Estimate. *J. Urol.* **2015**, *193*, 30–35. [CrossRef] [PubMed]
41. Smaldone, M.C.; Kutikov, A.; Egleston, B.; Canter, D.J.; Viterbo, R.; Chen, D.Y.T.; Jewett, M.A.; Greenberg, R.E.; Uzzo, R.G. Small renal masses progressing to metastases under active surveillance. *Cancer* **2011**, *118*, 997–1006. [CrossRef]
42. Thompson, R.H.; Kurta, J.M.; Kaag, M.; Tickoo, S.K.; Kundu, S.; Katz, D.; Nogueira, L.; Reuter, V.E.; Russo, P. Tumor Size is Associated With Malignant Potential in Renal Cell Carcinoma Cases. *J. Urol.* **2009**, *181*, 2033–2036. [CrossRef]

43. Soria, F.; Marra, G.; Allasia, M.; Gontero, P. Retreatment after focal therapy for failure. *Curr. Opin. Urol.* **2018**, *28*, 544–549. [CrossRef] [PubMed]
44. Uzosike, A.C.; Patel, H.D.; Alam, R.; Schwen, Z.R.; Gupta, M.; Gorin, M.A.; Johnson, M.H.; Gausepohl, H.; Riffon, M.F.; Trock, B.J.; et al. Growth Kinetics of Small Renal Masses on Active Surveillance: Variability and Results from the DISSRM Registry. *J. Urol.* **2018**, *199*, 641–648. [CrossRef]
45. Mir, M.C.; Capitanio, U.; Bertolo, R.; Ouzaid, I.; Salagierski, M.; Kriegmair, M.; Volpe, A.; Jewett, M.A.; Kutikov, A.; Pierorazio, P.M. Role of Active Surveillance for Localized Small Renal Masses. *Eur. Urol. Oncol.* **2018**, *1*, 177–187. [CrossRef] [PubMed]
46. Gupta, M.; Alam, R.; Patel, H.D.; Semerjian, A.; Gorin, M.A.; Johnson, M.H.; Chang, P.; Wagner, A.A.; McKiernan, J.M.; Allaf, M.E.; et al. Use of delayed intervention for small renal masses initially managed with active surveillance. *Urol. Oncol. Semin. Orig. Investig.* **2018**, *37*, 18–25. [CrossRef] [PubMed]
47. Bhindi, B.; Thompson, R.H.; Lohse, C.M.; Mason, R.J.; Frank, I.; Costello, B.A.; Potretzke, A.M.; Hartman, R.P.; Potretzke, T.A.; Boorjian, S.A.; et al. The Probability of Aggressive Versus Indolent Histology Based on Renal Tumor Size: Implications for Surveillance and Treatment. *Eur. Urol.* **2018**, *74*, 489–497. [CrossRef] [PubMed]
48. Wośkowiak, P.; Lewicka, K.; Bureta, A.; Salagierski, M. Active surveillance and focal ablation for small renal masses: A better solution for comorbid patients. *Arch. Med. Sci.* **2020**, *16*, 1111–1118. [CrossRef]
49. Aron, M.; Kamoi, K.; Remer, E.; Berger, A.; Desai, M.; Gill, I. Laparoscopic Renal Cryoablation: 8-Year, Single Surgeon Outcomes. *J. Urol.* **2010**, *183*, 889–895. [CrossRef] [PubMed]
50. Wah, T.M.; Irving, H.C.; Gregory, W.; Cartledge, J.; Joyce, A.D.; Selby, P.J. Radiofrequency ablation (RFA) of renal cell carcinoma (RCC): Experience in 200 tumours. *Br. J. Urol.* **2013**, *113*, 416–428. [CrossRef] [PubMed]
51. Yu, J.; Liang, P.; Yu, X.-L.; Cheng, Z.-G.; Han, Z.-Y.; Zhang, X.; Dong, J.; Mu, M.-J.; Li, X.; Wang, X.-H. US-guided Percutaneous Microwave Ablation versus Open Radical Nephrectomy for Small Renal Cell Carcinoma: Intermediate-term Results. *Radiology* **2014**, *270*, 880–887. [CrossRef] [PubMed]
52. Guan, W.; Bai, J.; Liu, J.; Wang, S.; Zhuang, Q.; Ye, Z.; Hu, Z. Microwave ablation versus partial nephrectomy for small renal tumors: Intermediate-term results. *J. Surg. Oncol.* **2012**, *106*, 316–321. [CrossRef] [PubMed]
53. Ward, R.D.; Tanaka, H.; Campbell, S.C.; Remer, E.M. 2017 AUA Renal Mass and Localized Renal Cancer Guidelines: Imaging Implications. *RadioGraphics* **2018**, *38*, 2021–2033. [CrossRef] [PubMed]
54. Campbell, S.C.; Uzzo, R.G.; Karam, J.A.; Chang, S.S.; Clark, P.E.; Souter, L. Renal Mass and Localized Renal Cancer: Evaluation, Management, and Follow-up: AUA Guideline: Part II. *J. Urol.* **2021**, *206*, 209–218. [CrossRef] [PubMed]
55. Ljungberg, B.; Albiges, L.; Abu-Ghanem, Y.; Bensalah, K.; Dabestani, S.; Fernández-Pello, S.; Giles, R.H.; Hofmann, F.; Hora, M.; Kuczyk, M.A.; et al. European Association of Urology Guidelines on Renal Cell Carcinoma: The 2018 Update. *Eur. Urol.* **2018**, *75*, 799–810. Available online: https://uroweb.org/guidelines/archive/renal-cell-carcinoma (accessed on 22 June 2020). [CrossRef] [PubMed]
56. Finelli, A.; Cheung, D.C.; Al-Matar, A.; Evans, A.J.; Morash, C.G.; Pautler, S.E.; Siemens, D.R.; Tanguay, S.; Rendon, R.A.; Gleave, M.E.; et al. Small Renal Mass Surveillance: Histology-specific Growth Rates in a Biopsy-characterized Cohort. *Eur. Urol.* **2020**, *78*, 460–467. [CrossRef] [PubMed]
57. Motzer, R.J.; Jonasch, E.; Agarwal, N.; Bhayani, S.; Bro, W.P.; Chang, S.S.; Choueiri, T.K.; Costello, B.A.; Derweesh, I.H.; Fishman, M.; et al. Kidney Cancer, Version 4.2018, NCCN Clinical Practice Guidelines in Oncology. *J. Natl. Compr. Cancer Netw.* **2017**, *15*, 804–834. [CrossRef] [PubMed]

MDPI
St. Alban-Anlage 66
4052 Basel
Switzerland
www.mdpi.com

*Biomedicines* Editorial Office
E-mail: biomedicines@mdpi.com
www.mdpi.com/journal/biomedicines

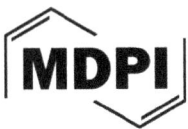

Disclaimer/Publisher's Note: The statements, opinions and data contained in all publications are solely those of the individual author(s) and contributor(s) and not of MDPI and/or the editor(s). MDPI and/or the editor(s) disclaim responsibility for any injury to people or property resulting from any ideas, methods, instructions or products referred to in the content.

www.ingramcontent.com/pod-product-compliance
Lightning Source LLC
LaVergne TN
LVHW070640100526
838202LV00013B/843